T0259314

A Practical Approach to the Spectrum of Alcoholic Liver Disease

Editor

DAVID BERNSTEIN

CLINICS IN LIVER DISEASE

www.liver.theclinics.com

Consulting Editor
NORMAN GITLIN

November 2012 • Volume 16 • Number 4

ELSEVIER

1600 John F. Kennedy Boulevard, Suite 1800 • Philadelphia, PA 19103-2899

http://www.theclinics.com

CLINICS IN LIVER DISEASE Volume 16, Number 4
November 2012 ISSN 1089-3261, ISBN-13: 978-1-4557-4917-1

Editor: Kerry Holland

Clinics in Liver Disease (ISSN 1089-3261) is published quarterly by Elsevier Inc., 360 Park Avenue South, New York, NY 10010-1710. Months of issue are February, May, August, and November. Business and Editorial Offices: 1600 John F. Kennedy Blvd., Ste. 1800, Philadelphia, PA 19103-2899. Customer Service Office: 3251 Riverport Lane, Maryland Heights, MO 63043. Periodicals postage paid at New York, NY and additional mailing offices. Subscription prices are $271.00 per year (U.S. individuals), $134.00 per year (U.S. student/resident), $365.00 per year (U.S. institutions), $360.00 per year (foreign individuals), $185.00 per year (foreign student/ resident), $440.00 per year (foreign instituitions), $313.00 per year (Canadian individuals), $185.00 per year (Canadian student/resident), and $440.00 per year (Canadian institutions). Foreign air speed delivery is included in all *Clinics* subscription prices. All prices are subject to change without notice. **POSTMASTER:** Send address changes to *Clinics in Liver Disease*, Elsevier Health Sciences Division, Subscription Customer Service, 3251 Riverport Lane, Maryland Heights, MO 63043. **Customer Service: Telephone: 1-800-654-2452 (U.S. and Canada); 314-447-8871 (outside U.S. and Canada). Fax: 314-447-8029. E-mail: journalscustomer service-usa@elsevier.com (for print support); journalsonlinesupport-usa@elsevier.com (for online support).**

Reprints. For copies of 100 or more of articles in this publication, please contact the Commercial Reprints Department, Elsevier Inc., 360 Park Avenue South, New York, NY 10010-1710. Tel.: 212-633-3812; Fax: 212-462-1935; E-mail: reprints@elsevier.com.

Clinics in Liver Disease is covered in *MEDLINE/PubMed (Index Medicus)*, Science Citation Index Expanded, Journal Citation Reports/Science Edition, and Current Contents/Clinical Medicine.

Printed and bound by CPI Group (UK) Ltd, Croydon, CR0 4YY

Transferred to digital print 2012

Contributors

CONSULTING EDITOR

NORMAN GITLIN, MD, FRCP (LONDON), FRCPE (EDINBURGH), FACG, FACP
Formerly, Professor of Medicine, Chief of Hepatology, Emory University; Currently,
Consultant, Atlanta Gastroenterology Associates, Atlanta, Georgia

GUEST EDITOR

DAVID BERNSTEIN, MD, AGAF, FACP, FACG
Professor of Medicine, Hofstra North Shore–LIJ School of Medicine; Chief of Hepatology,
North Shore University Hospital and Long Island Jewish Medical Center, Manhasset,
New York

AUTHORS

ANTHONY P. ALBANESE, MD, FACP, FASAM
Chief, Hepatology and Chemical Dependency, VA Northern California Healthcare System,
Health Sciences Clinical Professor of Medicine and Psychiatry, University of California
Davis School of Medicine, Sacramento, California

ARTHUR I. CEDERBAUM, PhD
Professor, Department of Pharmacology and Systems Therapeutics, Mount Sinai School
of Medicine, New York, New York

MICHAEL R. CHARLTON, MD
Division of Gastroenterology and Hepatology, Department of Internal Medicine, Mayo
Clinic, Rochester, Minnesota

JAMES M. CRAWFORD, MD, PhD
Professor and Chair, Department of Pathology and Laboratory Medicine, Hofstra North
Shore-LIJ School of Medicine; Senior Vice President, Laboratory Services, North
Shore-LIJ Health System, North Shore-LIJ Laboratories, Uniondale, New York

THIEN-LY DOAN, PharmD
Antibiotic Utilization Coordinator, Pharmacy Department, Long Island Jewish Medical
Center, New Hyde Park, New York

ANUPAMA T. DUDDEMPUDI, MD
Division of Gastroenterology, Hepatology and Nutrition, North Shore University Hospital,
Manhasset, New York

MARCIA E. EPSTEIN, MD
Associate Professor of Medicine, Division of Infectious Disease, Department of Medicine,
North Shore LIJ Health System, Manhasset, New York

PAUL J. GAGLIO JR
Rutgers University College of Arts and Sciences, New Brunswick, New Jersey

PAUL J. GAGLIO SR, MD, FACP, AGAF
Professor of Clinical Medicine, Department of Medicine, Montefiore Einstein Liver Center, Albert Einstein College of Medicine, Bronx, New York

PRANISHA GAUTAM-GOYAL, MD
Fellow in Infectious Diseases, Division of Infectious Disease, Department of Medicine, North Shore LIJ Health System, Manhasset, New York

PRIYA GREWAL, MD
Assistant Professor of Medicine, Division of Liver Diseases, Mount Sinai School of Medicine, New York, New York

GENE Y. IM, MD
Assistant Professor of Medicine, Division of Liver Diseases, Department of Medicine; Recanati/Miller Transplantation Institute, Mount Sinai School of Medicine, New York, New York

ANGELA C. KIM, MD
Assistant Professor of Medicine, Division of Infectious Disease, Department of Medicine, North Shore LIJ Health System, Manhasset, New York

KRIS V. KOWDLEY, MD
Clinical Professor of Medicine, University of Washington School of Medicine; Liver Center of Excellence, Virginia Mason Medical Center, Seattle, Washington

MAXIMILIAN LEE, MD, MPH
Liver Center of Excellence, Virginia Mason Medical Center, Seattle, Washington

JENNIFER LEONG, MD
Assistant Professor of Medicine, Division of Liver Diseases, Department of Medicine; Recanati/Miller Transplantation Institute, Mount Sinai School of Medicine, New York, New York

CHRISTOPHER O'BRIEN, MD, AGAF, FRCMI
Professor of Clinical Medicine, Divisions of Liver and GI Transplantation, Center for Liver Diseases, Miller School of Medicine, University of Miami, Miami, Florida

JOHN F. REINUS, MD
Division of Gastroenterology and Liver Diseases, Department of Medicine, Albert Einstein College of Medicine/Montefiore Medical Center, Bronx, New York

SANJAYA K. SATAPATHY, MBBS, MD, DM
Assistant Professor of Surgery, Transplant Hepatologist, Methodist University Hospital Transplant Institution, Department of Surgery, University of Tennessee Health Sciences Center, Memphis, Tennessee

JONATHAN M. SCHWARTZ, MD
Division of Gastroenterology and Liver Diseases, Department of Medicine, Albert Einstein College of Medicine/Montefiore Medical Center, Bronx, New York

ASHWANI K. SINGAL, MD
Division of Gastroenterology and Hepatology, Department of Internal Medicine, Mayo Clinic, Rochester, Minnesota

UMAIR SOHAIL, MD
Transplant Hepatology Fellow, University of Tennessee Health Sciences Center, Memphis, Tennessee

VIJAY ANAND VISWANATHEN, MD
Hepatology Fellow, Division of Liver Diseases, Mount Sinai School of Medicine, New York, New York

GARMEN A. WOO, MD
Center for Liver Diseases, Miller School of Medicine, University of Miami, Miami, Florida

Contents

> Alcoholic liver disease is a major cause of morbidity and mortality among people who drink excessive amounts of alcohol. There is a spectrum of liver injury that ranges from steatosis to varying stages of hepatic fibrosis and cirrhosis, with subsequent risk for hepatocellular carcinoma. Steato-hepatitis can occur at any stage of disease.

> This article describes the pathways and factors that modulate blood alcohol levels and metabolism and describes how the body disposes of alcohol. The various factors that play a role in the distribution of alcohol in the body, influence the absorption of alcohol, and contribute to first-pass metabolism of alcohol are described. Most alcohol is oxidized in the liver, and general principles and overall mechanisms for alcohol oxidation are summarized. The kinetics of alcohol elimination in-vivo and the various genetic and environmental factors that can modify the rate of alcohol metabolism are discussed.

> Hepatic fibrosis is a known consequence of long-term use of alcohol and is regarded as a turning point in alcohol-induced liver disease because it can lead to cirrhosis. The mechanisms of injury are not well understood, but recent studies have helped advance the understanding of the earliest events in the process that eventually leads to hepatic injury and, in some cases, fibrosis. It is hoped that increasing understanding of the role played by the immune system in the process will lead to the development of new therapies for these patients.

> The necessity of the liver being the organ responsible for metabolism of alcohol exposes it to many untoward toxic side effects. In the first instance of hepatic steatosis, fibrosis may occur indolently over years, slowly converting a greasy, steatotic liver into a cirrhotic liver. In the case of alcoholic hepatitis, brisk sinusoidal fibrosis may lead to more rapid development of cirrhosis, with the liver extensively subdivided by sublobular fibrous septa developing in the midst of extensive ongoing inflammation and hepatocellular destruction. Continued destruction of the parenchyma after cirrhosis

has developed may produce a densely fibrotic organ with little remaining parenchyma.

Alcoholic hepatitis is a form of severe, cholestatic liver disease that results from consumption of large amount of alcohol during a sustained period of time in a subset of alcoholics. Symptoms could be mild and nonspecific to more severe. The diagnosis of alcoholic hepatitis can be made with a thorough history, physical examination, and review of laboratory results. Liver biopsy is confirmatory but generally not indicated for the diagnosis. Abstinence is the key form of therapeutic intervention. Despite variable results in clinical trials, corticosteroids and pentoxifylline seem to provide moderate survival benefit. Liver transplantation in acute alcoholic hepatitis is contentious.

This article reviews the spectrum of alcohol use disorders. The pharmacologic properties of ethanol and its metabolism, and the historical, physical, and laboratory elements that may help diagnose an alcohol use disorder are examined. The concepts of motivational interviewing and stages of change are mentioned, along with the American Society of Addiction Medicine patient placement criteria, to determine the best level of treatment for alcoholism. Various therapeutic management options are reviewed, including psychological, pharmacologic, and complementary/ alternative choices. This article provides a basic understanding of available tools to diagnose and treat this cunning and baffling brain and multisystem disease.

Alcoholic liver disease is a major cause of morbidity and mortality worldwide. Patients with cirrhosis caused by alcohol are at risk for developing complications associated with a failing liver. The long-term management of alcoholic liver disease stresses the following: (1) Abstinence of alcohol (Grade 1A), with referral to an alcoholic rehabilitation program; (2) Adequate nutritional support (Grade 1B), emphasizing multiple feedings and a referral to a nutritionist; (3) Routine screening in alcoholic cirrhosis to prevent complications; (4) Timely referral to a liver transplant program for those with decompensated cirrhosis; (5) Avoid pharmacologic therapies, as these medications have shown no benefit.

Alcoholic individuals are at increased risk of infection in general, in part because of immune defects. In addition, associated situations, such as depressed mental status, increase risk to specific syndromes such as lung abscess related to depressed consciousness and aspiration. Social factors related to hygiene and living situations are also linked to specific microorganisms, such as *Mycobacteria tuberculosis, Bartonella quintana, Vibrio vulnificus,* and *Capnocytophaga canimorus.*

The liver plays an important role in the metabolism, synthesis, storage, and absorption of nutrients. Patients with cirrhosis are prone to nutritional deficiencies and malnutrition, with a higher prevalence among patients with decompensated disease. Mechanisms of nutritional deficiencies in patients with liver disease are not completely understood and probably multifactorial. Malnutrition among patients with cirrhosis or alcoholic liver disease correlates with poor quality of life, increased risk of infections, frequent hospitalizations, complications, mortality, poor graft and patient survival after liver transplantation, and economic burden. Physicians, including gastroenterologists and hepatologists, should be conversant with assessment and management of malnutrition and nutritional supplementation.

In addition to directly causing liver disease, alcohol consumption is a common comorbid condition with other chronic liver diseases and may exacerbate liver injury, particularly in nonalcoholic fatty liver disease, chronic viral hepatitis, hereditary hemochromatosis, and autoimmune liver diseases. This synergism can result in increased hepatic inflammation and accelerated rates of fibrosis, with more rapid and earlier development of cirrhosis, and also increase the risk for liver cancer and death from liver disease.

Annually, hepatocellular carcinoma is diagnosed in approximately a half-million people worldwide. Based on the association of alcohol with cancer, a International Agency for Research on Cancer working group recently deemed alcoholic beverages "carcinogenic to humans," causally related to occurrence of malignant tumors of the oral cavity, pharynx, larynx, esophagus, liver, colorectum, and female breast. Alcohol metabolism in the liver leads to reactive oxygen species production, induction of activity of cytochrome P450s, and reduction of antioxidants. This review analyzes the epidemiology and pathogenesis of alcohol in hepatocellular cancer.

Alcoholic liver cirrhosis is the second most common indication for liver transplantation in the United States. Studies have shown that these patients do as well as those transplanted for nonalcoholic liver disease.

CLINICS IN LIVER DISEASE

Preface
Alcoholic Liver Disease

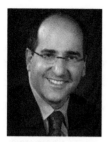

David Bernstein, MD, AGAF, FACP, FACG
Guest Editor

Alcohol is recognized by the general public as one of the most common causes of liver disease and, through the ages, its effects on the liver have been well described. Alcohol can cause a spectrum of liver diseases from fatty liver to acute hepatitis to cirrhosis and its complications. End-stage liver disease secondary to alcohol is a frequent indication for liver transplantation. This issue of *Clinics in Liver Disease* offers a comprehensive review of the broad spectrum of alcoholic liver disease from basic alcohol metabolism and immunology through the evaluation for liver transplantation and beyond.

In order to understand the scope of the problem, the prevalence and natural history of alcoholic liver disease are reviewed by Dr Reinus. This is followed by a detailed discussion of the biochemistry of alcohol metabolism and immunology by Drs Cederbaum and Duddempudi, respectively. Knowledge of the histological findings seen in alcoholic liver disease is essential for the determination of prognosis; these findings are reviewed by Dr Crawford. As alcohol can cause acute disease, the diagnosis and management of alcoholic hepatitis are reviewed by Dr Satapathy. An important component of care in patients with alcoholic liver disease is the management of their addiction and this vital, yet often neglected, aspect of care is discussed by Dr Albanese.

Alcohol use and abuse may lead to systemic effects. Certain infections are more commonly seen in patients with alcoholic liver disease; these are well reviewed by Drs Epstein and colleagues. Chronic use of alcohol may lead to nutritional deficiencies and these are reviewed in the issue by Dr Charlton.

Chronic alcohol use can lead to various complications of decompensated liver disease. Dr O'Brien reviews the long-term management of alcoholic liver disease and Dr Grewal discusses the relationship between alcohol and liver cancer. Selection criteria for liver transplantation are reviewed by Dr Leong and the management of specific issues in patients with alcoholic liver disease following liver transplantation is reviewed by Dr Gaglio.

Clin Liver Dis 16 (2012) xiii–xiv
http://dx.doi.org/10.1016/j.cld.2012.09.009
1089-3261/12/$ – see front matter © 2012 Elsevier Inc. All rights reserved.

liver.theclinics.com

This issue of *Clinics in Liver Disease* provides the reader with a soup-to-nuts review of the understanding of the mechanism of alcoholic liver disease as well the diagnosis and management of both acute and chronic alcoholic liver diseases and addiction management. It should be an excellent resource for any clinician caring for patients with this condition.

David Bernstein, MD, AGAF, FACP, FACG
Hofstra North Shore–LIJ School of Medicine
North Shore University Hospital and
Long Island Jewish Medical Center
300 Community Drive
Manhasset, NY 11030, USA

E-mail address:
dbernste@nshs.edu

Prevalence and Natural History of Alcoholic Liver Disease

Jonathan M. Schwartz, MD*, John F. Reinus, MD

KEYWORDS

- Alcoholic liver disease • Epidemiology • Alcoholism • Natural history

KEY POINTS

- Alcoholic liver disease is a chronic progressive illness in those who continue to drink, but often may improve or resolve in those who become abstinent.
- Because liver disease and other problems related to alcohol consumption are entirely the consequences of human behavior, programs that educate the public regarding the nature and dangers of alcohol toxicity and that support responsible consumption or abstinence when necessary can be expected to have a significant health and financial benefit.
- There is a spectrum of liver injury that ranges from steatosis to varying stages of hepatic fibrosis and cirrhosis, with subsequent risk for hepatocellular carcinoma.
- Although there are many variables that influence individual susceptibility to the toxic effects of alcohol on the liver, limitations on targeted advertising and easy availability of alcohol for the populations at highest risk may reduce the deleterious effects of alcohol on society.

INTRODUCTION

Humans have consumed alcoholic beverages for more than 10,000 years, primarily as indispensible sources of both water and calories. This fact has been especially true in the Western world, where bacterial contamination made most water supplies unsafe for millennia and where the practice of boiling water to make coffee, tea, and other drinks did not become prevalent until relatively recently. Fermented beverages, consumed by people of all ages as their most important daily drink, had low alcohol content because yeasts will not tolerate alcohol concentrations of more than 16%, likely limiting secondary morbidity. Such was the case until distillation of wine to produce spirits began in Europe around 1100 and subsequently became common practice in the sixteenth century after publication in 1500 of *Liber de Arte Destillandi* (The Book of the Art of Distillation).[1] After that, it is safe to assume, the risk of alcohol-related morbidity increased dramatically.

Division of Gastroenterology and Liver Diseases, Department of Medicine, Albert Einstein College of Medicine/Montefiore Medical Center, 111 East 210th Street, Bronx, NY 10467, USA
* Corresponding author.
E-mail address: jonschwa@montefiore.org

Clin Liver Dis 16 (2012) 659–666
http://dx.doi.org/10.1016/j.cld.2012.08.001
1089-3261/12/$ – see front matter © 2012 Elsevier Inc. All rights reserved.

In the present era, alcohol toxicity is the third most common worldwide cause of morbidity,[2] and alcohol-related morbidity is the third most common preventable cause of death in the United States.[3] Many of the harmful effects of alcohol are listed in **Table 1**. In the most recent data from the US Centers for Disease Control and Prevention (CDC) available between 2001 and 2005, 80,000 Americans died as a result of alcohol consumption. These deaths and the nonfatal morbid consequences of alcohol use were responsible for more than $257 billion in costs to the American economy in 2006.[3] The real costs of alcohol-induced morbidity are probably underestimated, owing to the social stigma associated with an admission of alcoholism and because of inaccurate diagnosis and underreporting of alcohol sales and consumption.

The National Epidemiologic Survey on Alcohol and Related Conditions (NESARC)[4] estimated the prevalence of alcohol abuse ("a maladaptive pattern of alcohol [consumption] leading to clinically significant impairment or distress"[5]) among United States adults in 2001-2002 to be 4.7% over the previous 12 months and 17% over a lifetime. The prevalence of alcohol dependence ("impaired control over drinking, preoccupation with alcohol, denial and continued use of alcohol despite adverse consequences"[5]) was 3.8% over the previous 12 months and 12.5% over a lifetime.

This article reviews the prevalence and natural history of alcoholic liver disease, including fatty-liver disease, alcoholic hepatitis, and alcoholic cirrhosis.

EPIDEMIOLOGY OF ALCOHOLIC LIVER DISEASE

In the most recent CDC Harmful Effects Summary,[3] liver disease was listed as the cause of death in 55% of alcohol-related fatalities. As might be expected, the prevalence of alcoholic liver disease throughout the world correlates with per capita alcohol consumption, with the greatest consumption and disease prevalence in eastern Europe, southern Europe, and the United Kingdom.[2] Countries with large Muslim populations have the lowest rates of alcohol consumption and alcoholic liver disease. In the United States, per capita alcohol consumption is 7.5 to 9.9 L per person-year, and disease prevalence is intermediate between that seen in countries with the lowest and countries with the highest consumption rates (**Fig. 1**).[2] It is the ethanol content of alcoholic beverages only, not their type, which is related to development of alcoholic liver disease and cirrhosis. The alcohol content of beverages differs among cultures

Table 1 Harmful effects of alcohol	
Pancreatitis (acute and chronic)	Ischemic heart disease
Cardiomyopathy	Oropharyngeal cancer
Polyneuropathy	Prostate cancer
Chronic liver disease	Psoriasis
Myopathy	Spontaneous abortion
Psychosis	Stroke
Breast cancer	Supraventricular Tachyarrhythmia
Epilepsy	
Esophageal cancer	
Fetal Alcohol Syndrome	
Gastrointestinal bleeding	
Hypertension	

Total adult (15+) per capita consumption, in litres of pure alcohol, 2005ᵃ

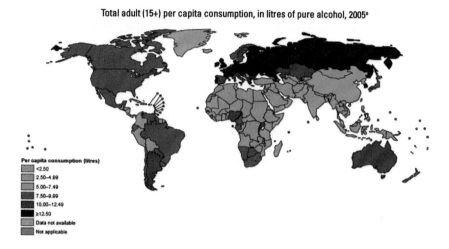

Per capita consumption (litres)
- <2.50
- 2.50–4.99
- 5.00–7.49
- 7.50–9.99
- 10.00–12.49
- ≥12.50
- Data not available
- Not applicable

ᵃ Best estimates of 2005 using average recorded alcohol consumption 2003–2005 (minus tourist consumption; see Appendix IV for details) and unrecorded alcohol consumption 2005.

Fig. 1. World Health Organization global status report, 2011. (*From* World Health Organization. Global status report on alcohol and health. Geneva: WHO Press; 2011; with permission.)

and localities; **Box 1** provides an estimate of the number of grams of alcohol in standard alcoholic beverages in the United States.[6]

Although the association between alcohol consumption and liver disease is well established, severe alcohol-related morbidity only develops in a small minority of heavy drinkers. The reasons for individual differences in susceptibility to the toxic effects of alcohol are discussed elsewhere in this issue. Rigorous study of the relationship between development of alcoholic liver disease and the quantity of alcohol consumed is almost impossible, because data collection always involves numerous broad assumptions and rough estimates. The Dionysos Study of a large Northern Italian cohort demonstrated that the risk of hepatotoxicity became significant with regular alcohol consumption in excess of 30 g daily; individuals who consumed more than 120 g of alcohol daily were most likely to have cirrhosis.[7] Only 2.2% of at-risk individuals in this study, however, had cirrhosis. The mortality rate from cirrhosis in France during the years 1925 to 1964 is estimated to have been 14 per 100,000 persons who drank less than 80 g of alcohol daily and 357 per 100,000 persons who drank more than 160 g of alcohol daily.[8] Overall, it appears that an individual must consume between 80 and 160 g of alcohol on a regular daily basis to be at

Box 1
Alcohol content in beverages in the United States
14 g of alcohol is the equivalent to:
1 12-oz (350 mL) beer or cooler (~5% alcohol)
1 5-oz (148 mL) glass of wine (~12% alcohol)
1.5 oz (44 mL) of hard liquor (40% alcohol)
Maximal daily quantities:
28 g/d for men
14 g/d for women

significant risk for developing alcoholic hepatitis and cirrhosis.[9] Because there are differences in susceptibility to alcohol, and there are benefits of moderate alcohol use, it is the recommendation of the National Institute of Alcohol Abuse and Alcoholism that men and women drink no more than 28 g and 14 g of alcohol each day, respectively.[10]

Age and Alcohol Consumption

Persons of all ages drink excessively; however, the majority of individuals admitted to hospitals with alcoholic liver disease are 45 to 64 years old.[11] Drinking often starts at a young age, as highlighted by the finding that underage individuals drank almost 20% of the total alcohol consumed in the United Kingdom in 2002.[12] On the other hand, a high proportion of individuals older than 65 years fulfill criteria for alcohol abuse and dependence.[13]

Gender and Alcohol-Related Liver Injury

As observed by the investigators of the Dionysos study,[7] men are far more likely than women to develop alcoholic liver disease. Women throughout the world generally consume less alcohol than do men; however, women appear to be more susceptible than men to the potential hepatotoxic effects of alcohol. For example, in a study of 13,000 Danes, women had higher rates of cirrhosis than men for given quantities of alcohol intake.[14] Reasons for female susceptibility to alcohol toxicity may include low levels of gastric alcohol dehydrogenase, high proportions of body fat and, possibly, an effect of estrogens.[15,16]

Ethnicity and Alcohol-Related Liver Disease

In 1979, the US National Center for Health Statistics published separate death rates for blacks. It reported 35.3 deaths from alcoholic liver disease per 100,000 black people and 19.2 similar deaths per 100,000 white people.[17] After the addition to the US Certificate of Death of the category Hispanic Ethnicity in 1989, Hispanic men were noted to have the highest cirrhosis mortality rates of those in any ethnic group between 1991 and 1997. Mortality rates from highest to lowest by ethnicity for men were: white Hispanic, black non-Hispanic, white non-Hispanic, and black Hispanic; and for women: black non-Hispanic, white Hispanic, white non-Hispanic, and black Hispanics.[17] Although data indicate that white Hispanics and African Americans drink more alcohol than do persons in other ethnic groups,[18] it is unclear whether the reported differences in rates of alcoholic liver disease and cirrhosis among people are related to socioeconomic patterns of consumption or genetic variables that predispose some individuals to develop more severe liver disease.

NATURAL HISTORY OF ALCOHOLIC LIVER DISEASE

Numerous histologic abnormalities (**Fig. 2**) are seen in the livers of people who drink potentially toxic amounts of alcohol; these include steatosis, steatohepatitis, fibrosis, cirrhosis, and hepatocellular carcinoma.

Hepatic Steatosis

More than 90% of heavy drinkers develop large-droplet (macrovesicular) steatosis unaccompanied by necrosis and inflammation, initially in zone 3 (those liver cells immediately surrounding the central vein) and, in more severe cases, throughout the liver.[19,20] Less commonly, alcoholics are found to have small-droplet (microvesicular) steatosis,[21] a distinct entity termed alcoholic foamy degeneration. Hepatic steatosis

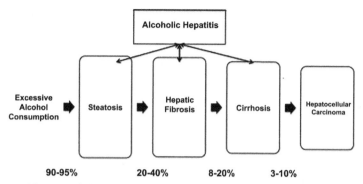

Fig. 2. Natural history of alcoholic liver disease.

may be found in individuals with previously normal livers after only 2 weeks of alcohol ingestion, which resolves rapidly after cessation of alcohol consumption.[22] Clinical manifestations of macrovesicular steatosis include asymptomatic hepatomegaly and nonspecific digestive complaints. Alcoholic foamy degeneration is associated with jaundice and marked elevations of serum aminotransferase levels in a pattern that is not typical of alcoholic steatohepatitis. Hepatic steatosis has been thought of as a benign reversible histologic abnormality. It has been demonstrated, however, that patients with steatosis who continue to drink may develop fibrosis and, in some cases, cirrhosis, without first developing clinical steatohepatitis.[23]

Steatohepatitis

Steatohepatitis (steatonecrosis), or simply alcoholic hepatitis, requires more time to develop than does simple steatosis and is not universally present in the livers of drinkers, even after years of alcohol consumption.[24] One study found that only one-third of heavy drinkers have clinical and histologic findings of alcoholic hepatitis.[25] In addition to the steatosis expected in the livers of all habitual alcohol drinkers, steatohepatitis is characterized by histologic features of inflammation and liver cell necrosis. Patients are likely to be clinically ill and to have abnormal results from biochemical liver tests. Symptomatic alcoholic hepatitis may occur several weeks after alcohol cessation.[26] The risk of ultimately developing cirrhosis is increased in patients with alcoholic hepatitis. In a Danish National Registry study, patients with steatohepatitis were far more likely to develop cirrhosis over a 5-year period than were those with steatosis only (16% vs 6.9%).[27] Forty percent of United States patients found to have alcoholic hepatitis had cirrhosis on liver biopsies that were repeated 5 years after the initial evaluation.[28] In general, 10% to 20% of patients with alcoholic hepatitis are likely to progress to cirrhosis per year, and up to 70% of patients with alcoholic hepatitis ultimately will become cirrhotic. On the other hand, a small proportion (up to 10%) of patients with alcoholic hepatitis has complete regression of liver injury with abstinence from alcohol. There are various models that are helpful in assessing short-term survival among patients with alcoholic hepatitis.[29,30]

Cirrhosis

Cirrhosis is defined as hepatic bridging fibrosis and nodular regeneration.[31] Cirrhotic changes develop progressively in persons with chronic hepatic necroinflammatory injury. The cirrhotic livers of alcoholics often also have features of alcoholic steatohepatitis, predominantly at the periphery of regenerative nodules. The regenerative nodules in alcoholic (Laennec) cirrhosis tend to be small (micronodular cirrhosis).

Although cirrhosis is a categorical diagnosis, in reality patients with alcoholic and other forms of chronic hepatitis have gradual worsening of hepatic fibrosis and growth of regenerative nodules. Several secondary factors may accelerate this process, including drinking patterns, cigarette smoking, body composition, gender, and the additional presence of chronic hepatitis B or hepatitis C virus infection. Daily drinking is more likely to cause severe alcoholic liver injury than is periodic binge drinking, and drinking with meals has been reported to be associated with a lower risk of alcoholic liver injury.[25,32] The combination of excessive alcohol consumption and obesity increases the risk of progression to advanced hepatic fibrosis, suggesting that individuals predisposed to develop nonalcoholic steatohepatitis are more susceptible to the hepatotoxic effects of alcohol.[33] The synergistic effects of alcohol and other chronic liver diseases are reviewed in detail in an article elsewhere in this issue.

Alcohol is the most common cause of cirrhosis in the developed world, and is responsible for 44% of all deaths from liver disease in the United States.[34] Furthermore, cirrhosis is the 12th most common cause of death in the United States.[35] Development of cirrhosis is associated with the gradual emergence of symptomatic (decompensated) liver disease. Five-year survival is approximately 70% in compensated cirrhotic patients who continue to drink, whereas it decreases to 30% in persistent drinkers with clinical decompensation (ascites, encephalopathy, or variceal bleeding).[23] Nevertheless, the long-term prognosis of patients with cirrhosis improves with alcohol abstinence: 5-year survival of patients with compensated and decompensated cirrhosis who stop drinking can be as great as 90% and 60%, respectively.[36] Cirrhosis of any etiology is a risk factor for development of hepatocellular carcinoma, with an incidence of approximately 1.5% annually.[37] Individuals with alcoholic cirrhosis should have liver cancer screening and surveillance, according to the recommendations of the American Association for the Study of Liver Diseases.[37]

SUMMARY

Disease caused by the toxic effects of alcohol on the liver is an important cause of morbidity and mortality worldwide, and imposes significant direct and indirect costs on national economies. Alcoholic liver disease is a chronic progressive illness in those who continue to drink, but often may improve or resolve in those who become abstinent. Because liver disease and other problems related to alcohol consumption are entirely the consequences of human behavior, programs that educate the public regarding the nature and dangers of alcohol toxicity and that support responsible consumption or abstinence when necessary can be expected to have a significant health and financial benefit. Although there are many variables that influence individual susceptibility to the toxic effects of alcohol on the liver, limitations on targeted advertising and easy availability of alcohol for the populations at highest risk may reduce the deleterious effects of alcohol on society.

REFERENCES

1. Brunschwig H. Liber de arte distillandi, de simplicibus: Das Buch der rechten Kunst zu distilieren die eintzige[n] Ding. Strassburg (Austria): Johan (Reinhard) Grüninger; 1500.
2. WHO global status report on alcohol. 2011.
3. Center for Disease Control and Prevention. Alcohol and public health: alcohol-related disease impact (ARDI). Center for Disease Control and Prevention; 2012.
4. Morse RM, Flavin DK. The definition of alcoholism. The Joint Committee of the National Council on Alcoholism and Drug Dependence and the American Society

of Addiction Medicine to study the definition and criteria for the diagnosis of alcoholism. JAMA 1992;268:1012–4.

5. American Psychiatric Association. Diagnostic criteria from DSM-IV-TR. Washington, DC: American Psychiatric Association; 2000.

6. What is a standard drink? National Institute of Alcohol Abuse and Alcoholism; 2012. http://pubs.niaaa.nih.gov/publications/Practitioner/pocketguide/pocket_guide2.htm

7. Bellentani S, Saccoccio G, Costa G, et al. Drinking habits as cofactors of risk for alcohol induced liver damage. The Dionysos Study Group. Gut 1997;41:845–50.

8. Pequignot G. About the geographical aspects of cirrhosis. Stuttgart (Germany): Schattauer Verlag; 1971.

9. Galambos JT. Cirrhosis. Philadelphia: WB Saunders; 1979.

10. National Institute on Alcohol Abuse and Alcoholism. The physicians' guide to helping patients with alcohol problems. Washington, DC: Government Printing Office; 1995.

11. Adams WL, Yuan Z, Barboriak JJ, et al. Alcohol-related hospitalizations of elderly people. Prevalence and geographic variation in the United States. JAMA 1993;270:1222–5.

12. Pincock S. Binge drinking on rise in UK and elsewhere. Government report shows increases in alcohol consumption, cirrhosis, and premature deaths. Lancet 2003;362:1126–7.

13. Adams WL, Magruder-Habib K, Trued S, et al. Alcohol abuse in elderly emergency department patients. J Am Geriatr Soc 1992;40:1236–40.

14. Becker U, Deis A, Sorensen TI, et al. Prediction of risk of liver disease by alcohol intake, sex, and age: a prospective population study. Hepatology 1996;23:1025–9.

15. Frezza M, di Padova C, Pozzato G, et al. High blood alcohol levels in women. The role of decreased gastric alcohol dehydrogenase activity and first-pass metabolism. N Engl J Med 1990;322:95–9.

16. Gao B, Bataller R. Alcoholic liver disease: pathogenesis and new therapeutic targets. Gastroenterology 2011;141:1572–85.

17. Stinson FS, Grant BF, Dufour MC. The critical dimension of ethnicity in liver cirrhosis mortality statistics. Alcohol Clin Exp Res 2001;25:1181–7.

18. Caetano R, Kaskutas LA. Changes in drinking patterns among whites, blacks and Hispanics, 1984-1992. J Stud Alcohol 1995;56:558–65.

19. Edmondson HA, Peters RL, Frankel HH, et al. The early stage of liver injury in the alcoholic. Medicine (Baltimore) 1967;46:119–29.

20. MacSween RN, Burt AD. Histologic spectrum of alcoholic liver disease. Semin Liver Dis 1986;6:221–32.

21. Uchida T, Kao H, Quispe-Sjogren M, et al. Alcoholic foamy degeneration—a pattern of acute alcoholic injury of the liver. Gastroenterology 1983;84:683–92.

22. Lane BP, Lieber CS. Ultrastructural alterations in human hepatocytes following ingestion of ethanol with adequate diets. Am J Pathol 1966;49:593–603.

23. Teli MR, Day CP, Burt AD, et al. Determinants of progression to cirrhosis or fibrosis in pure alcoholic fatty liver. Lancet 1995;346:987–90.

24. Lischner MW, Alexander JF, Galambos JT. Natural history of alcoholic hepatitis. I. The acute disease. Am J Dig Dis 1971;16:481–94.

25. Barrio E, Tome S, Rodriguez I, et al. Liver disease in heavy drinkers with and without alcohol withdrawal syndrome. Alcohol Clin Exp Res 2004;28:131–6.

26. Lucey MR, Mathurin P, Morgan TR. Alcoholic hepatitis. N Engl J Med 2009;360: 2758–69.
27. Deleuran T, Gronbaek H, Vilstrup H, et al. Cirrhosis and mortality risks of biopsy-verified alcoholic pure steatosis and steatohepatitis: a nationwide registry-based study. Aliment Pharmacol Ther 2012;35(11):1336–42.
28. Alexander JF, Lischner MW, Galambos JT. Natural history of alcoholic hepatitis. II. The long-term prognosis. Am J Gastroenterol 1971;56:515–25.
29. Maddrey WC, Boitnott JK, Bedine MS, et al. Corticosteroid therapy of alcoholic hepatitis. Gastroenterology 1978;75:193–9.
30. Dunn W, Jamil LH, Brown LS, et al. MELD accurately predicts mortality in patients with alcoholic hepatitis. Hepatology 2005;41:353–8.
31. Anthony PP, Ishak KG, Nayak NC, et al. The morphology of cirrhosis. Recommendations on definition, nomenclature, and classification by a working group sponsored by the World Health Organization. J Clin Pathol 1978;31:395–414.
32. Hatton J, Burton A, Nash H, et al. Drinking patterns, dependency and life-time drinking history in alcohol-related liver disease. Addiction 2009;104:587–92.
33. Naveau S, Giraud V, Borotto E, et al. Excess weight risk factor for alcoholic liver disease. Hepatology 1997;25:108–11.
34. Yoon YH. Surveillance report #75: liver cirrhosis mortality in the United States, 1970-2003. Bethesda (MD): National Institute of Alcohol Abuse and Alcoholism; 2006.
35. Murphy SL, Xu J, Kochanek KD. National vital statistics reports. vol. 2012. US Department of Health and Human Services. Centers for Disease Control and Prevention. National Center for Health Statistics, National Vital Statistics Systems; 2012.
36. Mandayam S, Jamal MM, Morgan TR. Epidemiology of alcoholic liver disease. Semin Liver Dis 2004;24:217–32.
37. Bruix J, Sherman M. Management of hepatocellular carcinoma: an update. Hepatology 2011;53:1020–2.

Alcohol Metabolism

Arthur I. Cederbaum, PhD

KEYWORDS

- Alcohol dehydrogenase • Cytochrome P4502E1 • Acetaldehyde metabolism
- Hepatic redox state • Alcohol absorption • Distribution and elimination
- Isoforms of alcohol dehydrogenase • Metabolic adaptation to alcohol

KEY POINTS

- The equilibrium concentration of alcohol in a tissue depends on the relative water content of that tissue.
- The rate of alcohol absorption depends on the rate of gastric emptying and the concentration of alcohol, and is more rapid in the fasted state.
- The blood alcohol concentration is determined by the amount of alcohol consumed, the presence or absence of food, and the rate of alcohol metabolism.
- First-pass metabolism of alcohol occurs in the stomach and is decreased in alcoholics.
- Liver alcohol dehydrogenase is the major enzyme system for metabolizing alcohol; this requires the cofactor nicotinamide adenine dinucleotide (NAD) and the products produced are acetaldehyde and reduced NAD (NADH).
- The acetaldehyde is further oxidized to acetate, the same final metabolite produced from all other nutrients (carbohydrates, fats, and proteins); the acetate can be converted to CO_2, fatty acids, ketone bodies, cholesterol, and steroids.
- Oxidation of alcohol by cytochrome P450 pathways, especially CYP2E1, which is induced by alcohol, are secondary pathways to remove alcohol, especially at high concentrations.
- Alcohol metabolism is regulated by the nutritional state, the concentration of alcohol, specific isoforms of alcohol dehydrogenase, the need to remove acetaldehyde and regenerate NAD, and induction of CYP2E1.
- Substrate shuttles and the mitochondrial respiratory chain are required to regenerate NAD from NADH, and this can limit the overall rate of alcohol metabolism.
- Metabolism of alcohol is increased in alcoholics without liver disease: this metabolic tolerance to alcohol may involve induction of CYP2E1, increased regeneration of NAD, or endotoxemia.

Disclosures: None to report.
Department of Pharmacology and Systems Therapeutics, Mount Sinai School of Medicine, One Gustave L Levy Place, New York, NY 10029, USA
E-mail address: arthur.cederbaum@mssm.edu

This article describes the pathways responsible for the metabolism of alcohol (ethanol) and discusses the factors that regulate this oxidation. Understanding pathways of alcohol oxidation is important because it allows clinicians to:

1. Learn how the body disposes of alcohol and its metabolites.
2. Discern some of the factors that influence this process.
3. Learn how alcohol influences the metabolism of nutrients and drugs.
4. Potentially learn how alcohol damages various organs.
5. Potentially identify individuals who are at increased or decreased risk for alcohol toxicity.

Some suggested causes for alcohol toxicity are linked to changes produced by the metabolism of ethanol, such as redox state changes in the nicotinamide adenine dinucleotide (NAD^+)/reduced NAD (NADH) ratio, acetaldehyde formation, oxidative stress, and mitochondrial function are shown in **Box 1** and are discussed later. General reviews on alcohol metabolism can be found in Refs.[1–9]

DISTRIBUTION OF ALCOHOL IN THE BODY

The equilibrium concentration of alcohol in a tissue depends on the relative water content of that tissue. Equilibration of alcohol within a tissue depends on the water content, rate of blood flow, and the tissue mass. Ethanol is practically insoluble in fats and oils, although, like water, it can pass through biologic membranes. Ethanol distributes from the blood into all tissues and fluids in proportion to their relative content of water. The concentration of ethanol in a tissue depends the relative water content of the tissue, and reaches equilibrium quickly with the concentration of ethanol in the plasma. There is no plasma protein binding of alcohol.

The same dose of alcohol per unit of body weight can produce different blood alcohol concentrations in different individuals because of the large variations in proportions of fat and water in their bodies, and the low lipid/water partition coefficient of ethanol. Women generally have a smaller volume of distribution for alcohol than men because of their higher percentage of body fat. Women have higher peak blood alcohol levels than men when given the same dose of alcohol as grams per kilogram body weight, but no differences occur when given the same dose per liter of body water. First-pass metabolism of alcohol by the stomach, which may be greater in men, may also contribute to the higher blood alcohol levels found in women.[10,11]

Box 1
Some suggested causes for alcohol toxicity

- Redox state changes in the NAD/NADH ratio
- Acetaldehyde formation
- Mitochondrial damage
- Cytokine formation (tumor necrosis factor α)
- Kupffer cell activation
- Membrane actions of ethanol
- Hypoxia
- Immune actions
- Oxidative stress

The breath analyzer test for estimating blood alcohol concentrations depends on the diffusion of ethanol from pulmonary arterial blood into the alveolar air. The ethanol vapor in breath is in equilibrium with the ethanol dissolved in the water of the blood at a blood/breath partition coefficient of about 2100:1. An excellent recent review summarizes many of these pharmacokinetic interactions.[12]

FACTORS AFFECTING ALCOHOL ABSORPTION

Box 2 describes some factors that affect the absorption of alcohol. Absorption of alcohol from the duodenum and jejunum is more rapid than from the stomach, hence the rate of gastric emptying is an important determinant of the rate of absorption of orally administered alcohol.

1. Alcohol crosses biologic membranes by passive diffusion, down its concentration gradient. Therefore, the higher the concentration of alcohol, the greater is the resulting concentration gradient, and the more rapid is the absorption.
2. Rapid removal of alcohol from the site of absorption by an efficient blood flow helps maintain the concentration gradient and thereby promote absorption.
3. Alcohol has irritant properties and high concentrations can cause superficial erosions, hemorrhages, and paralysis of the stomach smooth muscle, which decrease alcohol absorption.
4. Peak blood alcohol levels are higher if ethanol is ingested as a single dose rather than several smaller doses, probably because alcohol concentration gradient is higher in the former case.
5. In general, there is little difference in the rate of absorption of the same dose of alcohol administered in the form of different alcoholic beverages (ie, blood ethanol concentration is not significantly influenced by the type of alcoholic beverage consumed).
6. The presence of food in the stomach retards gastric emptying and thus reduces the absorption of alcohol; the concept of not drinking on an empty stomach. Meals high in fat, carbohydrate, or protein are equally effective in retarding gastric emptying. The major factor governing the absorption rate of alcohol is whether the drink is taken on an empty stomach, or together with or after a meal.[13–15]

The blood alcohol concentration is determined by the amount of alcohol consumed, by the presence or absence of food in the stomach, factors that affect gastric emptying, and the rate of alcohol oxidation.

FIRST-PASS METABOLISM OF ALCOHOL IN THE STOMACH

Some of the alcohol that is ingested orally does not enter the systemic circulation but may be oxidized in the stomach by alcohol dehydrogenase (ADH) isoforms such as

---

Box 2
Factors affecting alcohol absorption

- Concentration of alcohol
- Blood flow at site of absorption
- Irritant properties of alcohol
- Rate of ingestion
- Type of beverage
- Food

σADH and class I and class III ADH. This first-pass metabolism could modulate alcohol toxicity because its efficiency determines the bioavailability of alcohol. Ethanol is rapidly passed into the duodenum from the stomach in the fasted state, which minimizes first-pass metabolism and thereby plays a role in the higher blood alcohol concentrations observed in the fasted versus the fed state.

First-pass metabolism has been reported to be low in alcoholics, especially in alcoholic women, because of decreased ADH activity, which may be important in the increased sensitivity to alcohol and the higher blood alcohol concentrations in women than in men after an equivalent oral dose of ethanol. Several drugs, including H2 receptor blockers, such as cimetidine or ranitidine, or aspirin, inhibit stomach ADH activity. This inhibition decreases first-pass metabolism by the stomach and hence increases blood alcohol concentrations.

The overall significance of first-pass metabolism by the stomach is controversial. The speed of gastric emptying modulates gastric and hepatic first-pass metabolism of alcohol. Considering the greater levels of alcohol-metabolizing enzymes in the liver compared with the stomach, it is likely that liver plays the major role in alcohol metabolism.[16–18]

ALCOHOL METABOLISM: GENERAL PRINCIPLES

Box 3 describes some general principles of alcohol metabolism.[1–9]

The major enzyme system(s) responsible for the oxidation of ethanol, ADH, and, to a lesser extent, the cytochrome P450–dependent ethanol-oxidizing system, are present to the largest extent in the liver. Liver damage reduces the rate of alcohol oxidation and, hence, elimination from the body. Ethanol is a nutrient and has caloric value (about 7 kcal (29.3 kjoules)/g; carbohydrates and protein produce 4 kcal (16.7 kjoules)/g, whereas fat produces 9 kcal (37.7 kjoules)/g). However, unlike carbohydrates (glycogen in liver and muscle) and fat (triglycerides in adipose tissues and liver), which can be stored and used in time of need (eg, fasting), alcohol is not stored and remains in body water until eliminated. Although metabolism of the major nutrients is under hormonal control (eg, insulin/glucagon, leptin, catecholamine, thyroid hormones), generally there is little hormonal regulation to pace the rate of alcohol elimination. In view of these considerations, there is a major burden on the liver to oxidize alcohol to remove this agent from the body.

Animals with small body weight metabolize alcohol at faster rates than larger animals (eg, the rate of alcohol elimination in mice is 5 times greater than the rate in humans). These rates of alcohol metabolism correlate with the basal metabolic rate for that species, indicating that the capacity to oxidize ethanol parallels the capacity to oxidize the typical nutrients. However, alcohol-derived calories are produced at

---

Box 3
General principles of alcohol oxidation

- <10% of alcohol is excreted in breath, sweat, and urine.
- ~90% of alcohol is removed by oxidation.
- Most of this alcohol oxidation occurs in the liver.
- Alcohol cannot be stored in the liver.
- There are no major feedback mechanisms to pace the rate of alcohol metabolism to the physiologic conditions of the liver cell.

the expense of the metabolism of normal nutrients because alcohol is oxidized preferentially rather than other nutrients.[19–23]

KINETICS OF ALCOHOL ELIMINATION IN VIVO

Alcohol elimination was originally thought to be a zero-order process, meaning that alcohol was removed from the body at a constant rate, independent of the concentration of alcohol.[12–14] Because the Michaelis constant (K_m) of most ADH isozymes for ethanol is low (about 1 mM), ADH is saturated at low concentrations of alcohol; hence, the overall elimination process proceeds at maximal velocity and is independent of the alcohol concentration. However, linearity is not observed at low alcohol concentration because ADH is no longer saturated with ethanol. Alcohol elimination now follows Michaelis-Menten kinetics; the rate of change in the concentration of alcohol depends on the concentration of alcohol and the kinetic constants K_m and V_{max}.[23,24]

In addition, because the metabolism of alcohol by CYP2E1 and some ADH isozymes, such as ADH4, involves a high K_m for alcohol system, a concentration-dependent rate of ethanol elimination is observed, with higher rates of alcohol elimination at higher blood alcohol concentrations. Because of this concentration dependence, it is not possible to estimate a single rate of alcohol metabolism. Concentration-dependent metabolism of alcohol has been observed in some, but not all, studies on alcohol elimination.[25,26]

Although rates vary, the average metabolic capacity to remove alcohol is about 170 to 240 g per day for a person with a body weight of 70 kg. This capacity is equivalent to an average metabolic rate of about 7 g/h, which translates to about 1 drink per hour. Because alcoholics may consume 200 to 300 g of ethanol per day, equivalent to 1400 to 2100 kcal, consumption of normal nutrients is usually significantly decreased (typically, 2000–3000 kcal consumed per day in the absence of alcohol).

FACTORS MODIFYING THE ALCOHOL ELIMINATION RATE

There is a 3-fold to 4-fold variability in the rate of alcohol elimination by humans because of various genetic and environmental factors (described later).

Sex

There is a faster rate of alcohol elimination by women when rates are corrected for lean body mass. Because women have smaller body size and therefore smaller lean body mass, ethanol elimination per unit lean body mass is higher in women. Men and women generally have similar alcohol elimination rates when results are expressed as grams per hour or grams per liter liver volume. Because of first-pass metabolism by the stomach, it is possible that a given oral dose of alcohol may produce a higher blood ethanol concentration in women than in men.[11,15]

Age

Very young animals have low alcohol elimination rates because ADH (and CYP2E1) are not fully expressed. Fetal liver eliminates alcohol poorly, which may have consequences for fetal alcohol syndrome. There may be a small decline in alcohol elimination with aging, perhaps caused by decreased liver mass, or body water content.

Race

Alcohol elimination is reported to be higher in subjects expressing the β 3 class I ADH isoforms compared with individuals who only express the β1 isoform (discussed later). Some studies, but not all, suggest an increased rate of alcohol elimination by native

Americans compared with white people. Rates of alcohol elimination by Chinese people are similar to those of white people. Liver mass may explain ethnic and gender differences in alcohol elimination rates. More research on possible population differences in alcohol elimination is required.[27,28]

Food

Alcohol metabolism is higher in the fed nutritional state compared with the fasted state because ADH levels are higher, and the ability of substrate shuttle mechanisms (discussed later) to transport reducing equivalents into the mitochondria is increased. Food may also increase liver blood flow. The sugar fructose increases alcohol metabolism by providing substrates that help to convert NADH to NAD^+, and by enhancing mitochondrial oxygen uptake. The increase in the alcohol elimination rate by food was similar for meals of different compositions because there was no difference between carbohydrate, fat, and protein on alcohol metabolic rate.[29–31]

Biologic Rhythms

The rate of alcohol elimination varies with the time of day, being maximal at the end of the daily dark period. This variation may be related to a body temperature cycle.

Exercise

The literature is unclear, because most studies report a small increase in alcohol elimination rate, perhaps caused by increased body temperature or catecholamine release.

Alcoholism

Heavy drinking increases alcohol metabolic rate (discussed later). Advanced liver disease decreases the rate of ethanol metabolism.

Drugs

Agents that inhibit ADH (pyrazoles, isobutyramide) or compete with ethanol for ADH (methanol, ethylene glycol), or that inhibit the mitochondrial respiratory chain decrease the alcohol elimination rate. Antabuse (disulfiram) slows alcohol metabolism by inhibiting the elimination of acetaldehyde.

Scheme for Alcohol Metabolism

Fig. 1 summarizes the basic overall metabolism of alcohol.

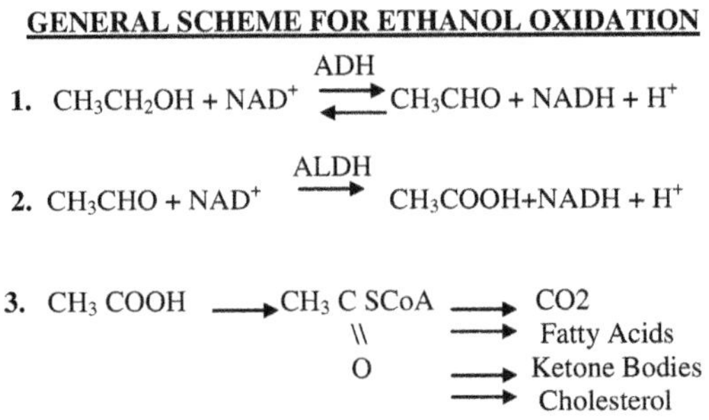

GENERAL SCHEME FOR ETHANOL OXIDATION

$$\textbf{1.} \quad CH_3CH_2OH + NAD^+ \underset{}{\overset{ADH}{\rightleftharpoons}} CH_3CHO + NADH + H^+$$

$$\textbf{2.} \quad CH_3CHO + NAD^+ \xrightarrow{ALDH} CH_3COOH + NADH + H^+$$

$$\textbf{3.} \quad CH_3COOH \longrightarrow CH_3 \underset{O}{\overset{\backslash\backslash}{C}} SCoA \longrightarrow \begin{array}{l} CO2 \\ Fatty\ Acids \\ Ketone\ Bodies \\ Cholesterol \end{array}$$

Fig. 1. Alcohol oxidation. Alcohol is oxidized by alcohol and aldehyde dehydrogenases eventually to acetyl CoA. Depending on the nutritional, hormonal, energetic status, the acetyl CoA is converted to the indicated products. ALDH, aldehyde dehydrogenase.

Step 1

Step 1 is catalyzed by the enzyme ADH, which is present largely in the liver and consists of a family of isoforms. A vitamin-related cofactor, NAD (derived from the vitamin niacin) is required to accept reducing equivalents (hydrogen atoms and electrons) from the alcohol. As a result, the ethanol is oxidized to the product acetaldehyde and the vitamin cofactor NAD^+ is reduced to the product $NADH + H^+$ (note that 2 hydrogens are removed from alcohol). The ADH reaction is reversible.

Step 2

Step 2 is catalyzed by the enzyme aldehyde dehydrogenase. Acetaldehyde is oxidized to acetate; NAD^+ is the cofactor, and is reduced to NADH. The aldehyde dehydrogenase (ALDH) reaction is irreversible. Much of the acetaldehyde produced from the oxidation of alcohol is oxidized in the liver to acetate; circulating levels of acetaldehyde are low under normal conditions.

Step 3

Much of the acetate produced by the oxidation of acetaldehyde leaves the liver and circulates to peripheral tissues where it is activated to a key metabolite acetyl coenzyme A (CoA). Acetyl CoA is also the key metabolite produced form the major nutrients (carbohydrate, fat, and excess protein). Thus, carbon atoms from alcohol become the same products produced from the oxidation of carbohydrate, fat, and protein, including CO_2, fatty acids, ketone bodies, and cholesterol; which products are formed depends on the energy state and the nutritional and hormonal conditions.

ADH

ADH is a zinc-containing enzyme consisting of 2 subunits of 40 kDa each.[4,32–34] It functions to oxidize endogenous alcohol produced by microorganisms in the gut, to oxidize exogenous ethanol and other alcohols consumed in the diet, and to oxidize substrates involved in steroid and bile acid metabolism. The enzyme has broad substrate specificity, oxidizing many primary or secondary alcohols. ADH is localized in the cytosolic fraction of the cell. ADH is found in greatest amount in the liver, followed by gastrointestinal tract, kidneys, nasal mucosa, testes, and uterus.

Multiple forms of ADH exist in human liver and their properties are reviewed in **Table 1**.

Class 1 ADH

Class 1 ADH contains 3 genes, ADH1, ADH2, and ADH3, which code for the following subunits: α(ADHIA), β1, β2, and β3(ADHIB), γ1, and γ2 (ADH1C). These different subunits and polymorphic forms can combine to produce a variety of homodimers or heterodimers (eg, αα, β1β1, αβ2). The forms are found primarily in the liver. The class I ADH forms are mainly responsible for the oxidation of alcohol. In a new classification,

Table 1
Kinetic constants for human liver ADH isoforms

Constant	αα	β1β1	β2β2	β3β3	γ1γ1	γ2γ2	ππ
K_m NAD$^+$, (μM)	13	7.4	180	530	7.9	8.7	14
K_m ethanol (mM)	4.2	0.049	0.94	24	1	0.63	34
K_i 4-methylpyrazole (μM)	1.1	0.13	—	2.1	0.1	—	2000
V_{max} (min^{-1})	27	9.2	400	300	87	35	20
pH (optimum)	10.5	10.5	8.5	7.0	10.5	10	10.5

the family members have been classified into 5 distinct classes, designated ADH1 to ADH5, from the structural and kinetic characteristics. Human ADH genes that encode the subunit polypeptides α, β_1, β_2, β_3, γ_1, γ_2, π, χ, and μ (or named σ) are designated ADH1A (old ADH1), ADH1B*1 (old ADH2*1), ADH1B*2 (old ADH2*2), ADH1B*3 (old ADH2*3), ADH1C*1 (old ADH3*1), ADH1C*2 (old ADH3*2), ADH2 (old ADH4), ADH3 (old ADH5), and ADH4 (old ADH7), respectively. The ADH5 (old ADH6)-encoding polypeptide has not been given a Greek letter.

Class II ADH

The ADH4 gene codes for the π subunit, which produces $\pi\pi$ homodimers in the liver and, to a lesser extent, in kidney and lung. The high K_m for alcohol may make this enzyme more important in metabolism of high concentrations of alcohol.

Class III ADH

The ADH5 gene codes for the χ subunit, which produces $\chi\chi$ homodimers. This isoform has a high K_m for alcohol (>2 M).

Class V ADH

The mRNA product produced by the ADH6 gene is present in liver and stomach, but the protein has not been characterized.

Class IV ADH

The ADH7 gene encodes the sigma subunit, which is efficient in oxidizing retinol to retinal. This form is present in the stomach.

The class I ADH isoforms play the most important role in alcohol oxidation.[33–37] ADH is present in low levels in fetal liver and the fetus eliminates ethanol slowly because of this late maturation of ADH genes. The ability to form many isoforms, with varying kinetic properties, probably contributes to the large variability in the capacity for metabolizing alcohol that human populations exhibit. The strong sensitivity of class I ADH to pyrazole inhibition explains the powerful inhibition of alcohol metabolism by these agents.

Control of ADH activity is complex:

1. Dissociation of the product NADH is the rate-limiting step
2. It is subject to product inhibition by NADH and acetaldehyde
3. It is subject to substrate inhibition by high concentrations of ethanol

Alcohol oxidation is generally limited by the maximum capacity of ADH. The amount of ADH in the liver is greater in the fed than the fasted state, which plays a major role in the increased rate of alcohol oxidation in the fed state.[38,39] Inhibitors of ADH inhibit ethanol oxidation in direct proportion to their potency as inhibitors of ADH. Hormonal effects on ADH are complex; some stimulation is found after treatment with growth hormone, epinephrine, or estrogens. Thyroid hormones and androgens inhibit ADH activity.

The polymorphic forms of ADH (class I ADH1B, ADH1C) vary to some extent in different racial groups, as shown in **Table 2**. To date, there are no clear associations between the various ADH isozymes and the development of alcoholic liver disease, or the susceptibility to alcohol actions, or the propensity to consume ethanol. Studies that have investigated the association between alcoholism and alcohol-induced liver damage with the ADH2, ADH3, CYP2E1, and ALDH2 polymorphisms are not conclusive. A large meta-analysis[36] showed that carriers of the ADH2*1 and ADH3*2 alleles, the less active ethanol-metabolizing ADHs, and the highly active ALDH2*1 allele had an increased risk of alcoholism. This finding likely reflects low accumulation of

Table 2
Frequency of ADH alleles in racial populations

	ADH1B*1 (%)	ADH1B*2 (%)	ADH1B*3 (%)	ADH1C*1 (%)	ADH1C*2 (%)
White American	>95	<5	<5	50	50
White European	85	15	<5	60	40
Japanese	15	85	<5	95	5
Black American	85	<5	15	85	15

acetaldehyde in these individuals. In liver disease, *ALDH2*1* is a protective factor because it removes toxic acetaldehyde. Neither the ADH2 nor the ADH3 polymorphism were implicated in the development of liver disease. Allelic variants of CYP2E1 were not involved in determining the risk of alcoholism or in alcoholic liver disease. Further research in this area is required, as is research on what other substrates the various ADH isoforms oxidize.

HEPATIC REDOX STATE

Because the ADH and ALDH2 reactions reduce NAD^+ to NADH, the cellular NAD^+/NADH redox ratio is reduced as a consequence of ethanol metabolism.[40–42] This reduction has profound effects on other liver metabolic pathways that require NAD^+ or are inhibited by NADH.

Because the ADH reactions occur in the cytosol, the cytosolic NAD^+/NADH redox ratio is reduced. This ratio is reflected by the pyruvate/lactate ratio because of the reaction:

$$Pyruvate + NADH^+ \overset{LDH}{\rightleftarrows} Lactate + NAD^+$$

Because the ALDH reaction occurs largely in the mitochondria, the mitochondrial NAD^+/NADH redox ratio is reduced. This reaction is reflected by the β-hydroxybutyrate/acetoacetate ratio because of the reaction:

$$Acetoacetate + NADH \overset{BOHBDH}{\rightleftarrows} \beta - Hydroxybutyrate + NAD^+$$

Important reactions inhibited because of this decreased NAD^+/NADH redox ratio are:

1. Glycolysis
2. Citric acid cycle (ketogenesis favored)
3. Pyruvate dehydrogenase
4. Fatty acid oxidation
5. Gluconeogenesis

REOXIDATION OF NADH GENERATED BY THE ADH REACTION

To maintain effective rates of alcohol oxidation by ADH, it is important to regenerate NAD^+ from the NADH produced by the ADH reaction. Under certain conditions, the rate of oxidation of alcohol is limited by the reoxidation of NADH. The major system for reoxidizing NADH is the mitochondrial electron transfer system. By coupling NADH reoxidation to this system, energy is produced from alcohol metabolism (7 kcal/g ethanol). **Fig. 2** shows the typical mitochondrial respiratory chain found in all tissues except the red blood cell. Note the 4 complexes that make up the chain.

Reoxidation of NADH Generated by

the ADH Reaction

- There is a need to reoxidize NADH back to NAD⁺.
- Cytosolic pathways are not sufficient.
- NADH must be reoxidized by the mitochondrial electron transfer pathway shown below.

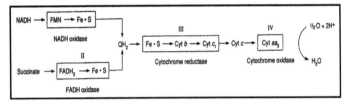

Fig. 2. The mitochondrial respiratory chain. Reducing equivalents (electrons) enter the respiratory chain either from NADH or from succinate and are passed through a series of electron carriers to cytochrome oxidase, which reacts with molecular oxygen to produce water. The NADH produced from the oxidation of alcohol by ADH is oxidized by the respiratory chain. Energy, in the form of ATP, is produced during this oxidation; hence, alcohol is of caloric value. Cyt, cytochrome; FMN, flavin mononucleotide.

As electrons or reducing equivalents pass through complexes I, III, and IV, an energized electrochemical and pH gradient is developed that is used to synthesize adenosine triphosphate (ATP) via complex V, the ATP synthase.[43,44]

SUBSTRATE SHUTTLES

Because intact mitochondria are not permeable to NADH, it is necessary to transfer the reducing equivalents of NADH present in the cytosol into the mitochondria by substrate shuttle mechanisms. The 2 major substrate shuttles are the á-glycerophosphate shuttle and the malate-aspartate shuttle (**Fig. 3**). The malate-aspartate shuttle plays the major role in transferring reducing equivalents into the mitochondria.[45–48] The rate of alcohol oxidation can be limited by the transfer of reducing equivalents into mitochondria or by the actual capacity of the respiratory chain to oxidize these reducing equivalents. Shuttle capacity may become limiting in fasting metabolic states as the levels of shuttle components decrease. This limitation may contribute to the reduced rates of alcohol oxidation (in addition to reduced ADH content) in the fasting metabolic state. Agents or conditions that enhance reoxidation of NADH by the respiratory chain can increase the rate of alcohol metabolism (eg, uncoupling agents can accelerate ethanol oxidation in the fed metabolic state).[38,39]

CATALASE-DEPENDENT OXIDATION OF ALCOHOL

$$CH_3CH_2OH + H_2O_2 \rightarrow CH_3CHO + 2H_2O \tag{a}$$

$$H_2O_2 + H_2O_2 \rightarrow 2H_2O + O_2 \tag{b}$$

Catalase, a heme-containing enzyme, is found in the peroxisomal fraction of the cell. This antioxidant enzyme is important because it normally catalyzes the removal of

Substrate Shuttles

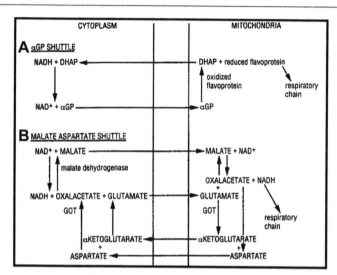

Fig. 3. Substrate shuttle mechanisms for the reoxidation of NADH by the mitochondrial respiratory chain. The ADH reaction oxidizes alcohol in the liver cytosol and therefore produces NADH in the cytosol. This NADH cannot directly enter the mitochondria for oxidation (see **Fig. 2**) and therefore has to be transported into the mitochondria by either the α-glycerophosphate (A) or the malate-aspartate (B) shuttle. DHAP, dihydroxyacetone phosphate; GOT, glutamate oxalacetate transaminase.

H_2O_2 (reaction b shown earlier) but it can also oxidize alcohol as shown in reaction (a) earlier. This pathway is limited by the low rates of H_2O_2 generation produced under physiologic cellular conditions (less than 4 μmol/g liver/h, only 2% that of alcohol oxidation) and seems to have an insignificant role in alcohol oxidation by the liver.

Several central nervous system effects of ethanol are mediated by acetaldehyde. Because circulating acetaldehyde levels are low, the metabolism of alcohol to acetaldehyde by the brain has been a major area of alcohol research. Catalase is present throughout the brain, in the peroxisomes. Inhibitors of catalase were reported to depress oxidation of alcohol to acetaldehyde by the brain. Acetaldehyde derived from catalase-dependent oxidation of alcohol in the brain has been suggested to play a role in the development of tolerance to alcohol, to voluntary ethanol consumption, and to the positive reinforcing actions of ethanol, perhaps via interaction with catecholamines to produce various condensation products.[49–51]

MICROSOMAL (CYTOCHROME P450) OXIDATION OF ETHANOL

$$NADPH + H^+ + CH_3CH_2OH + O_2 \rightarrow NADP^+ + CH_3CHO + 2H_2O$$

Cytochrome P450s are a family of heme enzymes that are involved in the oxidation of steroids, fatty acids, and numerous xenobiotics ingested from the environment. Highest levels of cytochrome P450 are in the liver, where they are present mainly in the endoplasmic reticulum (microsomal fraction). Some P450s are also found in mitochondria. P450 functions in conjunction with other microsomal enzymes such as NADPH–cytochrome P450 reductase and cytochrome b5.[52–54]There are many isoforms of P450; more than 100 gene families have been identified. The P450s are arranged in families based on sequence homologies. CYP2E1 is a P450 that has the highest activity for oxidizing alcohol to acetaldehyde. Besides ethanol, CYP2E1 can oxidize many other compounds including acetone, benzene, and other alcohols. A clear physiologic function for CYP2E1 has not been identified. Some of the significant properties of CYP2E1 are listed in **Box 4**.[55–58]

The K_m of CYP2E1 for alcohol is 10 mM,10-fold higher than the K_m of ADH for ethanol but still within the range of alcohol concentrations seen in social drinking. At low alcohol concentrations, CYP2E1 may account for about 10% of the total alcohol-oxidizing capacity of the liver. However, in view of its higher K_m, the relevance of CYP2E1 in ethanol oxidation increases as blood alcohol concentrations increase. Alcohol oxidation increases at higher ethanol concentrations, and much of this increase is caused by CYP2E1 metabolism of alcohol.

Many P450s are induced by their substrates; this helps to remove the xenobiotic from the body. CYP2E1 levels are increased by chronic ethanol administration by a mechanism largely involving protection of the enzyme against proteolysis by the macromolecular proteasome complex. CYP2E1 is also induced in diabetics, in the fasted nutritional state, and by certain drugs. Because of its inducibility, CYP2E1 may play an important role in alcohol metabolism after chronic ethanol consumption (ie, in alcoholics). Thirteen different CYP2E1 polymorphisms have been identified. Some of these may be important as risk factors for carcinogenicity of tobacco or certain toxins; however, there is no evidence linking any of these polymorphisms to the frequency of alcohol liver damage.

ALCOHOL-DRUG INTERACTIONS

Because ethanol and certain drugs compete for metabolism by CYP2E1, active drinkers often display an enhanced sensitivity to certain drugs as alcohol inhibits the metabolism of the drug and thereby prolongs its half-life. In contrast, because CYP2E1 is induced after chronic alcohol consumption, metabolism of drugs that are also substrates for CYP2E1 is increased, which decreases the half-life of the drug, and thus decreases the effectiveness of the drug when ethanol is not present. CYP2E1 is active in oxidizing many chemicals to reactive intermediates (eg, carbon tetrachloride, benzene, nitrosamines, acetaminophen, halothane). Toxicity of these agents is enhanced in alcoholics.[55,57–59]

Box 4
Cytochrome P4502E1 (CYP2E1)

- A minor pathway for alcohol metabolism
- Produces acetaldehyde, 1-hydroxyethyl radical
- Responsible for alcohol-drug interactions
- Activates toxins such as acetaminophen, CCl4, halothane, benzene, and halogenated hydrocarbons to reactive toxic intermediates
- Activates procarcinogens such as nitrosamines and azo compounds to active carcinogens
- Activates molecular oxygen to reactive oxygen species such as superoxide radical anion, H_2O_2, and hydroxyl radical

The CYP2E1 catalytic turnover cycle results in the production of large amounts of reactive oxygen intermediates such as the superoxide radical and hydrogen peroxide. This production may be important in mechanisms of alcoholic liver injury involving oxidative stress.[60] Regulation of CYP2E1 is complex, involving transcription, translation, and protein turnover mechanisms.

METABOLIC ADAPTATION (TOLERANCE)

Besides central nervous system adaptation, alcoholics (in the absence of liver disease) often display an increased rate of blood ethanol clearance. This increase is metabolic tolerance or adaptation. Suggested mechanisms for this metabolic tolerance are shown in **Box 5**.[55,61–63]

1. Class I ADH is not inducible. Further work with the many human isoforms is needed.
2. Substrate shuttle capacity and transport of reducing equivalents into the mitochondria is not altered by chronic alcohol consumption.
3. A major theory to explain metabolic adaptation, the hypermetabolic state hypothesis, postulates that changes in thyroid hormone levels increases ($Na^+ + K^+$) activated ATPase, with the subsequent increase of adenosine diphosphate (ADP) levels, which increases the state 3 mitochondrial oxygen consumption, therefore increasing NADH reoxidation. Increased oxygen consumption may cause hypoxia, especially to hepatocytes of zone 3 of the liver acinus, the region where alcohol toxicity originates (centrilobular hypoxia hypothesis).
4. CYP2E1 levels are enhanced after alcohol treatment. Because CYP2E1 is the most active P450 for oxidizing alcohol, this may play an important role in metabolic tolerance.
5. Ethanol, perhaps via increasing endotoxin levels, may activate nonparenchymal cells such as Kupffer cells to release mediators (cytokines and prostaglandins) that stimulate oxygen consumption, and thereby NADH reoxidation, by parenchymal cells.

The so-called swift increase in alcohol metabolism (SIAM) refers to an increased rate of ethanol metabolism within a few hours after alcohol administration in vivo or in vitro. Mechanisms responsible for SIAM are complex and seem to involve 3 major pathways: the mitochondria, the peroxisome, and endotoxin activation of Kupffer cells.[64]

ZONAL METABOLISM OF ALCOHOL IN THE HEPATIC ACINUS

Liver injury after chronic alcohol treatment originates in the perivenous zone of the hepatic lobule.[65–67] Possible factors to explain this include:

Box 5
Suggested mechanisms for metabolic tolerance to alcohol

- Induction of ADHs
- Increased shuttle capacity
- Increased reoxidation of NADH by mitochondria
- Induction of CYP2E1
- Hypermetabolic state
- Increased release of cytokines or prostaglandins, which increase oxygen consumption by hepatocytes

1. Oxygenation is low in this zone because there is an oxygen gradient across the liver lobule and less oxygen reaches the hepatocytes in the perivenous zone. This gradient is exacerbated after chronic alcohol administration, which increases hepatic oxygen uptake, so even less oxygen reaches perivenous hepatocytes

2 and 3. ADH and ALDH2, and rates of alcohol and acetaldehyde metabolism, are evenly distributed across the liver lobule. However, because of the reduced oxygen tension, there is a more pronounced reduction of the hepatic redox state produced by ethanol in the perivenous zone

4. CYP2E1 is largely in the perivenous zone, which explains why toxicity of drugs metabolized by CYP2E1 to reactive metabolites (eg, CCl4 or acetaminophen) occurs in the perivenous zone.

5. Level of antioxidants, such as glutathione, are reduced in the perivenous zone.

OTHER PATHWAYS OF ALCOHOL METABOLISM
Conjugation Reactions

Ethanol can react with glucuronic acid to form ethylglucuronide. Such soluble conjugates are readily excreted. Cofactor availability and the poor affinity for alcohol of most conjugation enzymes limit these pathways. Ethyl glucuronide[68] is a nonvolatile, water-soluble direct metabolite of ethanol. It can be detected in body fluids, tissue, sweat, and hair for an extended time after alcohol has been eliminated from the body. These properties led to the suggestion that ethyl glucuronide may be a marker for alcohol consumption or for the detection of relapse of alcoholics. Ethyl glucuronide is not detectable in abstinent patients, nondrinkers, or teetotalers and is thus specific for alcohol consumption.

Fatty Acyl Synthases

Fatty acid ethyl ester synthases catalyze the reaction between ethanol and a fatty acid to produce a fatty acyl ester. These synthases are present in most tissues, especially the liver and pancreas, which are the organs most susceptible to alcohol toxicity.[69] These esters are synthesized in the endoplasmic reticulum, and transported to the plasma membrane and then removed from the cell by binding to lipoproteins and albumin and transported in the circulation. Fatty acid ethyl esters can be toxic, inhibiting DNA and protein synthesis. When oxidative metabolism of ethanol is blocked, there is an increase in ethanol metabolism to the fatty acid ethyl ester. These esters can be detected in the blood after alcohol is no longer detectable and therefore detection of fatty acid ethyl esters may serve as a marker of alcohol intake.

ACETALDEHYDE METABOLISM

The balance between the various ADH and ALDH isoforms regulates the concentration of acetaldehyde, which is important as a key risk factor for the development of alcoholism.[70–74] Most of the acetaldehyde produced from the oxidation of alcohol is further oxidized in the liver by a family of ALDH isoforms. Major ALDH isoforms exist in the mitochondrial, microsomal, and cytosolic compartments. Mitochondria contain a low K_m ALDH in the matrix space (class II ALDH) and a high K_m ALDH in the outer membrane, microsomes contain a high K_m ALDH, whereas the cytosol contains an intermediate-K_m (class I ALDH) and a high K_m (class III ALDH) ALDH. Acetaldehyde can also be oxidized by aldehyde oxidase, xanthine oxidase, and by CYP2E1, but these are insignificant pathways. The low K_m mitochondrial ALDH oxidizes most of the acetaldehyde produced from the oxidation of alcohol, although, in human liver, the class I cytosolic ALDH may also contribute.[75] The class I and II ALDHs are tetra-meric enzymes with subunit molecular weights of 54 kDa.

In general, the capacity of ALDH to remove acetaldehyde exceeds the capacity of acetaldehyde generation by the various pathways of alcohol oxidation. Therefore, circulating levels of acetaldehyde are usually low. Chronic alcohol consumption decreases acetaldehyde oxidation, either because of decreased ALDH2 activity or impaired mitochondrial function. Acetaldehyde generation is increased by chronic alcohol consumption because of metabolic adaptation. As a result, circulating levels of acetaldehyde are usually increased in alcoholics because of increased production, decreased removal, or both.

The basis of action for certain alcohol-aversive drugs such as disulfiram (Antabuse) or cyanamide is to inhibit ALDH, and therefore alcohol oxidation. The resulting accumu-lation of acetaldehyde causes a variety of effects such as nausea, sweating, vomiting, and increased heart rate if ethanol is consumed with these drugs. Certain individuals, usually of Asian extraction, have an inactive mitochondrial ALDH2 because of a single amino acid substitution. Glutamate 487 is converted to a lysine residue, which causes a large decrease in affinity for the NAD$^+$ cofactor. Thus inactive enzyme can be found in 15% to 40% of the population of east Asia and, when these individuals consume ethanol, blood levels of acetaldehyde are 5-fold to 20- fold higher than those found in individuals with the active ALDH allele. Individuals with the inactive ALDH show marked vasodilation, nausea, and dysphasia when consuming alcohol, and are virtual abstainers if homozygous for the *ALDH2*2* allele. Acetaldehyde is poorly eliminated by these individuals and, as a consequence, little alcohol is consumed. ALDH2-deficient individuals are at reduced risk for alcoholism. They may have possible increased risk for liver damage if alcohol continues to be consumed.

Acetaldehyde is a reactive compound and can interact with thiol and amino groups of amino acids in proteins. Formation of acetaldehyde adducts with proteins may cause inhibition of that protein's function and/or cause an immune response.[73,74] ALDH is important not only for removing acetaldehyde but also for the removal of other aldehydes, including biogenic aldehydes and lipid peroxidation–derived aldehydes. Effective removal of acetaldehyde is important not only to prevent cellular toxicity but also to maintain efficient removal of alcohol (eg, acetaldehyde is a product inhibitor of ADH). The class I ALDH can oxidize retinal to retinoic acid; the possibility that high levels of acetaldehyde compete with retinal for oxidation by class I ALDH may be of developmental significance.[75]

CONCLUSIONS AND FUTURE CONSIDERATIONS

Although much has been learned about the pathways of ethanol metabolism and how these pathways are regulated, there are many critical questions remaining. For example:

- What limits and regulates alcohol metabolism in vivo?
- What is the mechanism(s) responsible for metabolic tolerance?
- Is it alcohol per se, or alcohol-derived metabolites, that play a key role in organ damage? What might be the consequences of attempting to accelerate ethanol metabolism?
- What is the role, if any, of the various ADH isoforms in oxidation of endogenous substrates, alcohol metabolism, and alcohol toxicity? The hypothesis that alcohol or acetaldehyde inhibit the oxidation of physiologically important endog-enous substrates of ADH or ALDH2 and that this may contribute to the adverse action of ethanol requires further study.

- Can the various ADH and ALDH isozymes or polymorphic forms of CYP2E1 be of predictive value or serve as markers to identify individuals who are susceptible to developing alcoholism? Can noninvasive probes be developed to measure the various isoforms present?
- Are there population and gender differences in rates of alcohol elimination and, if so, are such differences explained by the varying isoforms present in that population?
- What controls the expression of the various isoforms at the transcriptional level, and are there posttranscriptional modifications? What dictates the turnover of these enzymes, which may be important in regulating the amount of active enzyme present in the cells (eg, CYP2E1)?
- Why are calories from alcohol not as efficient in providing energy as are calories from typical nutrients? What is the mechanism by which food increases alcohol metabolism?
- What role, if any, does acetate play in the metabolic actions of alcohol?
- Can appropriate models and rate equations be built to kinetically describe the process of alcohol elimination under various conditions?

REFERENCES

1. Khanna JM, Israel Y. Ethanol metabolism. Int Rev Physiol 1980;21:275–315.
2. Crabb DW, Bosron WF, Li TK. Ethanol metabolism. Pharmacol Ther 1987;34: 59–73.
3. Kennedy NP, Tipton KF. Ethanol metabolism and alcoholic liver disease. Essays Biochem 1990;25:137–95.
4. Riveros-Rosas H, Julian-Sanchez A, Pina E. Enzymology of ethanol and acetalde-hyde metabolism in mammals. Arch Med Res 1997;28:453–71.
5. Kalant H. Pharmacokinetics of ethanol: absorption, distribution and elimination. In: Begleiter H, Kissin B, editors. The pharmacology of alcohol and alcohol dependence. New York: Oxford University Press; 1996. p. 15–58.
6. Cederbaum A. Metabolism of ethanol, acetaldehyde and condensation products. In: Begleiter H, Kissin B, editors. The pharmacology of alcohol and alcohol dependence. New York: Oxford University Press; 1996. p. 59–109.
7. Lands WE. A review of alcohol clearance in humans. Alcohol 1998;15:147–60.
8. Zakhari S. Overview: how is alcohol metabolized by the body. Alcohol Res Health 2006;29:245–54.
9. Zakhari S, Li TK. Determinants of alcohol use and abuse: impact of quantity and frequency patterns on liver disease. Hepatology 2007;46:2032–9.
10. Frezza M, Di Padova C, Pozzato G, et al. High blood alcohol levels in women. N Engl J Med 1990;322:95–9.
11. Cole-Harding S, Wilson JR. Ethanol metabolism in men and women. J Stud Alcohol 1987;48:380–7.
12. Norberg A, Jones WA, Hahn RG, et al. Role of variability in explaining ethanol pharmacokinetics. Clin Pharmacokinet 2003;42:1–31.
13. Wilkinson PK, Sedman AJ, Sakmar E, et al. Pharmacokinetics of ethanol after oral administration in the fasting state. J Pharmacokinet Biopharm 1977;5:207–24.
14. Baraona E, Abittan CS, Dohmen K, et al. Gender differences in pharmacokinetics of alcohol. Alcohol Clin Exp Res 2001;25:502–7.
15. Kwo PY, Ramchandanl VA, O'Connor S, et al. Gender differences in alcohol metabolism: relationship to liver volume and effect of adjusting for body mass. Gastroenterology 1998;115:1552–7.

16. DiPadova C, Worner TM, Julkunen RJ, et al. Effects of fasting and chronic alcohol consumption on the first pass metabolism of ethanol. Gastroenterologist 1987;92: 1169–73.
17. Levitt MD, Furne J, DeMaster E. First pass metabolism of ethanol is negligible in rat gastric mucosa. Alcohol Clin Exp Res 1997;21:293–7.
18. Lee SL, Chau GY, Yao CT, et al. Functional assessment of human alcohol dehydrogenase family in ethanol metabolism: significance of first-pass metabolism. Alcohol Clin Exp Res 2006;30:1132–42.
19. Morgan MY, Levine JA. Alcohol and nutrition. Proc Nutr Soc 1988;47:85–98.
20. Lieber CS. Perspectives: do alcohol calories count? Am J Clin Nutr 1991;54: 976–82.
21. Lands WE. Alcohol and energy intake. Am J Clin Nutr 1995;62:1101S–6S.
22. Addolorato G, Capristo E, Greco AL, et al. Energy expenditure, substrate oxidation and body composition in subjects with chronic alcoholism: new findings from metabolic assessment. Alcohol Clin Exp Res 1997;21:962–7.
23. Salaspuro MP, Lieber CS. Non-uniformity of blood ethanol elimination: its exaggeration after chronic consumption. Ann Clin Res 1978;10:294–7.
24. Matsumoto H, Fukui Y. Pharmacokinetics of ethanol: a review of the methodology. Addict Biol 2002;7:5–14.
25. Holford NG. Clinical pharmacokinetics of ethanol. Clin Pharmacokinet 1987;13: 273–92.
26. Ramchandani VA, Bostron WF, Li TK. Research advances in ethanol metabolism. Pathol Biol 2001;49:676–82.
27. Reed TE, Kalant H, Gibbins RJ, et al. Alcohol and acetaldehyde metabolism in Caucasians, Chinese and Amerinds. Can Med Assoc J 1976;6:851–5.
28. Bennion LJ, Li TK. Alcohol metabolism in American Indians and Whites. N Engl J Med 1976;294:9–13.
29. Passanati GT, Wolff CA, Vesell E. Reproducibility of individual rates of ethanol metabolism in fasting subjects. Clin Pharmacol Ther 1990;47:389–96.
30. Wissel PS. Dietary influences on ethanol metabolism. Drug Nutr Interact 1987;5: 161–8.
31. Ramchandani VA, Kwo PY, Li TK. Effect of food and food composition on alcohol elimination rates in healthy men and women. J Clin Pharmacol 2001;41:1345–50.
32. Edenberg H. The genetics of alcohol metabolism. Alcohol Res Health 2007;30:5–13.
33. Crabb DW. Ethanol oxidizing enzymes: roles in alcohol metabolism and alcoholic liver disease. Prog Liver Dis 1995;13:151–72.
34. Bosron W, Ehrig T, Li TK. Genetic factors in alcohol metabolism and alcoholism. Semin Liver Dis 1993;13:126–35.
35. Eriksson CJ, Fukunaga T, Sarkola T, et al. Functional relevance of human ADH polymorphism. Alcohol Clin Exp Res 2001;25:157S–63S.
36. Zintzaras E, Stefanidis I, Santos M, et al. Do alcohol-metabolizing enzyme gene polymorphisms increase the risk of alcoholism and alcoholic liver disease. Hepatology 2006;43:352–61.
37. Kimura M, Miyakawa T, Matsushita S, et al. Gender differences in the effects of ADHIB and ALDH2 polymorphisms in alcoholism. Alcohol Clin Exp Res 2011; 35:1923–7.
38. Meijer AJ, Van Wuerkom GM, Williamson JR, et al. Rate-limiting factors in the oxidation of ethanol by isolated rat liver cells. Biochem J 1975;150:205–9.
39. Cederbaum AI, Dicker E, Rubin E. Transfer and reoxidation of reducing equivalents as the rate-limiting steps in the oxidation of ethanol by liver cells isolated from fed and fasted rats. Arch Biochem Biophys 1977;183:638–46.

40. Gordon ER. The effect of chronic consumption of ethanol on the redox state of the rat liver. Can J Biochem 1972;50:949–57.

41. Stubbs M, Veech RL, Krebs HA. Control of the redox of the nicotinamide-adenine-dinucleotide couple in rat liver cytoplasm. Biochem J 1972;126:59–65.

42. Veech RL, Guynn R, Veloso D. The time course of the effects of ethanol in the redox and phosphorylation states of rat liver. Biochem J 1972;127:387–97.

43. Szabo G, Hoek JB, Darley-Usmar V, et al. Alcohol and mitochondrial metabolism: at the crossroads of life and death. Alcohol Clin Exp Res 2005;29:1749–52.

44. Teplova VV, Belosludtsev KN, Belosludtseva NV, et al. Role of mitochondria in hepatotoxicity of ethanol. Cell Biophys 2010;55:951–8.

45. Cederbaum AI, Lieber CS, Beattie DS, et al. Characterization of shuttle mechanisms in the transport of reducing equivalents into mitochondria. Arch Biochem Biophys 1973;158:763–81.

46. Dawson AG. Rapid oxidation of NADH via the reconstituted malate-aspartate shuttle in systems containing mitochondrial and soluble fractions of rat liver: implications for ethanol metabolism. Biochem Pharmacol 1982;31:2733–8.

47. Cederbaum AI, Lieber CS, Toth A, et al. Effect of ethanol and fat on the transport of reducing equivalents into rat liver mitochondria. J Biol Chem 1973;248:4977–86.

48. Sugano T, Handler JA, Yoshihara H, et al. Acute and chronic ethanol treatment in vivo increases malate-aspartate shuttle capacity in perfused rat liver. J Biol Chem 1990;265:21549–53.

49. Zimatkin SM, Liopo AV, Deitrich RA. Distribution and kinetics of ethanol metabolism in rat brain. Alcohol Clin Exp Res 1998;22:1623–7.

50. Thurman RG, Handler JA. New perspectives in catalase-dependent ethanol metabolism. Drug Metab Rev 1989;20:679–88.

51. Deng XS, Deitrich RA. Putative role of brain acetaldehyde in ethanol addiction. Curr Drug Abuse Rev 2008;1:3–8.

52. Guengerich FR. Mammalian cytochrome P450. Boca Raton (FL): CRC Press; 1987.

53. Nelson DR, Koymans L, Kamataki T, et al. P450 superfamily: update on new sequences, gene mapping, accession numbers and nomenclature. Pharmacogenomics 1996;6:1–42.

54. Lewis DF, Pratt JM. The P450 catalytic cycle and oxygenation mechanism. Drug Metab Rev 1998;30:739–86.

55. Lieber CS. Cytochrome P4502E1: its physiological and pathological role. Physiol Rev 1997;77:517–44.

56. Caro AA, Cederbaum AI. Oxidative stress, toxicology and pharmacology of CYP2E1. Annu Rev Pharmacol Toxicol 2004;44:27–42.

57. Bolt M, Koos PH, Their H. The cytochrome P450 isoenzyme CYP2E1 in the biological processing of industrial chemicals. Int Arch Occup Environ Health 2003;76:174–85.

58. Koop DP. Oxidative and reductive metabolism by cytochrome P4502E1. FASEB J 1992;6:724–30.

59. Gonzalez FJ. Roles of cytochromes P450 in chemical toxicity and oxidative stress: studies with CYP2E1. Mutat Res 2005;569:101–10.

60. Lu Y, Cederbaum AI. CYP2E1 and oxidative liver injury by alcohol. Free Radic Biol Med 2008;44:723–38.

61. Bernstein J, Videla L, Israel Y. Role of the sodium pump in the regulation of liver metabolism in experimental alcoholism. Ann N Y Acad Sci 1974;242:560–72.

62. Cederbaum AI, Dicker E, Lieber CS, et al. Ethanol oxidation by isolated hepatocytes from ethanol-treated and control rats; factor contributing to the metabolic

adaptation after chronic ethanol consumption. Biochem Pharmacol 1978;27: 7–15.

63. Videla L, Israel Y. Factors that modify the metabolism of ethanol in rat liver and adaptive changes produced by its chronic administration. Biochem J 1970; 118:275–81.

64. Bradford BU, Rusyn I. Swift increase in alcohol metabolism (SIAM): understanding the phenomenon of hypermetabolism in liver. Alcohol 2005;35:13–7.

65. Kashiwagi T, Ji S, Lemasters JJ, et al. Rates of alcohol dehydrogenase-dependent ethanol metabolism in periportal and pericentral regions of the perfused rat liver. Mol Pharmacol 1982;21:438–43.

66. Vaananen H, Lindros KO. Comparison of ethanol metabolism in isolated periportal or perivenous hepatocytes: effects of chronic ethanol treatment. Alcohol Clin Exp Res 1985;9:315–21.

67. Chen L, Sidner RA, Lumeng L. Distribution of alcohol dehydrogenase and the low K_m form of aldehyde dehydrogenase in isolated perivenous and periportal hepatocytes in rats. Alcohol Clin Exp Res 1992;16:23–9.

68. Seidl S, Wurst FM, Alt A. Ethyl glucuronide - a biological marker for recent alcohol consumption. Addict Biol 2001;6:205–12.

69. Laposata M. Fatty acid ethyl esters: non oxidative metabolites of ethanol. Addict Biol 1998;3:5–14.

70. Agarwal DP, Goedde HW. Human aldehyde dehydrogenases: their role in alcoholism. Alcohol 1989;6:517–23.

71. Goedde HW, Agarwal DP. Pharmacogenetics of aldehyde dehydrogenase. Pharmacol Ther 1990;45:345–71.

72. Lindros KO, Eriksson CJ. The role of acetaldehyde in the action of ethanol. Finnish Foundation Stud Alc 1975;23.

73. Niemela O. Acetaldehyde adducts of proteins: diagnostic and pathogenic implications in diseases caused by excessive alcohol consumption. Scand J Clin Lab Invest Suppl 1993;53:45–54.

74. Sorrell MF, Tuma DJ. Hypothesis: alcoholic liver injury and the covalent binding of acetaldehyde. Alcohol Clin Exp Res 1989;9:306–9.

75. Sophos NA, Vasiliou V. Aldehyde dehydrogenase gene superfamily: the 2002 update. Chem Biol Interact 2002;143–144:5–22.

Immunology in Alcoholic Liver Disease

Anupama T. Duddempudi, MD

KEYWORDS

- Immunology • Kupffer cell • Alcoholic liver disease • Inflammation • Immune system

KEY POINTS

- The progression of alcohol-induced liver damage involves complex interactions of the immune system and hepatocytes.
- Elevated endotoxin levels lead to the Kupffer cells activation and internalization of the endotoxin leads to the transcription of pro-inflammatory cytokines such as tumor necrosis factor-α and production of superoxides.
- The production of cytokines and superoxides leads to hepatic injury and in some cases fibrosis.
- Hepatic fibrosis is regarded as a turning point in alcohol induced liver disease because it can lead to cirrhosis.
- Understanding the role that the immune system plays in alcohol-induced liver injury is instrumental in leading to development of new therapies. For example, these new insights could help develop applications that prevent endotoxemia which would modulate the interleukin-17 pathway to decrease neutrophils in the liver.

INTRODUCTION

Chronic alcohol consumption is known to cause significant liver damage, resulting in fibrosis and, eventually, cirrhosis. The mechanisms by which alcohol exerts the damaging effects on the hepatocytes have not been well understood, but recent advancements have been made in the delineation of the earliest events in the injury pattern. Understanding the mechanisms of alcohol-induced liver damage may open the door to new therapeutic alternatives for the treatment of these patients.

Alcohol is primarily metabolized by alcohol dehydrogenase or cytochrome P450 pathways. During the metabolization of alcohol by the cytochrome P450 pathway, there is release of highly reactive oxygen species (ROS). ROS can damage the liver by altering the degradation of fat molecules, resulting in oxidative stress and free radical build up.[1] Recently it has been shown that immune mechanisms are partially responsible for the onset and progression of alcoholic liver disease. It appears that several

There is no financial disclosure.
Division of Gastroenterology, Hepatology and Nutrition North Shore University Hospital, 300 Community Drive, Manhasset, NY 11030, USA
E-mail address: aduddempudi@nshs.edu

Clin Liver Dis 16 (2012) 687–698
http://dx.doi.org/10.1016/j.cld.2012.08.003
1089-3261/12/$ – see front matter © 2012 Elsevier Inc. All rights reserved.

components of the immune system are involved in the process to varying degrees (**Table 1**).

The main events whereby the activation of immune system plays a role in pathogenesis of alcoholic liver disease are activation of the innate immune system, specifically the activation of Kupffer cells via toll-like receptor (TLR)-4 by endotoxin and fatty acids, complement activation, alteration in natural killer (NK) and NK T-cell number, and activity and activation of the adaptive immune system.

INNATE IMMUNE SYSTEM

The innate immune response is the first line of defense against invading pathogens. It includes mainly phagocytic cells such as macrophages and neutrophils, as well as nonspecific cytotoxic T cells and NK cells. The liver is the first to encounter bacteria and bacterial cell-wall components from the intestine. The innate immune response reacts toward a few highly conserved antigens present on microorganisms, including endotoxin, but acts nonspecifically and with no memory.

Endotoxin

Gut microbiota is the major source of lipopolysaccharides (LPS) or endotoxin. Endotoxin is a component of the outer wall of gram-negative bacteria that has been implicated in sepsis, organ failure, and shock. With chronic alcohol use endotoxin is found in high levels in the portal circulation, but under normal conditions only a small quantity of LPS can translocate into the portal blood to reach the liver.[2,3] Gut-barrier dysfunction ("leaky gut"), altered clearance of endotoxins, or changes in the composition of gut microbiota are some of the mechanisms that may explain the high levels of

Table 1
Components of the immune system and their role in alcohol-induced liver injury

Immune Cell Type	Role in Innate Immune Response	Role in Alcoholic Liver Disease
Kupffer cell	Primary effector cell. Activation of oxidant and cytokine production. Phagocytosis of bacterial antigens and clearance from circulation.	Activated by recognition of endotoxin through ligation of TLR 4. Produces large amounts of superoxide and TNF-α which leads to liver injury.
Neutrophil	Recruited to site of oxidant and cytokine secretion. Phagocytosis of bacterial antigens and leads to release of proteolytic enzymes. Production of additional oxidants and chemotactic mediators to perpetuate inflammation.	Recruited by chemotactic gradients and up-regulated adhesion molecule expression. Leads to phagocytosis of bacterial antigens and dead or dying hepatocytes. Also produces additional oxidants and chemotactic mediators.
NK cell	Activated by cytokines and mitogenic mediators produced during inflammation. Immune surviellance for potential tumor cells.	Activated by TNF-α and IFN-γ produced within the inflamed liver. Leads to production of additional inflammatory mediators.
T cell/NK T cell	Activated by cytokines and mitogenic mediators produced during inflammation. Accessory function to augment phagocytic cell activity/recruitment and cytokine secretion.	Activated and recruited nonspecifically by inflammation in the liver. Produce additional inflammatory mediators including TNF-α.

endotoxin after exposure to alcohol. Numerous studies have shown that alcohol might increase gut permeability, but the exact mechanism of alcohol-induced gut-barrier dysfunction is not clear.[4–8] Studies have shown that when bacterial colonization is reduced with antibiotics or Lactobacillus GG, liver injury that is usually induced by continuous enteral alcohol administration in rats is prevented (Tsukamoto model of experimental alcoholic liver disease).[9,10] The improvement in histology was associated with reduced plasma endotoxin levels. A recent study showed that intestinal barrier dysfunction and endotoxemia preceded hepatic injury induced by intragastric ethanol administration twice a day in rats.[4] Endotoxin levels appear to correlate with severity of alcohol-induced liver injury.[11] Endotoxin is also known to activate isolated Kupffer cells. The mechanisms by which alcohol increases Kupffer-cell activation by endotoxin is not completely clear, but it is believed that leaky gut plays a key role.

Kupffer Cell

The Kupffer cell has been studied extensively in the course of examining the mechanisms of alcohol-induced liver injury. Its main function is as a primary effector cell of the innate immune response. Cell development begins in the bone marrow with the genesis of promonocytes and monoblasts into monocytes, and then on to peripheral blood monocytes, finally completing their differentiation into Kupffer cells. Several studies suggested that Kupffer cells have a key role in the pathogenesis of alcohol-induced liver injury. Depletion of Kupffer cells by the use of gadolinium chloride blunted increases in serum transaminase levels, steatosis, and necroinflammation.[12] Furthermore, destruction of Kupffer cells blocks formation of alcohol-derived free radicals, which points toward these cells being a source of the damaging oxidants.[12] Kupffer cells from female rats fed ethanol had a significantly greater response to LPS than did male rats.[13] The females produced more tumor necrosis factor (TNF)-α in response to chronic alcohol use than did male rats, suggesting that Kupffer cells in females are more active when alcohol is consumed. This finding shows that Kupffer cells are important in alcohol-induced liver injury.

LPS/TLR-4 signaling pathway

Recognition of endotoxin by Kupffer cells occurs via the pattern recognition receptor TLR-4 and its coreceptors CD14, MD-2, and LPS-binding protein (LBP).[5] TLRs are a family of receptors that are specific for the recognition of bacterial and viral components. TLRs are activated by bacterial lipoproteins, viral RNA/DNA, endotoxin, and lipoteichoic acid.[14] In liver disease TLR-2, -4, and -9 respond to gram-positive and gram-negative bacterial products and bacterial DNA.[1] Studies have shown that mice in which LBP, CD14 receptor, or TLR-4 receptor are knocked out are protected from alcohol-induced liver damage.[15,16]

CD14 is the first described receptor involved in the recognition and responses to LBP.[17] It is present on the cell surface of monocytes and macrophages but also in a soluble form. The severity of alcoholic liver disease in humans correlates with a polymorphism in the CD14 promoter that coffered an increase in CD14 levels.[12] Serum from patients with severe alcoholic hepatitis contained higher levels of soluble CD14 compared with healthy controls.[18] Exactly how CD14 is regulated is not completely clear, but it appears to be an important factor in the development of therapies for alcoholic liver disease.

TLR-4 is a membrane pattern-recognition receptor that plays a key role in the endotoxin-induced innate immune system activation.[19,20] TLR-4 triggers intracellular signaling through recruitment of intracellular factors such as myeloid differentiation factor 88 (MyD88), which results in production of inflammatory cytokines and interferons.[21] MD-2 is a soluble protein anchored to the cell membrane via the association with TLR-4.[22]

The LPS/TLR-4 signaling transduction pathway consists of activation of various transcription factors such as nuclear factor κB (NF-κB) or activator protein 1 (AP-1), which induces the proinflammatory cytokine gene expression in the Kupffer cell: TNF-α and interleukin (IL)-1β. Serum TNF-α is increased in persons with alcoholic liver disease and correlates with mortality.[23] Recently it has been shown that genetic factors determining increased TNF-α release have been linked to susceptibility to develop acute severe hepatitis in humans.[24] TNF-α and IL-1β further increase production of proinflammatory cytokines such as IL-6 and IL-8, which then leads to attraction of other immune cells: neutrophils, monocytes, and lymphocytes.[25,26]

Reactive oxygen species

Kupffer cells also can make large amounts of potentially damaging free radicals such as superoxide. One potential source of superoxide is the phagocytic nicotinamide adenine dinucleotide phosphate (NADPH) oxidase system. The role of the NADPH oxidase system was tested using mice deficient in p47phox, a regulatory subunit of the oxidase.[12] After 4 weeks of enteral alcohol feeding, the mice had significantly reduced liver injury with lower serum transaminase levels and by histopathological assessment of tissue damage.[12] In addition to generation of free radicals, cytokine production was significantly blunted. This finding showed a strong link between oxidant production and cytokine generation in this model of alcoholic liver disease.

Chronic alcohol feeding of mice and rats induces high intestinal oxidative stress.[27,28] Nitric oxide is overproduced and reacts with superoxide anions to form peroxynitrite, which can oxidatively damage the microtubules inducing gut barrier dysfunction.[29] The ROS can also release zinc, which plays a key role in free radical defense and leads to cellular zinc deficiency.[5] Zinc deficiency may also sensitize intestinal epithelium to alcohol-induced hyperpermeability, as suggested by a recent study showing that alcohol feeding induced zinc deficiency in the ileum of mice.[28]

Fibrosis

It is thought that steatosis and the observed inflammatory cell activation and infiltration promote the activation of hepatic stellate cells. The stellate cells are fibroblast-like and can make large amounts of collagen when activated. Oxidants and cytokines can activate the stellate cells. A recent study showed that stellate cells can also be directly activated by endotoxin through the CD14/TLR-4 pathway,[30] suggesting that stellate cells also participate in the innate immune system.

ADAPTIVE IMMUNE SYSTEM

Adaptive immunity consists of cell types designed to induce memory to specific antigens. It is characterized by the presentation of antigen to T cells and clonal expansion of these cells to increase specificity to proteins, further increasing disposal of foreign agents. The liver contains significant number lymphocytes including NK T cells, T cells, and B cells, with the largest subset being the NK T cells. These lymphocytes are characterized by the expression of both NK cell markers and the αβ T-cell receptor. Such lymphocytes control the immune system to be in either an inflammatory or tolerant state as they make both T-helper 1 (Th1)- and Th2-associated cytokines. T cells and NK T cells have been implicated in the development of alcoholic liver disease by the increased numbers found in human livers following ethanol injury.[31]

With chronic alcohol consumption, there is a change in hepatic T-cell function and the number of cells. The immediate level of alcohol consumption in addition to severity of alcoholic liver disease also correlates with the numbers of CD4 and CD8 T cells expressing inflammatory mediators such as TNF-α and IL-4.[32] T cells from alcoholic patients express markers associated with activation and memory phenotypes including CD45RO, CD11b, and CD54.[33] The ability of these cells to produce cytokines is thought to be induced by alcohol.[33]

Another study implicating lymphocytes in alcoholic liver disease showed that T cells from alcohol-fed rats given to healthy rats damaged the healthy livers.[34] Cytotoxic T cells can be generated in response to acetaldehyde-modified spleen cells,[35] giving aldehyde-modified proteins a role in the activation of these cells. It has been shown that aldehyde-modified proteins at high levels (nonphysiologic) can cause cell death and apoptosis in these cells.[36] Therefore, the buildup of these adducts in the liver could increase the level of cell death/apoptosis, increase cytokine production, and increase inflammation in the liver, eventually leading to cirrhosis.

Malondialdehyde-acetaldehyde (MAA) adducts have been found to be significantly increased in patients with alcoholic liver disease, and correlates with the severity of liver damage.[37] MAA-adducted proteins are immunogenic without the use of adjuvants.[38] It is thought that metabolites of alcohol hepatic self antigens may induce an autoimmune response against the liver.[39] Experimental animal models have shown that reactive cytotoxic T cells or the production of antibody could aid in damaging the liver.[40,41] It appears that the presence of alcohol metabolites increases the immune response in the liver, which then leads to macrophages and neutrophils, cleaning up cellular debris. The self proteins from hepatocytes can become modified with acetaldehyde, malondialdehyde, or both. These self proteins could bind to and be taken up by macrophages, endothelial cells, or dendritic cells, and be presented to T cells. When this occurs the reactive T cells can damage the liver.

One other factor to support the adaptive immune system is seen in alcoholic patients who have received a liver transplant. If these individuals start consuming ethanol, hepatic fibrosis or cirrhosis occurs much more quickly than the years it took to develop before the transplant.[42] This quick memory response to the liver suggests that the adaptive immune system is involved.

Interleukins

Activation of NF-κB in rats can induce the expression of IL-1β, which increases the expression of proinflammatory molecules.[25,43] A recent study showed that IL-1β alone or in association with IL-6 was essential for the induction of Th17 lymphocyte differentiation from human naïve CD4$^+$ T cells.[44] Furthermore, LPS-stimulated human monocytes induced Th17 polarization of naïve CD4$^+$ T cells in an IL-1β-signaling–dependent manner.

The Th17 cells are the main source of IL-17, which plays a key role in enhancing host immune response against microorganisms as well as in autoimmune diseases.[45] IL-17 stimulates multiple types of nonparenchymal hepatic cells to produce proinflammatory cytokines and chemokines.[46] Recently it was shown that patients with alcoholic liver disease had higher IL-17 plasma levels compared with healthy subjects.[47]

The role of IL-6 in alcoholic liver disease is complex and is not well understood. It appears to have some beneficial effects on the liver. IL-6 may protect against hepatocyte apoptosis and participate in mitochondrial DNA repair after alcoholic liver injury.[48,49] However, the IL-6 pathway may significantly contribute to the induction and promotion of liver inflammation. A recent study reported that blockade of IL-6 trans-signaling in mice reduced neutrophil and mononuclear cell infiltration to the site of inflammation.[50] IL-6 may also promote human Th17 differentiation and IL-17 production, thus contributing to ethanol-induced liver inflammation. Therefore it appears that when endotoxin activates Kupffer cells, it creates the conditions (IL-1β

and IL-6 secretion) for IL-17 secretion in the liver, which in turn maintains and amplifies the inflammatory process already initiated by TNF-α and IL-1β production.

The functions of Th17 cells are also mediated via the production of IL-22. IL-22 is a member of the IL-10 family of cytokines, and plays an important role in promoting hepatocyte survival and proliferation.[46] Recently it was shown that the use of IL-22 can improve alcoholic liver injury in a murine model of chronic binge alcohol use.[51]

IL-17 is also known to enhance neutrophil recruitment. A recent study showed that in vitro IL-17 stimulation of human hepatic stellate cells induced neutrophil recruitment in a dose-dependent manner through IL-8 and growth-related oncogene α (GRO-α) secretion.[46]

Hepatic neutrophil infiltration and activation

Neutrophils play a key role in host defense against pathogenic microorganisms, but also contribute to the generation of tissue injury. Neutrophils accumulate in the hepatic sinusoids in response to cytokines and chemokines released by Kupffer cells as well as by hepatocytes and hepatic stellate cells, in response to TNF-α, IL-1β, or endotoxin stimulation.[30,52,53] Studies in patients with alcoholic hepatitis have shown that the neutrophils have a significantly higher resting activation status than patients with cirrhosis or healthy subjects, and that the increased activation is dependent on endotoxins.[54]

The migration of neutrophils in the sinusoids through the endothelium into the liver parenchyma is essential for the development of alcohol-induced hepatic inflammation. For the neutrophil to adhere to the endothelium, interaction of integrin CD11b/CD18 (on the neutrophil surface) with intercellular adhesion molecule ICAM-1 (on the endothelial cell surface) has to occur.[55] This idea is supported by a study showed that ICAM-1 deficiency significantly reduces hepatic injury and neutrophil infiltration in a mouse model of continuous enteral alcohol feeding.[56]

Once neutrophils reach the liver parenchyma, they undergo further activation via the proinflammatory cytokines present. The activated neutrophils release additional proinflammatory cytokines and chemokines, which potentate the liver inflammation through the recruitment of other inflammatory cells: neutrophils, lymphocytes, and monocytes. However, ROS production and proteolytic enzyme release are the major mechanisms of neutrophil-induced hepatic damage.[57]

COMPLEMENT PATHWAY

The complement system is also thought to play a role in alcohol-induced liver disease. It bridges innate and adaptive immunity systems, and can be activated via the classical, lectin, or alternative pathways (**Fig. 1**). Complement activation leads to increased expression of inflammatory cytokines and chemokines, and plays an important role in host defense, wound healing, and response to tissue injury.[58] Dysregulation of the complement pathway is also linked to pathogenesis of alcohol-induced liver disease.[59] In mice, it was shown that acute alcohol exposure can activate complement within 2 to 4 days as well as after chronic exposure within 4 to 6 weeks.[59–61]

C3a levels in animal models are increased with alcohol use, which reflects activation of the common complement pathway. Recent studies have shown that C3 activation is an early step that coincides with release of the proinflammatory cytokines and precedes oxidative stress and liver injury.[61] However, the C5 gene is needed for increased cytokine release and liver injury.[59] It has been shown that deficiency in C3 or C5 protected mice from chronic alcohol-induced liver injury.[59] This finding leads to the thought that while alcohol is necessary for C3a activation, the increase in TNF-α levels is dependent on both C3a and C5a receptors.

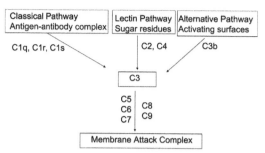

Fig. 1. Overview of the Complement Pathways. The three activating pathways are shown. The lectin pathway is initiated when one or more recognition molecules bind to patterns of carbohydrates or patterns of acetyl groups on the surface of, for example, bacteria or viruses. The classical pathway is activated by C1q in complex with C1s and C1r upon binding of antibody-antigen complexes. The alternative pathway is constitutively activated and inhibited on self-surfaces, but is allowed to proceed on foreign surfaces. The three pathways converge on C3 and C5 and the common terminal pathway leading to formation of the membrane attack complex.

The mechanisms by which ethanol activates complement were recently investigated. The classical pathway of complement is activated on the binding of C1q, the recognition subunit of first component (C1) to immune complexes and to cell-surface markers on apoptotic cells.[62,63] The binding of C1q to apoptotic cells likely plays a dual role in mediating the clearance of apoptotic cells. First, C1q binding leads to activation of the C1/classical pathway and production of C3 fragments that opsonize apoptotic cells and mark them for clearance.[64] Second, C1q on the surface of apoptotic cells likely serves as a bridging molecule, interacting with receptors on the surface of macrophages involved in the clearance of apoptotic cells.[65] One of the hallmarks of alcoholic-induced liver injury is hepatocellular apoptosis; ethanol sensitizes hepatocytes to apoptosis both in vivo[66,67] and in vitro.[68,69]

Through the use of wild-type and C1q knock-out mice, it was shown that C1q-deficient mice were protected from chronic ethanol-induced liver injury, indicated by a reduced accumulation of hepatic triglycerides, hepatocellular apoptosis, and reduced activity of serum transaminases.[70] This finding suggests that alcohol exposure activates the classical complement pathway through C1q, which contributes to the development of alcohol-induced liver injury in mice.

ANTI-INFLAMMATORY FACTORS

Endotoxin stimulation of Kupffer cells also causes release of anti-inflammatory factors, which help to limit tissue damage. For example, IL-10 is an anti-inflammatory cytokine, mainly produced by activated monocytes and macrophages, that activates the activation of signal transducer and activator of transcription 3 (STAT3) protein.[71] It has been shown that alcohol downregulates IL-10, and IL-10 deficiency also enhances alcohol-induced hepatic damage in mice.[72] A recent study showed that monocyte/macrophage STAT3-deficient mice have increased hepatic and serum levels of proinflammatory cytokines and chemokines following oral ethanol feeding, in comparison with wild-type mice.[73]

Another example is glucocorticoid-induced leucine zipper (GILZ), which is a major mediator of glucocorticoid, anti-inflammatory, and immunosuppressive effects.[74] GILZ inhibits the NF-κB nuclear translocation and essentially downregulates inflammatory gene expression in immune cells. GILZ mRNA expression level was found to be lower in patients with alcoholic hepatitis than in healthy subjects.[75] Interestingly, Kupffer cells were the main source of GILZ in both normal and alcoholic human livers.[75]

SUMMARY

It is well known that there are numerous factors that result in the development and progression of alcoholic liver disease. However, the immune system appears to play a large role. The progression of alcohol-induced liver damage involves complex interactions of several immune cells and hepatocytes through the release of cytokines and chemokines. Kupffer cells are activated early in alcohol-induced liver injury. Activation of TLR-4 and CD14, receptors on the Kupffer cell that internalize endotoxin, leads to the transcription of proinflammatory cytokines such as TNF-α and production of superoxides. This process then leads to hepatic injury and, potentially fibrosis.

The enhancement in understanding the pathogenesis of alcoholic liver disease is key to developing new approaches to its treatment. For instance, therapeutic applications from these new insights could prevent alcoholic liver intestinal barrier disruption and endotoxemia, or induce GILZ to upregulate anti-inflammatory and immunosuppressive effects. However, we are far from using these potential therapies. Further studies are necessary.

REFERENCES

1. Wu D, Cederbaum AI. Alcohol, oxidative stress, and free radical damage. Alcohol Res Health 2003;27:277–84.
2. Tamai H, Kato S, Horie Y, et al. Effect of acute ethanol administration on the intestinal absorption of endotoxin in rats. Alcohol Clin Exp Res 2000;24:390–4.
3. Fukui H, Brauner B, Bode JC, et al. Plasma endotoxin concentrations in patients with alcoholic and non-alcoholic liver disease: reevaluation with an improved chromogenic assay. J Hepatol 1991;12:162–9.
4. Keshavarzian A, Farhadi A, Forsyth CB, et al. Evidence that chronic alcohol exposure promotes intestinal oxidative stress, intestinal hyperpermeability and endotoxemia prior to development of alcoholic steatohepatitis in rats. J Hepatol 2009; 50:538–47.
5. Voican CS, Perlemuter G, Naveua S. Mechanisms of the inflammatory reaction implicated in alcoholic hepatitis: 2011 update. Clin Res Hepatol Gastroenterol 2011;35(6–7):465–74.
6. Mathurin P, Deng QG, Keshavarzian A, et al. Exacerbation of alcoholic liver injury by enteral endotoxin in rats. Hepatology 2000;32:1008–17.
7. Parlesak A, Schäfer C, Schütz T, et al. Increased intestinal permeability to macromolecules and endotoxemia in patients with chronic alcohol abuse in different stages of alcohol-induced liver disease. J Hepatol 2000;32:742–7.
8. Rao R. Endotoxemia and gut barrier dysfunction in alcoholic liver disease. Hepatology 2009;50:638–44.
9. Adachi Y, Moore LE, Bradford BU, et al. Antibiotics prevent liver injury in rats following long-term exposure to ethanol. Gastroenterology 1995;108:218–24.
10. Nanji AA, Khettry U, Sadrzadeh SM. Lactobacillus feeding reduces endotoxemia and severity of experimental alcoholic liver (disease). Proc Soc Exp Biol Med 1994;205:243–7.
11. Nanji AA, Khettry U, Sadrzadeh SM, et al. Severity of liver injury in experimental alcoholic liver disease. Correlation with plasma endotoxin, prostaglandin E2, leukotriene B4, and thromboxane B2. Am J Pathol 1993;142:367–73.

12. Wheeler MD, Kono H, Yin M, et al. The role of Kupffer cell oxidant production in early ethanol-induced liver disease. Free Radic Biol Med 2001;31:1544–9.
13. Yin M, Ikejima K, Wheeler MD, et al. Estrogen is involved in early alcohol-induced liver injury in a rat enteral feeding model. Hepatology 2000;31:117–23.
14. Stadlbauer V, Mookerjee RP, Wright GAK, et al. Role of Toll-like receptors 2, 4, and 9 in mediating neutrophil dysfunction in alcoholic hepatitis. Am J Physiol Gastrointest Liver Physiol 2009;296(1):G15–22.
15. Uesugi T, Froh M, Arteel GE, et al. Toll-like receptor 4 is also involved in the mechanism of early alcohol-induced liver injury in mice. Hepatology 2001;32:101–8.
16. Yin M, Bradford BU, Wheeler MD, et al. Reduced early alcohol-induced liver injury in CD14-deficient mice. J Immunol 2001;166:4737–42.
17. Wright SD, Ramos RA, Tobias PS, et al. CD14, a receptor for complexes of lipopolysaccharide (LPS) and LPS binding protein. Science 1990;249:1431–3.
18. Schafer C, Parlesak A, Schutt C, et al. Concentration of lipopolysaccharide-binding protein, bactericidal/permeability-increasing protein, soluble CD14 and plasma lipids in relation to endotoxaemia in patients with alcoholic liver disease. Alcohol 2002;37:81–6.
19. Chow JC, Young DW, Golenbock DT, et al. Toll-like receptor-4 mediates lipopolysaccharide-induced signal transduction. J Biol Chem 1999;274:10689–92.
20. Poltorak A, He X, Smirnova I, et al. Defective LPS signaling in C3H/HeJ and C57BL/10ScCr mice: mutations in Tlr4 gene. Science 1998;282:2085–8.
21. Valenti L, Fracanzani AL, Fargion S. The immunopathogenesis of alcoholic and nonalcoholic steatohepatitis: two triggers for one disease? Semin Immunopathol 2009;31:359–69.
22. Shimazu R, Akashi S, Ogata H, et al. MD-2, a molecule that confers lipopolysaccharide responsiveness on toll-like receptor 4. J Exp Med 1999;189:1777–82.
23. Wheeler MD, Kono H, Yin M, et al. Delivery of Cu/Zn-superoxide dismutase gene with adenovirus reduces early alcohol-induced liver injury in rats. Gastroenterology 2001;120:1241–50.
24. Grove J, Daly AK, Bassendine MF, et al. Association of a tumor necrosis factor promoter polymorphism with susceptibility to alcoholic steatohepatitis. Hepatology 1997;26:143–6.
25. Nanji AA, Jokelainen K, Rahemtulla A, et al. Activation of nuclear factor kappa B and cytokine imbalance in experimental alcoholic liver disease in the rat. Hepatology 1999;30:934–43.
26. Takeda K, Akira S. TLR signaling pathways. Semin Immunol 2004;16:3–9.
27. Tang Y, Forsyth CB, Farhadi A, et al. Nitric oxide-mediated intestinal injury is required for alcohol-induced gut leakiness and liver damage. Alcohol Clin Exp Res 2009;33:1220–30.
28. Zhong W, McClain CJ, Cave M, et al. The role of zinc deficiency in alcohol-induced intestinal barrier dysfunction. Am J Physiol Gastrointest Liver Physiol 2010;298:G625–33.
29. Banan A, Fields JZ, Decker H, et al. Nitric oxide and its metabolites mediate ethanol-induced microtubule disruption and intestinal barrier dysfunction. J Pharmacol Exp Ther 2000;294:997–1008.
30. Paik YH, Schwabe RF, Bataller R, et al. Toll-like receptor 4 mediates inflammatory signaling by bacterial lipopolysaccharide in human hepatic stellate cells. Hepatology 2003;37:1043–55.
31. Sakai Y, Izumi N, Marumo F, et al. Quantitative immunohistochemical analysis of lymphocyte subsets in alcoholic liver disease. J Gastroenterol Hepatol 1993;8:39–43.

32. Laso FJ, Iglesias-Osma C, Ciudad J, et al. Chronic alcoholism is associated with an imbalanced production of Th-1/Th-2 cytokines by peripheral blood T cells. Alcohol Clin Exp Res 1999;23:1306–11.

33. Song K, Coleman RA, Zhu X, et al. Chronic ethanol consumption by mice results in activated splenic T cells. J Leukoc Biol 2002;72:1109–16.

34. Cao Q, Batey R, Pang G, et al. Altered T-lymphocyte responsiveness to polyclonal cell activators is responsible for liver cell necrosis in alcohol-fed rates. Alcohol Clin Exp Res 1998;22:723–9.

35. Terabayashi H, Kolber MA. The generation of cytotoxic T lymphocytes against acetaldehyde-modified syngeneic cells. Alcohol Clin Exp Res 1990;14:893–9.

36. Willis MS, Klassen LW, Tuma DJ, et al. Malondialdehyde-acetaldehyde-haptenated protein induces cell death by induction of necrosis and apoptosis in immune cells. Int Immunopharmacol 2002;2:519–35.

37. Rolla R, Vay D, Mottaran E, et al. Detection of circulating antibodies against malondialdehyde-acetaldehyde adducts in patients with alcohol-induced liver disease. Hepatology 2000;31:878–84.

38. Thiele GM, Tuma DJ, Willis MS, et al. Soluble proteins modified with acetaldehyde and malondialdehyde are immunogenic in the absence of adjuvant. Alcohol Clin Exp Res 1998;22:1731–9.

39. Willis MS, Klassen LW, Tuma DJ, et al. Adduction of soluble proteins with malondialdehyde-acetaldehyde (MAA) induces antibody production and enhances T-cell proliferation. Alcohol Clin Exp Res 2002;26:94–106.

40. Lohse AW. Experimental models of autoimmune hepatitis. Semin Liver Dis 1991; 11:241–7.

41. Thiele GM, Freeman TL, Willis MS, et al. Identification of liver cytosolic proteins associated with malondialdehyde-acetaldehyde (MAA) adducted liver cytosol induced autoimmune hepatitis. Hepatology 2003;38:488A.

42. Bonet H, Manez R, Kramer D, et al. Liver transplantation for alcoholic liver disease: survival of patients transplanted with alcoholic hepatitis plus cirrhosis as compared with those with cirrhosis alone. Alcohol Clin Exp Res 1993;17: 1102–6.

43. Jura J, Wegrzyn P, Korostynski M, et al. Identification of interleukin-1 and interleukin-6-responsive genes in human monocyte-derived macrophages using microarrays. Biochem Biophys Acta 2008;1779:383–9.

44. Acosta-Rodriguez EV, Napolitani G, Lanzavecchia A, et al. Interleukins 1beta and 6 but not transforming growth factor beta are essential for the differentiation of interleukin 17- producing human T helper cells. Nat Immunol 2007;8:942–9.

45. Weaver CT, Hatton RD, Mangan PR, et al. IL-17 family cytokines and the expanding diversity of effector T cell lineages. Annu Rev Immunol 2007;25:821–52.

46. Lafdil F, Miller AM, Ki SH, et al. Th17 cells and their associated cytokines in liver diseases. Cell Mol Immunol 2010;7:250–4.

47. Lemmers A, Moreno C, Gustot T, et al. The interleukin-17 pathway is involved in human alcoholic liver disease. Hepatology 2009;49:646–57.

48. Sheron N, Bird G, Goka J, et al. Elevated plasma interleukin-6 and increased severity and mortality in alcoholic hepatitis. Clin Exp Immunol 1991;84:449–53.

49. Hong F, Kim WH, Tian Z, et al. Elevated interleukin-6 during ethanol consumption acts as a potential endogenous protective cytokine against ethanol-induced apoptosis in the liver: involvement of induction of Bcl-2 and Bcl-xL proteins. Oncogene 2002;21:32–43.

50. Rabe B, Chalaris A, May U, et al. Transgenic blockade of interleukin 6 trans-signaling abrogates inflammation. Blood 2008;111:1021–8.

51. Ki SH, Park O, Zheng M, et al. Interleukin-22 treatment ameliorates alcoholic liver injury in a murine model of chronic-binge ethanol feeding: role of signal transducer and activator of transcription 3. Hepatology 2010;52:1291–300.

52. Thornton AJ, Strieter RM, Lindley I, et al. Cytokine-induced gene expression of a neutrophil chemotactic factor/IL-8 in human hepatocytes. J Immunol 1990; 144:2609–13.

53. Paik YH, Lee KS, Lee HJ, et al. Hepatic stellate cells primed with cytokines upregulate inflammation in response to peptidoglycan or lipoteichoic acid. Lab Invest 2006;86:676–86.

54. Mookerjee RP, Stadlbauer V, Lidder S, et al. Neutrophil dysfunction in alcoholic hepatitis superimposed on cirrhosis is reversible and predicts the outcome. Hepatology 2007;46:831–40.

55. Woodfin A, Voisin MB, Nourshargh S. Recent developments and complexities in neutrophil transmigration. Curr Opin Hematol 2010;17:9–17.

56. Kono H, Uesugi T, Froh M, et al. ICAM-1 is involved in the mechanism of alcohol-induced liver injury: studies with knockout mice. Am J Physiol Gastrointest Liver Physiol 2001;280:G1289–95.

57. Banerjee A, Apte UM, Smith R, et al. Higher neutrophil infiltration mediated by osteopontin is a likely contributing factor to the increased susceptibility of females to alcoholic liver disease. J Pathol 2006;208:473–85.

58. Gasque P. Complement: a unique innate immune sensor for danger signals. Mol Immunol 2004;41:1089–98.

59. Pritchard MT, McMullen MR, Stavitsky AB, et al. Differential contributions of C3, C5 and decay-accelerating factor to ethanol-induced fatty liver in mice. Gastroenterology 2007;132:1117–26.

60. Jarvelainen HA, Vakeva A, Lindros KO, et al. Activation of complement components and reduced regulator expression in alcohol-induced liver injury in the rat. Clin Immunol 2002;105:57–63.

61. Roychowdhury S, McMullen MR, Pritchard MT, et al. An early complement-dependent and TLR-4-independent phase in the pathogenesis of ethanol-induced liver injury in mice. Hepatology 2009;49:1326–34.

62. Paidassi H, Tacnet-Delorme P, Garlatti V, et al. C1q binds phosphatidylserine and likely acts as a multiligand-bridging molecule in apoptotic cell recognition. J Immunol 2008;180:2329–38.

63. Elward K, Griffiths M, Mizuno M, et al. CD46 plays a key role in tailoring innate immune recognition of apoptotic and necrotic cells. J Biol Chem 2005;280:36342–54.

64. Mevorach D, Mascarenhas JO, Gershov D, et al. Complement-dependent clearance of apoptotic cells by human macrophages. J Exp Med 1998;188:2313–20.

65. Trouw LA, Blom AM, Gasque P. Role of complement and complement regulators in the removal of apoptotic cells. Mol Immunol 2008;45:1199–207.

66. Higuchi H, Kurose I, Kato S, et al. Ethanol-induced apoptosis and oxidative stress in hepatocytes. Alcohol Clin Exp Res 1996;20:340A–6A.

67. Cohen JI, Roychowdhury S, Dibello PM, et al. Exogenous thioredoxin prevents ethanol-induced oxidative damage and apoptosis in mouse liver. Hepatology 2009;49:1709–17.

68. Pastorino JG, Shulga N, Hoek JB. TNF-alpha-induced cell death in ethanol-exposed cells depends on p38 MAPK signaling but is independent of Bid and caspase-8. Am J Physiol Gastrointest Liver Physiol 2003;285:G503–16.

69. McVicker BL, Tuma DJ, Kubik JL, et al. Ethanol-induced apoptosis in polarized hepatic cells possibly through regulation of the Fas pathway. Alcohol Clin Exp Res 2006;30:1906–15.

70. Cohen JI, Roychowdhury S, McMullen MR, et al. Complement and alcoholic liver disease: role of C1q in the pathogenesis of ethanol-induced liver injury in mice. Gastroenterology 2010;139:664–74.

71. Sabat R, Grütz G, Warszawska K, et al. Biology of interleukin-10. Cytokine Growth Factor Rev 2010;21:331–44.

72. Hill DB, D'Souza NB, Lee EY, et al. A role for interleukin-10 in alcohol-induced liver sensitization to bacterial lipopolysaccharide. Alcohol Clin Exp Res 2002;26:74–82.

73. Horiguchi N, Wang L, Mukhopadhyay P, et al. Cell type dependent pro- and anti-inflammatory role of signal transducer and activator of transcription 3 in alcoholic liver injury. Gastroenterology 2008;134:1148–58.

74. Ayroldi E, Riccardi C. Glucocorticoid-induced leucine zipper (GILZ): a new important mediator of glucocorticoid action. FASEB J 2009;23:3649–58.

75. Hamdi H, Bigorgne A, Naveau S, et al. Glucocorticoid-induced leucine zipper: a key protein in the sensitization of monocytes to lipopolysaccharide in alcoholic hepatitis. Hepatology 2007;46:1986–92.

Histologic Findings in Alcoholic Liver Disease

James M. Crawford, MD, PhD*

KEYWORDS

- Steatosis • Alcoholic hepatitis • Cirrhosis • Mallory bodies • Fibrosis

KEY POINTS

The key histologic features of alcoholic liver disease are:

- *Steatosis,* arising from diversion of metabolic reducing equivalents from conversion of ethanol into acetate and thence into fatty acids and triglyceride synthesis.
- *Ballooning degeneration,* owing to loss of osmoregulatory control at the level of the plasma membrane.
- *Mallory body formation,* resulting from condensation of intracellular cytokeratin microfilaments into skeins of clumped intracellular protein.
- *Inflammation,* which is predominantly neutrophilic within the parenchyma but may also include mixed inflammation within portal tracts.
- *Regeneration,* usually less evident in alcoholic liver disease (especially alcoholic hepatitis) than in other forms of hepatitis. But with progression to alcoholic cirrhosis, such hepatocellular regeneration can create small nodular parenchymal islands of hepatocytes.
- *Fibrosis with progression to cirrhosis.* The bridging fibrosis that may occur in steatotic alcoholic liver disease may be very indolent and progress only over many years, in contrast to the brisk fibrosis that occurs in alcoholic hepatitis, putting the patient at risk for development of cirrhosis within a few short years.
- The morphologic features of alcoholic liver disease are therefore grouped into: steatosis; alcoholic hepatitis (hepatocellular ballooning degeneration and Mallory body formation, with neutrophilic parenchymal inflammation and sinusoidal fibrogenesis); and cirrhosis. In the last instance, development of hepatocellular carcinoma is a consideration in the histologic evaluation of liver tissue from a patient with alcoholic liver disease.

As the world's most prevalent psychotropic chemical, ethyl alcohol is woven into human history at virtually every recorded time point. Whatever the reason for alcohol consumption, the liver has the dubious honor of being responsible for its disposition. Arguably alcohol is food, with a caloric equivalent of 7 kcal/g. With approximately 14 g

Disclosure: The author has no conflicts of interest to disclose.
Department of Pathology and Laboratory Medicine, Hofstra North Shore-LIJ School of Medicine, Uniondale, NY, USA
* North Shore-LIJ Laboratories, 10 Nevada Drive, Lake Success, NY 11042.
E-mail address: jcrawford1@nshs.edu

of alcohol in a "drink," there are about 200 food calories in 1 oz (28 g) of pure spirits, and about 150 calories in 12 oz (340 g) of beer, of which 100 calories are attributable to alcohol. Consuming a 6-pack of beer constitutes 900 calories of food consumption; two 6-packs are 1800 calories. The alcoholic who consumes a pint of 86-proof spirits has imbibed about 2700 calories of alcohol. Hence, alcoholics can easily consume well over half of their daily caloric equivalent in alcohol. Although the individual who drinks only 2 glasses of wine a day may be subject to less disapprobation, he or she may still be consuming 10% of their daily caloric intake in alcohol.

The problem is that alcohol also is a toxin. Both by generating a metabolic burden and oxidative by-products, and by being an organic solvent and direct physiologic regulator, alcohol has an extraordinary ability to become the dominant cause of disease in individuals who come under its influence.[1] This article examines the morphologic features of alcoholic liver disease. The histologic features of alcoholic liver disease are presented in the context of the underlying pathophysiologic mechanisms. The morphologic features of liver damage induced by alcohol[2] are:

- Steatosis: Accumulation of lipid droplets within the hepatocellular cytoplasm.
- Hepatocyte ballooning: Single or scattered foci of cells undergo swelling (ballooning, also called oncosis). The swelling results from the accumulation of fat and water, as well as proteins that normally are exported.
- Mallory bodies: Scattered hepatocytes accumulate tangled skeins of cytokeratin intermediate filaments such as cytokeratin 8 and 18, complexed with other proteins such as ubiquitin.
- Inflammation: In alcoholic hepatitis, neutrophils permeate the hepatic lobule and accumulate around degenerating hepatocytes, particularly those having Mallory bodies. Lymphocytes and macrophages also enter portal tracts and spill into the parenchyma.
- Hepatocellular necrosis and apoptosis: Ballooned hepatocytes undergo oncotic necrosis, whereby the swollen hepatocytes rupture. Hepatocellular apoptosis also may occur.
- Regeneration: In the midst of ongoing injury, liver regeneration and repair may occur.
- Fibrosis: Alcoholic hepatitis is almost always accompanied by prominent activation of sinusoidal stellate cells and portal tract fibroblasts, giving rise to sinusoidal and perivenular, separating parenchymal cells.
- Cirrhosis: Long-standing alcohol-induced liver disease culminates in cirrhosis. Although cirrhosis usually evolves slowly and insidiously, it may develop in 1 or 2 years when alcoholic hepatitis is rampant.

Table 1 indicates how these features occur in the 3 forms of alcoholic liver disease.

LIPID ACCUMULATION AND HEPATIC STEATOSIS

Alcohol must be metabolized, and it must be metabolized by the liver. There are 3 metabolic pathways for its disposition.

- Cytosolic dehydrogenases: The normal metabolic pathway utilizes cytosolic alcohol dehydrogenase, which converts alcohol to acetaldehyde; and acetaldehyde dehydrogenase, which completes the conversion to acetate.
- Cytochromes: Cytochrome P450 enzymes in the endoplasmic reticulum are induced during sustained alcohol exposure.
- Peroxisomes: Peroxisomal catalase can use alcohol as a substrate.

Table 1
The 3 forms of alcoholic liver disease

Feature	Fatty Liver Disease	Alcoholic Hepatitis	Cirrhosis
Steatosis	•••	••	••• to •[a]
Hepatocyte ballooning	—	•••	•
Mallory bodies	—	••	•
Inflammation	—	•••	•
Hepatocyte necrosis	—	•••	••
Regeneration	—	•	••
Fibrosis	—	••	••••

The relative proportions of 7 morphologic findings are given as the number of dots.
[a] The degree of steatosis in alcoholic cirrhosis depends on whether the cirrhosis developed in the absence (•••) or presence (••) of alcoholic hepatitis. Regardless, with the passage of time steatosis in the cirrhotic liver may diminish to a minimal value (•).

Via the usual cytosolic pathway, complete alcohol metabolism to acetate generates abundant oxidative energy, because acetate is activated by acetyl–coenzyme A (CoA) synthase and enters into the heart of oxidative metabolism, the tricarboxylic acid cycle. However, even this innocuous entry point into intermediary metabolism begins the process of liver toxicity, and with it morphologic changes in the liver. Starting with the reduced nicotinamide adenine dinucleotide (NADH) + H^+ equivalents generated by both acetate dehydrogenase and acetaldehyde dehydrogenase, the NAD phosphate (NADPH) + H^+ generated by conversion of isocitric acid to oxalosuccinic acid, the NADH + H^+ generated by oxidation of α-ketoglutaric acid to succinyl CoA, the $FADH_2$ as succinic acid is converted to fumaric acid, and the final NADH + H^+ generated by the final step of the cycle, conversion of malic acid to oxaloacetic acid, routine oxidation of alcohol spins off 6 pairs of reducing equivalents. To the extent that these reducing equivalents are not oxidized by mitochondria, they have to be diverted elsewhere.

The most important side pathway is fatty acid synthesis, which in the simplest sense for diversion of reducing equivalents involves ligation of acetate molecules into fatty acids, which are then esterified with glycerol to form triglycerides. Thus are created the cytosolic lipid droplets of hepatic steatosis, containing not only triglycerides but also free fatty acids, monoglycerides, and diglycerides. The liver does not normally store lipids. However, after even moderate intake of alcohol, within a matter of hours microvesicular lipid droplets accumulate in hepatocytes, consisting of a core of triglycerides coated with amphiphilic phospholipids at the cytosolic interface.

Chronic alcohol exposure induces expression of cytochromes P450, especially CYP2E1, which increases catabolism of alcohol in the endoplasmic reticulum. Cytochrome P450 metabolism produces reactive oxygen species that induce lipid peroxidation and formation of acetaldehyde protein adducts.[3] As a solute at millimolar concentrations, alcohol directly affects microtubular and mitochondrial function and membrane fluidity. Alcohol-induced impaired hepatic metabolism of methionine leads to decreased intrahepatic glutathione (GSH) levels, thereby sensitizing the liver to the oxidative injury arising from microsomal and peroxisomal metabolism of alcohol. Lastly, alcohol metabolism by peroxisomal catalase generates hydrogen peroxide, a potent oxidant in its own right.

Among the intracellular protein and membrane machinery that is disrupted by oxidative damage to proteins and membranes is intracellular vesicular transport. Included among the vesicular cargo is very low-density lipoprotein (VLDL), a mechanism by which hepatocytes export their burden of lipid. Alcohol exposure impairs intracellular delivery of VLDL-containing vesicles from the Golgi apparatus to the hepatocyte basolateral plasma membrane for release into the circulation. This process leads to accumulation of lipoprotein lipid with a distended Golgi apparatus,[4] further contributing to the accumulation of steatosis within the hepatocyte. Moreover, the presence of lipid droplets within the cytoplasm provides ample fatty substrate for oxidative generation of lipid peroxidation by-products such as malondialdehyde.[5]

Regardless of location, the lipid droplets that accumulate initially within hepatocytes are only about 1 to 2 μm in diameter (microvesicular), with a high surface/volume ratio. These droplets are thus amenable to rapid dissolution through the action of lipases, which occurs at the cytoplasmic interface. A purely microvesicular form of alcoholic steatosis is unusual.[2] Over time (most likely days), the droplets coalesce, forming droplets exceeding 20 μm in diameter (macrovesicular), displacing the hepatocyte nucleus (**Fig. 1**). As the surface/volume ratio of these larger droplets is exceedingly low, the action of surface lipases is of minimal impact. These macrovesicular lipid droplets can thus remain for months, even in the absence of further alcohol exposure. Rupture of hepatocytes containing fat may also result in lipogranuloma formation.[5]

Hepatocellular steatosis per se does not induce inflammation. In an otherwise uninjured liver, steatosis will subside on sustained abstinence. It is the addition of both hepatocellular degeneration and necrosis, and hepatic inflammation that constitutes alcoholic hepatitis. With progression to alcoholic hepatitis, the number of steatotic hepatocytes may actually diminish, as the hepatic parenchyma becomes a battleground of hepatocellular destruction, inflammation, fibrosis, and regeneration in the midst of ongoing injury.

BALLOONING DEGENERATION AND ONCOTIC NECROSIS

Hepatocyte volume change ("swelling") is part of normal physiology, and plays a critical role in regulation of hepatocellular metabolism and gene regulation, in response to environmental changes such as ambient osmolarity changes, oxidative stress, intracellular substrate accumulation, and hormones such as insulin.[6] However, deranged

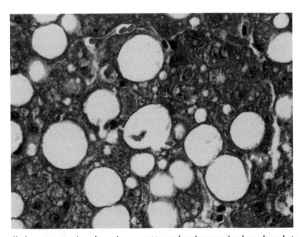

Fig. 1. Hepatocellular steatosis, showing scattered microvesicular droplets, which do not displace the hepatocyte nucleus, and macrovesicular droplets, which displace the nucleus (trichrome stain, original magnification ×400).

cellular swelling is a fundamental feature of cellular injury, and is termed oncosis. In the lexicon of liver pathology, "ballooning degeneration" is the term used. Hepatocytes are massively swollen, usually with clumped cytoplasmic proteins with clarified intracellular spaces (**Fig. 2**). Hepatocyte ballooning is the result of severe cell injury, involving depletion of adenosine triphosphate (ATP) and an increase in intracellular Ca^{2+}, leading to loss of plasma membrane volume control and disruption of the hepatocyte intermediate filament network.[7] If severe enough, cell death occurs. Ballooning degeneration is not specific to alcoholic liver disease, and occurs in ischemic liver cells, cholestasis, and many other forms of hepatic toxicity including alcoholic hepatitis.[8]

The end point of ballooning degeneration is oncotic necrosis, whereby the cell swelling leads to vacuolation, karyolysis, and release of cellular contents; this is considered to be a hallmark of steatohepatitis.[9] In addition to cellular swelling en route to plasma membrane rupture and cell death, plasma membrane blebs form, which are devoid of organelles. Both with fragmentation of the membrane blebs and outright cell rupture, there is complete release of cellular contents into the extracellular environment, quite distinct from apoptosis.

Oncotic necrosis is the predominant mode of death in states of extreme depletion of ATP, such as occurs during oxidative stress with formation of reactive oxygen species,[10] precisely what occurs in alcoholic hepatitis.[11] The resultant oxidative damage disrupts cytoplasmic and nuclear proteins, organelle membranes and proteins, and DNA. Mitochondrial oxygen reduction becomes impaired, leading to the mitochondrial dysfunction, characterized by permeability of both the outer and inner mitochondrial membranes.[12] This process is termed the mitochondrial permeability transition (MPT), and contrasts with apoptosis, which is associated with selective permeabilization only of the outer mitochrondrial membrane. Loss of the inner mitochrondrial membrane barrier leads to collapse of ion gradients and loss of the mitochrondrial membrane potential that drives oxidative phosphorylation.

Cellular ATP levels then collapse, precipitating an increase in intracellular Ca^{2+}, owing to decreased active extrusion of Ca^{2+} from the cell by Ca^{2+}-ATPase, and an opening of voltage-dependent Ca^{2+} channels caused by membrane depolarization owing to decreased activity of the Na^+, K^+-ATPase (the latter of which consumes approximately

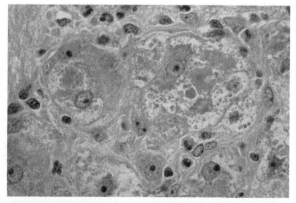

Fig. 2. Hepatocyte ballooning degeneration. Hepatocytes are massively swollen, and contain clumped and disorganized cytoplasmic elements, some of which have coalesced into Mallory bodies. Inflammatory cells, including neutrophils, are present in the vicinity of these ballooned hepatocytes (hematoxylin and eosin [H&E] stain, ×400).

25% of cellular ATP under normal conditions).[13] The increase in intracellular Ca^{2+} destroys the cytoskeleton,[14] and plays a critical role in the opening of the MPT pore, thereby stimulating the mitochondrial pathway of apoptotic cell death.[15,16]

The morphologic manifestation of hepatocellular ballooning degeneration is hepatocellular swelling, vacuolization of the cytoplasm, clumping of intermediate filaments (manifest in tissue sections as clumped strands of eosinophilic cytoplasmic material), swelling of mitochondria, and blebbing of the cell membrane. These features, which affect the entirety of the hepatocyte cytoplasm, are to be distinguished from the well-delineated spherical lipid vacuoles of the steatotic hepatocyte.

MALLORY BODIES

Cytokeratins are the intermediate filaments of epithelial cells and are present in hepatocytes and, in greater amounts, in bile-duct epithelium. In hepatocytes, they are located predominantly just inside the plasma membrane, and are particularly condensed as a pericanalicular sheath that extends into desmosomes. Cytokeratins are linked to desmosomes on the lateral plasma membrane of hepatocytes, in so doing providing scaffolding for the bile canalicular region. Cytokeratins also attach to other components of the cytoskeleton, for example serving as anchors for the contractile activities of microfilaments. Cytokeratins also attach to organelles such as the rough endoplasmic reticulum and vesicles.

Cytokeratins function as "the mechanical integrators of cellular space," because their firm attachment to desmosomes, and the latter to desmosomes on adjacent hepatocytes, provides an integrated continuity of stable 3-dimensional architecture across a multicellular region.[17] Cytokeratins maintain structural polarity, provide scaffolding for the bile canaliculus, and provide a framework for the distribution of actin and endocytotic vesicles along the plasma membrane. Differentiated hepatocytes exhibit a simple cytokeratin expression pattern: the type I cytokeratin CK8, and the type II cytokeratin CK18.[18] In keeping with the requirement that proper assembly of cytokeratins requires the presence of at least one type I and one type II peptide, CK8 and CK18 assemble in equimolar ratios into intermediate filaments (IF), which form a filamentous network within the cytoplasm of hepatocytes. In a variety of disease conditions, alterations in assembly of hepatocellular cytokeratin occur. Ballooning of hepatocytes is accompanied by a reduced density or even loss of the cytoplasmic IF network. Misfolded and aggregated keratins can accumulate, forming Mallory bodies.[19] Mallory bodies exhibit aberrant cross-linking, increased phosphorylation, partial proteolytic degradation, and an increase of β-sheet conformation.[20] Mallory bodies accumulate in alcoholic and nonalcoholic steatohepatitis, Wilson disease, cholestatic conditions such as primary biliary cirrhosis, and following exposure to certain drugs (such as amiodarone). A key degradation pathway for misfolded proteins is the ubiquitination-proteasome pathway. By mass spectrometry, Mallory bodies consist of keratin, ubiquitinated keratin, the stress-induced and ubiquitin-binding protein p62, heat-shock proteins (HSPs) 70 and 25, and other peptides.[21] Hence, antibodies to ubiquitin and p62 highlight Mallory bodies in tissue sections. Of interest, cytokeratins are able to modulate tumor necrosis factor (TNF) signaling pathways and the apoptosis pathway. Specifically, cytokeratins can bind to the TNF receptor 2 (TNFR2), thereby influencing TNF-α–induced activation of the death signaling pathway.[22] TNF-α is a potent inducer of neutrophilic inflammation, and ballooned hepatocytes containing Mallory bodies are frequently surrounded by neutrophils. Thus, the accumulation of Mallory bodies may not simply be a by-product of hepatocellular toxic damage, but may also contribute to the perpetuation or advancement of inflammatory injury. Mallory bodies are visible as skeins of eosino-philic material in the cytoplasm of hepatocytes (**Fig. 3**).

INFLAMMATION (STEATOHEPATITIS)

The lobular inflammatory infiltrate of alcoholic hepatitis consists of neutrophils admixed with lymphocytes, often wrapped around ballooned hepatocytes containing Mallory bodies for the reasons already noted (**Fig. 4**). Usually, but not always, this occurs against a background of steatosis (therefore, alcoholic "steatohepatitis"). Neutrophil infiltration into the liver contributes significantly to the damage of alcoholic liver disease.[23] The inflammation and hepatocellular damage of alcoholic hepatitis is much more severe than the occasional ballooned hepatocytes and the rare Mallory bodies and apoptotic hepatocytes observed in nonalcoholic fatty liver disease.

Regarding mononuclear inflammatory cells, it is worth considering the cellular makeup of the liver. Whereas hepatocytes constitute 80% of the cells in the liver, bile-duct epithelial cells comprise only 1%, with the remainder made up of sinusoidal endothelial cells at 10%, Kupffer cells (the resident macrophages of the liver) at 4%, and lymphocytes at 5%. The last include cells of the adaptive immune system (T and B lymphocytes) and of the innate immune system: natural killer (NK) and natural killer T (NKT) cells. In the latter case, NK cells comprise 31% of hepatic lymphocytes, and NKT cells 26%. The liver is thus particularly enriched with cells of the innate immune system in comparison with other parenchymal organs. In addition to the detri-mental recruitment of neutrophils to the liver as part of an adaptive immune response, activation of the innate immune system also contributes significantly to the progres-sion of alcoholic liver disease. Specifically, this involves Kupffer cells and endothelial cells, cytotoxic T cells, and hepatic stellate cells,[24,25] as will become evident.

Kupffer cells play a role in all forms of hepatitis, as an obligate anatomic companion. Indeed, hepatic Kupffer cells comprise 80% of the systemic host mononuclear phago-cytic system.[26] These cells reside normally on the luminal aspect of the sinusoidal endothelium, so as to engulf particulate material and microorganisms that arrive via the splanchnic circulation from the gut.[27] Kupffer cells are potent scavengers for systemic and gut-derived inflammatory mediators and cytokines.[28] Alcohol ingestion increases gut permeability, either from acute binges or on a chronic basis. The liver is

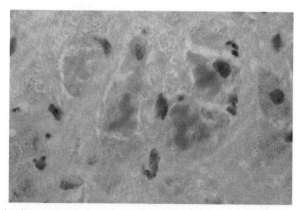

Fig. 3. Mallory bodies, present densely eosinophilic skeins of cytokeratin filaments within the cytoplasm of hepatocytes. In this image from a cirrhotic liver, the hepatocytes are en-trapped in fibrous tissue (H&E stain, original magnification ×400).

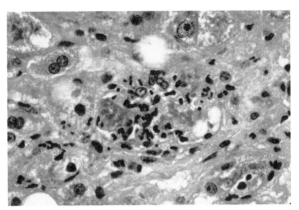

Fig. 4. Parenchymal neutrophilic inflammation in alcoholic hepatitis. The neutrophils are clustered around hepatocytes that contain Mallory bodies (H&E stain, original magnification ×400).

thus exposed to an increased burden of gut-derived bacterial degradation products, especially endotoxin.[29] Endotoxin is a potent activator of Kupffer cells, which in turn release the proinflammatory mediators TNF-α, interleukin (IL)-2, IL-12 and leukotriene B3. These mediators are involved in the hepatic recruitment of neutrophils and cytotoxic T lymphocytes (CTL). Kupffer cells also rapidly engulf hepatocellular debris arising from hepatocellular death of any sort, oncotic or apoptotic.[30] The parenchyma in alcoholic hepatitis, in particular, thus also includes hepatocellular debris with increased numbers of macrophages (**Fig. 5**). The end result is that Kupffer cells may be, at the same time, targets and effectors of different, self-perpetuating events that involve endotoxin, proinflammatory cytokines, fat metabolism, and generation of free radicals in the perpetuation of alcoholic liver disease.[31]

Portal-tract inflammation is also a component of alcoholic hepatitis, and is most likely the result of recruitment of circulating inflammatory cells to the liver as part of an adaptive immune response. For those leukocytes (mononuclear and otherwise) that

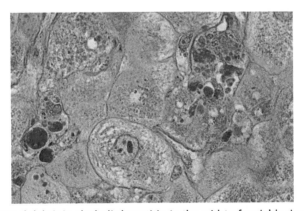

Fig. 5. Parenchymal debris in alcoholic hepatitis. In the midst of variably sized hepatocytes, cellular debris also is present, derived from apoptosis (the eosinophilic spheroid material, *lower left*) and necrosis (the more disorganized granular material, *upper right*). Both forms of debris are engulfed by Kupffer cells as part of the host response (trichrome stain, original magnification ×400).

accumulate within portal tracts during chronic hepatitis, a mixture of lymphocytes, plasma cells, macrophages, neutrophils, eosinophils, and even mast cells may occupy an expanded mesenchymal space within the portal tract. The stimuli for their retention are presumably chemotactic factors, although this is a presumption. Regardless of mechanism, portal-tract inflammation is present as a mute background element in alcoholic liver disease, compared with the dramatic changes occurring in the parenchyma.

APOPTOSIS AND NECROSIS

Arguably the reason alcoholic hepatitis is of such great concern is the hepatocellular destruction and fibrosis that occur. As alluded to earlier, the irreversible toxic injury of alcohol-induced damage is intertwined with steatosis, ballooning degeneration, formation of Mallory bodies, and inflammation. The predominant form of hepatocellular destruction is necrosis: the result of loss of osmotic regulation of cell size; extensive damage to all cellular membranes; swelling of lysosomes; vacuolization of mitochondria; and extensive catabolism of cellular membranes, proteins, ATP, and nucleic acid. Necrosis is the predominant mode of death in states of oxidative stress, as occurs in alcoholic hepatitis,[32] although apoptosis also may contribute.[33] Alcohol-induced oxidative damage disrupts cytoplasmic and nuclear proteins, organelle membranes and proteins, and DNA.[11] The cytoskeleton also undergoes proteolysis, and mitochondrial oxygen reduction is also impaired. The reactive oxygen species also act as intracellular second messengers, inducing cascade reactions through the transcriptional factors nuclear factor κB and activator protein 1. As the liver has the greatest amount of macrophages of any organ in the body, these macrophages also can secrete oxygen radicals as well as tissue-toxic cytokines such as TNF-α and IL-1. The recruitment of inflammatory cells further exacerbates the tissue injury.

Nitric oxide (NO) is generated by endothelial cells, including sinusoidal endothelial cells, which are activated during tissue injury and inflammation.[34] In necrotic death, NO potentiates hepatocellular necrosis, which appears to be mediated by an NO-induced decrease in intracellular ATP.[35] Hence, the sinusoidal endothelium can be yet another contributor to hepatic injury.

In the case of apoptosis, hepatocytes exhibit cytoplasmic shrinkage, cell-membrane blebbing, chromatin condensation, and cellular fragmentation into small membrane-bound "apoptotic bodies."[36] These characteristic changes are the result of activation of caspases and endonucleases, which induce the cleavage of structural proteins and DNA, respectively.[37] In the liver, apoptotic bodies have long been referred to as acidophilic bodies or Councilman bodies (**Fig. 6**).[38,39] Identification of apoptotic bodies indicates current and ongoing hepatocellular apoptosis, because apoptotic hepatocytes are engulfed within a matter of hours by Kupffer cells or other macrophages.

Apoptosis is triggered by cytotoxic T cells, which induce a characteristic sequence of downstream events: translocation of phosphatidylserine to the outer leaflet of the cell plasma membrane; caspase activation; activation of the MPT; cytochrome c release from the mitochondrion; and DNA fragmentation. Exposure of phosphatidylserine on the outer leaflet of the cell membrane is an early stimulus for phagocytosis of the apoptotic body. A role for activation of complement C3 and C1q also has been proposed, especially in the inducement of apoptosis in alcoholic liver disease.[40,41] In the end, whether by oncotic necrosis or apoptosis, hepatocytes are eliminated.

REGENERATION

The phenomenon of liver regeneration has been studied for almost a century, as the liver is an organ with one of the greatest propensities to restore tissue mass and

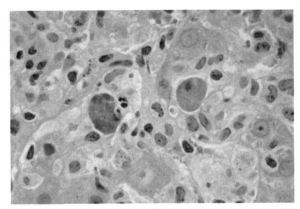

Fig. 6. Hepatocellular apoptosis. Two apoptotic hepatocytes are present in the midst of an otherwise inflamed parenchyma. The apoptotic hepatocyte on the left exhibits extruded nuclear material to its immediate right (H&E stain, original magnification ×400).

function after its destruction. This topic has been reviewed extensively elsewhere,[41] and only brief mention is made here. Mild injury to hepatocytes with limited hepatocellular destruction stimulates neighboring differentiated hepatocytes to undergo division and replication, usually within hours, and therefore responding quickly to liver damage. More extensive liver destruction, particularly that occurring at the interface between portal tracts and the parenchyma, stimulates proliferation of periportal progenitor cells. Unfortunately, there are mitigating factors in alcoholic liver disease.

First, hepatic regeneration depends on the availability of the basic nutrient building blocks that are usually supplied via the portal venous blood from intestinal digestion and absorption.[42] Dietary protein does enhance regeneration, as increased mitotic activity can be demonstrated in hepatocytes when experimental animals are transferred from low-protein to normal or high-protein diets.[43] Unfortunately, alcoholic individuals may be malnourished and have insufficient nutritive resources to stimulate the hepatocellular regeneration necessary to respond to more severe hepatic injury, as in alcoholic hepatitis. Unlike other forms of hepatic injury (such as viral hepatitis), mitotic figures are difficult to identify in alcoholic hepatitis.

Second, the parenchymal fibrosis that develops in alcoholic liver disease can put severe spatial constraints on the ability of hepatocytes to replicate, and this holds particularly true as alcoholic hepatitis progresses toward cirrhosis. Hence, even if alcohol intake subsides and the liver becomes more able to reconstitute its mass through regeneration, deposition of fibrous tissue may render the regenerative response insufficient.

FIBROSIS AND PROGRESSION TO CIRRHOSIS

Steatosis per se is not a strong stimulus for fibrogenesis. Unfortunately, the individual who continually exposes her or his liver to nontrivial doses of alcohol is unlikely to develop only steatosis. The more toxic effects of alcohol, especially its propensity to cause oxidative parenchymal damage and induce inflammation, induce activation of the cells that deposit connective tissue within the liver. It is the progression of fibrogenesis that constitutes the greatest risk to sustenance of homeostasis.

The key events in hepatic fibrogenesis involve activation of perisinusoidal (hepatic) stellate cells, deposition of extracellular matrix, and alteration of the parenchymal microvasculature. In the normal liver parenchyma, extracellular matrix may be produced by perisinusoidal stellate cells, hepatocytes, and the sinusoidal endothelial cells.[44] The normally fat-storing stellate cells are present in the subendothelial space of Disse and sometimes in the perisinusoidal recess between hepatocytes. Stellate cells comprise fewer than 10% of total resident liver cells under normal conditions, and are regularly spaced along the sinusoids (approximately 40 μm from nucleus to nucleus).[45] Despite their relative scarcity, they have long cytoplasmic processes that can cover the entire perisinusoidal area.[46] With repeated injury to the liver paren-chyma, stellate cells become activated and transform into myofibroblast-like cells. The key features of stellate cell activation are[47]: (1) robust mitotic activity in areas developing new parenchymal fibrosis; (2) a shift from the resting-state lipocyte pheno-type to a transitional myofibroblast phenotype; and (3) increased capacity for synthesis and secretion of extracellular matrix. It is predominantly the cytokines secreted by activated Kupffer cells and other inflammatory cells that stimulate the stel-late cells to divide and to secrete large amounts of extracellular matrix.

The contractile properties of stellate cells have a major impact on liver blood flow and modification of portal vascular resistance during fibrosis and cirrhosis. Endothelin-1 (ET-1) is the key contractile stimulus for activated stellate cells.[46] This system acts in an auto-crine loop of stimulation whereby ET-1 synthesis is upregulated in activated stellate cells, as is expression of its 2 receptors, ET-A and ET-B.[48] In the normal liver, ET-1–induced vasoconstriction is in balance with NO-mediated vasodilatation (via antago-nism of ET-1). During liver fibrosis, there is an increase in ET-1 expression and a decrease in NO generation by the sinusoidal endothelium, shifting the balance toward stellate cell (myofibroblast) contractility.[49]

The greatest activation of stellate cells is in areas of severe hepatocellular necrosis and inflammation.[50] The activation of stellate cells may exhibit a zonal pattern. Perive-nular (centrilobular) sinusoidal fibrosis has been well documented in the early stages of liver injury from alcohol,[51] and is accompanied by a decrease in sinusoidal density in the perivenular region.[52] There is an increase in perisinusoidal stellate cells in the peri-venular region before the development of fibrous septa.[53] These findings indicate that simultaneous alterations in perisinusoidal stellate cells, extracellular matrix, and the parenchymal microvasculature occur during the evolution of cirrhosis. Put differently, microvascular changes are not merely the consequence of fibrosis and nodule forma-tion, but are part and parcel of the evolution of cirrhosis.[54]

In the normal liver, the extracellular matrix comprises less than 3% of the relative area on a tissue section.[55] As the liver progresses toward cirrhosis, all types of colla-gens, glycoproteins, and proteoglycans can increase to 3 times or even more the amounts normally found in the liver. Aberrant deposition of extracellular matrix within the hepatic parenchyma produces an environment in which: (1) scarring with type I collagen develops; and (2) extracellular matrix proteins normally present in basement membranes are deposited within the space of Disse, creating a major barrier for solute exchange between hepatocytes and sinusoidal blood.[56] Studies in rats have shown that, on a percentage-area basis, total extracellular matrix components can increase to 25% to 40% in cirrhosis.[57] In humans, this has been measured at 30% of area by the time of liver transplantation for alcoholic liver disease.[58] The total matrix in the space of Disse can increase and change its character to the extent that these struc-tural changes can be identified by routine light microscopy. In particular, the change of the space of Disse from containing delicate interspersed strands of fibrillar collagen (types III and IV) to one containing a dense matrix of basement membrane–type matrix proteins closes the space of Disse to protein exchange between hepatocytes and plasma. In combination with the loss of fenestrations in the sinusoidal endothelium, this process is called capillarization of the sinusoids.[59] In general, abnormal matrix deposition within the space of Disse occurs in those parts of the parenchyma where cell injury and inflammation are greatest. The changes in the extracellular matrix have a profound effect on regeneration of liver cells and vascular redistribution.

Although the predominant source of abnormal extracellular matrix in the cirrhotic liver derives from stellate cells, particularly the alcoholic liver, portal-tract fibrogenesis must also be considered.[60–63] Cells that can contribute to portal-tract fibrosis include the periductular fibroblasts that can surround bile ducts, myofibroblasts loosely placed around the portal vein and hepatic artery, and fibroblasts and in the loose connective tissue of the portal field, especially at the interface between the portal tract and parenchyma. Smooth muscle cells in the wall of the portal-tract blood vessels and second-layer fibroblasts of the terminal hepatic vein are also capable of synthesizing extracellular matrix proteins, in keeping with the general observation that the main contributors to hepatic matrix production are mesenchymal cells. The generalized inflammatory environment of alcoholic hepatitis, in particular, can activate portal-tract fibrogenesis as well, further contributing to the brisk fibrogenesis that can occur in this condition.

In what might otherwise be considered a "purely" steatotic liver, delicate strands of fibrous tissue may nevertheless be deposited over time within the subendothelial space of Disse by activated stellate cells; this becomes manifest as fibrous septa traversing parenchymal sinusoids. A perivenous location for these fibrous septa is most common (**Fig. 7**A), although periportal sinusoidal fibrosis also may develop (**Fig. 7**B). Even in a predominantly steatotic liver, ongoing parenchymal damage may be present, as evidenced by the formation of Mallory bodies and occasional inflammatory cells (**Fig. 8**). This damage is sufficient to stimulate sinusoidal fibrogenesis, eventually creating a steatotic liver subdivided by bridging fibrous septa (**Fig. 9**).

The indolent progression of fibrogenesis over many years in the steatotic form of alcoholic liver disease is to be contrasted with the aggressive progression of fibrosis in alcoholic hepatitis. The extensive hepatocellular damage and parenchymal inflammation that occur in alcoholic hepatitis stimulate brisk fibrogenesis. Virtually every sinusoid is subject to deposition of abnormal extracellular matrix, encasing hepatocytes in dense fibrous tissue (**Fig. 10**A). The cirrhosis that can develop out of this environment constrains hepatocyte cords to a tomb-like fibrous environment. The parenchyma in turn is subdivided by fibers at the sublobular level, leaving little spatial room for hepatocellular regeneration and hepatic recovery (**Fig. 10**B). With time and some element of hepatocellular regeneration, parenchymal islands can emerge in

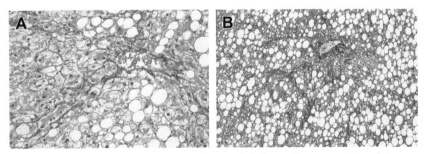

Fig. 7. Sinusoidal fibrosis in steatotic liver disease. (*A*) The perivenous region of the parenchyma is shown, with delicate blue fibrous sinusoidal strands extending into the parenchyma. (*B*) The region around this portal tract also exhibits deposition of sinusoidal fibrous septa (trichrome stain, original magnification ×200 [*A*], ×100 [*B*]).

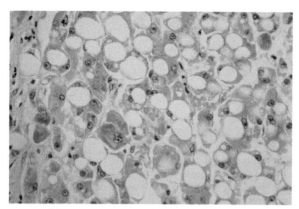

Fig. 8. Steatotic liver disease in an alcoholic, with scattered parenchymal inflammatory cells (*far left*) and one hepatocyte containing a Mallory body (H&E stain, original magnification ×200).

the midst of dense fibrous septa, creating the characteristic "micronodular" cirrhosis of alcoholic liver disease (**Fig. 11**). Of note, both alcoholic hepatitis and the cirrhosis developing from alcoholic hepatitis may exhibit little to no steatosis.[64]

In the alcoholic patient, at first the cirrhotic liver is yellow-tan, fatty, and enlarged, usually weighing more than 2 kg. Over the span of years it is transformed into a brown, shrunken, nonfatty organ, sometimes less than 1 kg in weight. Initially, the developing fibrous septae are delicate and extend through sinusoids from central to portal regions as well as from portal tract to portal tract. Regenerative activity of entrapped parenchymal hepatocytes generates nodules 1–3 mm in diameter or smaller. With time, the nodularity becomes more prominent; scattered larger nodules create a "hobnail" appearance on the surface of the liver. As fibrous septae dissect and surround nodules, the liver becomes more fibrotic, loses fat, and shrinks progressively in size. Parenchymal islands are engulfed by ever wider bands of fibrous tissue, and the liver is converted into a mixed pattern of small (micronodular) and larger (macronodular) parenchymal nodules, embedded in dense fibrous tissue. Ongoing ischemic

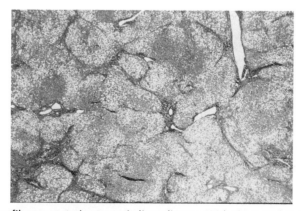

Fig. 9. Bridging fibrous septa in steatotic liver disease. With time, and in the absence of substantive inflammation, the steatotic liver may nevertheless develop progressive fibrosis. In this liver, bridging fibrous septa partially subdivide an otherwise severely steatotic liver. This liver is not yet cirrhotic (trichrome stain, original magnification ×40).

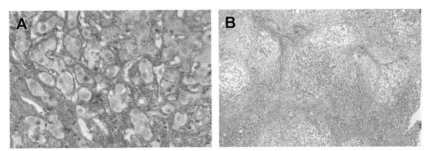

Fig. 10. Fibrosis in alcoholic hepatitis. (*A*) Sinusoidal fibrosis encases every hepatocyte cord. Some neutrophilic inflammation is present. (*B*) Alcoholic hepatitis progressing to cirrhosis. A parenchyma that is extensively subdivided by sublobular sinusoidal fibrosis also exhibits broader fibrous septa that partially isolate islands of hepatocellular parenchyma (trichrome stain, original magnification ×400 [*A*], ×40 [*B*]).

necrosis and fibrous obliteration of nodules eventually create broad expanses of tough, pale scar tissue (Laennec cirrhosis). The tell-tale residua of alcoholic liver disease may still be evident, such as solitary hepatocytes containing Mallory bodies and embedded in dense fibrous tissue, as shown in **Fig. 3**.

DIFFERENTIAL DIAGNOSIS

As in many forms of liver disease, the morphologic features of alcoholic liver disease are not specific to this condition. In part because individuals with excessive alcohol exposure may also be subject to other forms of liver injury, both pathologist and treating physician must keep in mind other potential causes of liver damage. In brief, these are[2]:

- Steatosis, macrovesicular: Alcohol, obesity, diabetes, hyperlipidemia, corticosteroid therapy, protein-calorie malnutrition
- Steatosis, microvesicular: Alcoholic foamy degeneration, drug hepatotoxicity (eg, nucleoside analogues), acute fatty liver of pregnancy, urea-cycle defects, mitochondriopathies

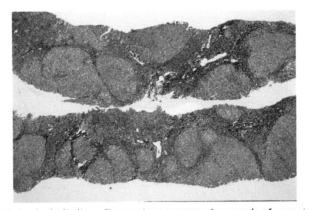

Fig. 11. Cirrhosis in alcoholic liver disease. Low-power micrograph of percutaneous needle biopsy tissue sections showing micronodular cirrhosis, whereby the bridging fibrous septa are at a lobular or sublobular level, isolating islands of hepatocytes that are the size of a lobule, or smaller (trichrome stain, original magnification ×40).

- Steatohepatitis: Alcoholic hepatitis, nonalcoholic steatohepatitis such as from obesity, diabetes, hyperlipidemia, insulin resistance/metabolic syndrome, drug hepatotoxicity (eg, tamoxifen, nifedipine)

The patient with cirrhosis arising from alcoholic liver disease also is at risk for development of hepatocellular carcinoma, which must be kept in mind both during general evaluation and by biochemical and noninvasive imaging studies, and in examination of liver biopsy tissue.

REFERENCES

1. Bosra S, Anand BS. Definition, epidemiology and magnitude of alcoholic hepatitis. World J Hepatol 2011;3:108–13.
2. Lefkowitch JH. Morphology of alcoholic liver disease. Clin Liver Dis 2005;9: 37–53.
3. Niemelä O, Parkkila S, Ylä-Herttuala S, et al. Covalent protein adducts in the liver as a result of ethanol metabolism and lipid peroxidation. Lab Invest 1994;70:537–46.
4. Peters TJ, Cairns SR. Analysis and subcellular localization of lipid in alcoholic liver disease. Alcohol 1985;2:447–51.
5. Christoffersen P, Braendstrup O, Juhl E, et al. Lipogranulomas in human liver biopsies with fatty change. A morphological, biochemical and clinical investigation. Acta Pathol Microbiol Scand A 1971;79:150–8.
6. Schiless F, Häussinger D. Osmosensing and signaling in the regulation of liver function. Contrib Nephrol 2006;152:190–209.
7. Farber JL, Kyle ME, Coleman JB. Mechanisms of cell injury by activated oxygen species. Lab Invest 1990;762:670–9.
8. Ficker P, Trauner M, Fuchsbichler A, et al. Oncosis represents the main type of cell death in mouse models of cholestasis. J Hepatol 2005;42:378–85.
9. Lackner C, Gogg-Kamerer M, Zatloukal K, et al. Ballooned hepatocytes in steatohepatitis: the value of keratin immunohistochemistry for diagnosis. J Hepatol 2008;48:821–8.
10. Jaeschke H, LeMasters JJ. Apoptosis versus oncotic necrosis in hepatic ischemia/reperfusion injury. Gastroenterology 2003;125:1246–57.
11. Zhu H, Jia Z, Misra H, et al. Oxidative stress and redox signaling mechanisms of alcoholic liver disease. Updated experimental and clinical evidence. J Dig Dis 2012;13:133–42.
12. Malhi H, Gores GH, LeMasters JJ. Apoptosis and necrosis in the liver: a tale of two deaths? Hepatology 2006;43:S31–44.
13. Buck LT, Hochachka PW. Anoxic suppression on Na^+-K^+-ATPase and constant membrane potential in hepatocytes: support for channel arrest. Am J Physiol 1993;265:R1020–5.
14. LeMasters JJ, Stemkowski CJ, Ji S, et al. Cell surface changes and enzyme release during hypoxia and reoxygenation in the isolated, perfused rat liver. J Cell Biol 1983;97:778–86.
15. Gateau-Roesch O, Pavlov E, Lazareva AV, et al. Calcium-binding properties of the mitochondrial channel-forming hydrophobic component. J Bioenerg Biomembr 2000;32:105–10.
16. Kim JS, He L, Qian T, et al. Role of the mitochondrial permeability transition in apoptotic and necrotic death after ischemia/reperfusion injury to hepatocytes. Curr Mol Med 2004;3:527–35.
17. Lazarides E. Intermediate filaments as mechanical integrators of cellular space. Nature 1980;283:249–56.

18. Schachter D. The hepatocyte plasma membrane: organization and differentiation. In: Arias IM, Jakoby WB, Popper H, et al, editors. The liver: biology and pathobiology. New York: Raven Press; 1988. p. 131–40.

19. Denk H, Stumptner C, Zatloukal K. Mallory bodies revisited. J Hepatol 2000;32: 689–702.

20. Stumptner C, Omary MB, Fickert P, et al. Hepatocyte cytokeratins are hyperphosphorylated at multiple sites in human alcoholic hepatitis and in a Mallory body mouse model. Am J Pathol 2000;156:77–90.

21. Zatloukal K, Stumptner C, Fuchsbichler A, et al. The keratin cytoskeleton in liver diseases. J Pathol 2004;204:367–76.

22. Caulin C, Ware CF, Magin TM, et al. Keratin-dependent, epithelial resistance to tumor necrosis factor-induced apoptosis. J Cell Biol 2000;149:17–22.

23. Ramaiah S, Jaeschke H. Role of neutrophils in the pathogenesis of acute inflammatory liver injury. Toxicol Pathol 2007;35:757–66.

24. Suh YG, Jeong WI. Hepatic stellate cells and innate immunity in alcoholic liver disease. World J Gastroenterol 2011;17:2543–51.

25. Gao B, Seki E, Brenner DA, et al. Innate immunity in alcoholic liver disease. Am J Physiol Gastroenterol Liver Physiol 2011;300:G516–25.

26. Saba TM. Physiology and physiopathology of the reticuloendothelial system. Arch Intern Med 1970;126:1031–52.

27. Sakaguchi S, Takahashi S, Sasaki T, et al. Progression of alcoholic and non-alcoholic steatohepatitis: common metabolic aspects of innate immune system and oxidative stress. Drug Metab Pharmacokinet 2011;26:30–46.

28. Monshouwer M, Hoebe KH. Hepatic (dys-)function during inflammation. Toxicology. In Vitro 2003;17:681–6.

29. Nagata K, Suzuki H, Sakaguchi S. Common pathogenic mechanism in development progression of liver injury caused by non-alcoholic or alcoholic steatohepatitis. J Toxicol Sci 2007;5:453–68.

30. Gores G, Ren Y, Savill J. Apoptosis: the importance of being eaten. Cell Death Differ 1998;5:563–9.

31. Casini A. Alcohol-induced fatty liver and inflammation: where do Kupffer cells act? J Hepatol 2000;32:1026–30.

32. LeMasters JJ, Qian T, He L, et al. Role of mitochondrial inner membrane permeabilization in necrotic cell death, apoptosis, and autophagy. Antioxid Redox Signal 2002;4:769–81.

33. Day CP. Apoptosis in alcoholic hepatitis: a novel therapeutic target? J Hepatol 2001;34:330–3.

34. Lin HI, Wang D, Leu FJ, et al. Ischemia and reperfusion of liver induces eNOS and iNOS expression: effects of a NO donor and NOS inhibitor. Chin J Physiol 2004;47:121–7.

35. Lee VG, Johnson ML, Baust J, et al. The roles of iNOS in liver ischemia-reperfusion injury. Shock 2001;16:355–60.

36. Kerr JF. History of the events leading to the formulation of the apoptosis concept. Toxicology 2002;181:471–4.

37. Jaeschke H, Gujral JS, Bajt ML. Apoptosis and necrosis in liver disease. Liver Int 2004;24:85–9.

38. Bai J, Odin JA. Apoptosis and the liver: relation to autoimmunity and related conditions. Autoimmunity Rev 2003;2:36–42.

39. Roychowdhury S, McMullen MR, Pritchard MT, et al. An early complement-dependent and TLR-4 independent phase in the pathogenesis of ethanol-induced liver injury. Hepatology 2009;49:1326–34.

40. Cohen JI, Roychowdhury S, McMullen MR, et al. Complement and alcoholic liver disease: role of C1q in the pathogenesis of ethanol-induced liver injury in mice. Gastroenterology 2010;139:664–74.
41. Riehle KJ, Dan YY, Campbell JS, et al. New concepts in liver regeneration. J Gastroenterol Hepatol 2011;26(Suppl 1):203–12.
42. Stirling GA, Laughlin J, Washington SL. Effects of starvation on the proliferative response after partial hepatectomy. Exp Mol Pathol 1973;19:44–52.
43. Rigotti P, Peters JC, Tranberg KG, et al. Effects of amino acid infusions on liver regeneration after hepatectomy in the rat. JPEN J Parenter Enteral Nutr 1986; 10:17–20.
44. Novo E, di Bonzo LV, Canito S, et al. Hepatic myofibroblasts: a heterogeneous population of multifunctional cells in liver fibrogenesis. Int J Biochem Cell Biol 2009;41:2089–93.
45. Zhao L, Burt AD. The diffuse stellate cell system. J Mol Histol 2007;38:53–64.
46. Frideman SL. Hepatic stellate cells: protean, multifunctional, and enigmatic cells of the liver. Physiol Rev 2008;88:125–72.
47. Friedman SL. Hepatic fibrosis—overview. Toxicology 2008;254:120–9.
48. Housset C, Rockey DC, Bissell DM. Endothelin receptors in rat liver: lipocytes as a contractile target for endothelin 1. Proc Natl Acad Sci U S A 1993;90: 9266–70.
49. Kawada N, Tran-Thi TA, Klein H, et al. The contraction of hepatic stellate (Ito) cells stimulated with vasoactive substances: possible involvement of endothelin 1 and nitric oxide in the regulation of sinusoidal tonus. Eur J Biochem 1993;213: 815–23.
50. Enzan H, Himeno H, Iwamura S, et al. Sequential changes in human Ito cells and their relation to postnecrotic liver fibrosis in massive and submassive hepatic necrosis. Virchows Arch 1995;426:95–101.
51. Worner TM, Lieber CS. Perivenular fibrosis as precursor lesion of cirrhosis. J Am Med Assoc 1985;254:627–30.
52. Vollmar B, Siegmund S, Menger MD. An intravital fluorescence microscopic study of hepatic microvascular and cellular derangements in developing cirrhosis in rats. Hepatology 1998;27:1544–53.
53. Yokoi Y, Namihisa T, Matsuzaki K, et al. Distribution of Ito cells in experimental hepatic fibrosis. Liver 1988;8:48–52.
54. Sherman IA, Pappas SC, Fisher MM. Hepatic microvascular changes associated with development of liver fibrosis and cirrhosis. Am J Physiol 1990;258:H460–5.
55. Lin XZ, Horng MH, Sun YN, et al. Computer morphometry for quantitative measurement of liver fibrosis: comparison with Knodell's score, colorimetry and conventional description reports. J Gastroenterol Hepatol 1998;13:75–80.
56. Martinez-Hernandez A, Martinez J. The role of capillarization in hepatic failure: studies in carbon tetrachloride-induced cirrhosis. Hepatology 1991;14:864–74.
57. James J, Bosch KS, Zuyderhoudt FM, et al. Histophotometric estimation of volume density of collagen as an indication of fibrosis in rat liver. Histochemistry 1986;85:129–33.
58. Hall A, Germani G, Isgrò G, et al. Fibrosis distribution in explanted cirrhotic livers. Histopathology 2012;60:270–7.
59. Mori T, Okanoue T, Sawa Y, et al. Defenestration of the sinusoidal endothelial cell in a rat model of cirrhosis. Hepatology 1993;17:891–7.
60. Tuchweber B, Desmoulière A, Bochaton-Piallat ML, et al. Proliferation and pheno-typic modulation of portal fibroblasts in the early stages of cholestatic fibrosis in the rat. Lab Invest 1996;74:265–78.

61. Desmouliere A, Darby I, Costa AMA, et al. Extracellular matrix deposition, lysyl oxidase expression, and myofibroblastic differentiation during the initial stages of cholestatic fibrosis in the rat. Lab Invest 1997;76:765–78.

62. Bhunchet E, Wake K. Role of mesenchymal cell populations in porcine serum-induced rat liver fibrosis. Hepatology 1992;16:1452–73.

63. Kinnman N, Francoz C, Barbu V, et al. The myofibroblast conversion of peribiliary fibrogenic cells distinct from hepatic stellate cells is stimulated by platelet-derived growth factor during liver fibrogenesis. Lab Invest 2003;83:163–73.

64. Yerian L. Histopathological evaluation of fatty and alcoholic liver diseases. J Dig Dis 2011;12:17–24.

Diagnosis and Management of Alcoholic Hepatitis

Umair Sohail, MD[a], Sanjaya K. Satapathy, MBBS, MD, DM[b],*

KEYWORDS

- Alcoholic hepatitis • Aminotransferases • Maddrey's discriminant function
- Liver biopsy • Steroids in alcoholic hepatitis • Enteral nutrition in alcoholic hepatitis
- Pentoxifylline • Liver transplantation

KEY POINTS

- The diagnosis of alcoholic hepatitis is based on the appropriate alcohol intake history and is supported with clinical features such as fever, jaundice, ascites, elevated white blood cells, generally aspartate aminotransferase <500 IU/mL, and alanine aminotransferase <200 IU/ml. Elevated aspartate aminotransferase-to-alanine aminotransferase ratio (usually >2:1) is also associated with alcoholic liver disease.
- A liver biopsy may help confirm the diagnosis, it is generally not recommended. The biopsy may demonstrate hepatocyte ballooning, Mallory hyaline, neutrophilic infiltration, and perisinuosidal fibrosis.
- The spectrum of severity ranges from mild to severe, mortality for severe alcoholic hepatitis is quite high, in the range of 30% to 50% during a 28-day period.
- Assessment of disease severity can be made using the Maddrey Discriminant Function, Model for End-Stage Liver Disease score, Glasgow Alcoholic Hepatitis Score, and the Lillie Model.
- Steroids are the main stay of treatment in absence of contraindications in patients with severe alcoholic Hepatitis (MDF >32) with Pentoxifylline used as an alternative to steroids.
- Early studies have shown some promise for aggressive interventions such as molecular adsorbent recirculating system, but more studies are needed. Liver transplantation in acute alcoholic hepatitis is debatable because of the 6-month abstinence rule, ethical concerns, risk of recidivism, and potential for poor post-transplant graft and patient survival.

The authors have no disclosures.
[a] University of Tennessee Health sciences center, Suite 340, 1211 Union Avenue, Memphis, TN 38104, USA; [b] Methodist University Hospital Transplant Institution, Department of Surgery, University of Tennessee Health Sciences Center, Suite 340, 1211 Union Avenue, Memphis, TN 38104, USA
* Corresponding author.
E-mail address: ssatapat@uthsc.edu

INTRODUCTION

Alcoholic hepatitis (AH) is an acute form of alcohol induced liver injury that is seen in patients who consume large quantities of alcohol during a prolonged period of time. It includes a spectrum of severity ranging from asymptomatic derangement of liver chemistry results to fulminant liver failure and even death. Although AH is most likely seen in people who drink heavily for many years, the relationship between drinking and AH is complex. Not all heavy drinkers develop AH, and the disease has been seen in people who drink moderately.

PREVALENCE AND RISK FACTORS

The prevalence of alcoholic liver disease (ALD) is influenced by many factors, including genetic factors (eg, tendency of alcohol abuse, gender) and environmental factors (eg, availability of alcohol, social acceptability of alcohol use, concomitant hepatotoxic insults), and it is therefore difficult to outline. In general, the risk of liver disease increases with the quantity and duration of alcohol intake.[1,2] Possible factors that affect the development of liver injury include the dose, duration, and type of alcohol consumption; drinking patterns; gender; and ethnicity. Other associated risk factors include obesity, iron overload, concomitant infection with viral hepatitis, and genetic factors.

Different alcoholic beverages contain varying quantities of alcohol. Based on a study of series of autopsies, a threshold daily alcohol intake of 40 g is necessary to produce pathologic changes consistent with AH. An increase in severity of AH is associated with consumption of more than 80 g/d.[1] A daily intake of more than 60 g of alcohol in men and 20 g in women significantly increases the risk of cirrhosis. In addition, persistent daily drinking, compared with binge drinking, has been shown to be more harmful.[3] Another factor that has been acknowledged is the pattern of drinking. It has been reported that drinking alcohol outside of mealtimes increases the risk of ALD by 2.7-fold compared with those who consumed alcohol only at mealtimes.[4]

SIGNS AND SYMPTOMS

AH is a syndrome with a spectrum of severity and, therefore, manifesting symptoms vary. Symptoms may be nonspecific and mild, which may include fever, anorexia, weight loss, abdominal pain, distention, or nausea and vomiting. Alternatively, more severe symptoms can include encephalopathy and hepatic failure. Physical findings include hepatomegaly, jaundice, ascites, spider angiomas, and encephalopathy.[5]

DIAGNOSIS

The diagnosis of AH is established on a thorough history, physical examination, and review of laboratory tests.[6] Characteristically the ratio of aspartate aminotransferase to alanine aminotransferase (AST/ALT) is approximately 2:1. In severe AH, serum AST is typically elevated to a level of 2 to 6 times the upper limits of normal. Levels of ALT of more than 200 IU/L or of AST of more than 500 IU/L are less commonly seen with AH (other than alcoholic foamy degeneration or concomitant acetaminophen overdose)[7] and should suggest an alternate cause. In about 70% of patients, the AST/ALT ratio is higher than 2, but this may be of greater value in patients without cirrhosis.[8–10] If the ratio is greater than 3, it is highly suggestive of ALD.[11]

Anemia and leukocytosis are other common and nonspecific laboratory abnormalities. Leukocytosis is caused by hepatitis and generally parallels hepatic tissue neutrophilic infiltration. Even if alcohol use is discontinued, 10% to 20% of patients with persistent leukocytosis progress to subfulminant hepatic failure.

Gamma glutamyl transpeptidase (GGT) has been evaluated in several settings, including large population surveys.[12,13] Unfortunately, the usefulness of elevated GGT is limited by its low sensitivity and specificity to diagnose alcohol abuse.[14–16] The levels of GGT may fluctuate with extensive liver injury.[17] Lower levels of GGT (<100) or a total bilirubin/GGT ratio of greater than 1 (expressed as mumoles per liter and GGT in IU per liter) has been reported as a predictor of 1-year mortality in patients with alcoholic cirrhosis,[17] although, this has not consistently added prognostic ability to other laboratory tests.[18] In combination with other biomarkers, however, GGT may add independent information in diagnosing alcohol abuse or problem drinking.

Measurement of carbohydrate deficient transferrin (CDT) is another potential tool for the diagnosis of ALD. The sensitivity and specificity for significant alcohol intake are in the range of 60% to 70% and of 80% to 90%, respectively.[9] Unfortunately, the utility of CDT is compounded by the its elevation in sepsis, anorexia nervosa, and airway disease.[19] Additionally, values of CDT are lower in patients with iron overload.[20] The usefulness of CDT, thus, depends on associated medical conditions and may not be useful in detection of chronic alcohol abuse in an unselected population.[21]

Direct ethanol metabolites, such as ethyl glucuronide (EtG), phosphatidyl ethanol, and fatty acid ethyl esters, and sialic acid index of plasma apolipoprotein J have proved to be promising biomarkers for active alcohol consumption and could be useful in special circumstances, such as in patients who deny ethanol intake as part of an evaluation for liver transplantation or in legal cases. Although the utility of these biomarkers are still under evaluation, EtG, a direct metabolite of ethanol formed by conjugation of ethanol to glucuronic acid, has shown potential utility in clinical practice.[22] EtG can be detected in various body fluids, tissue, and hair up to 80 hours after the complete elimination of alcohol from the body.[22] An enzyme-linked immunosorbent EtG test yields a serum sensitivity and specificity rate of 92% and 91%, respectively.[23]

Role of Liver Biopsy in the Diagnosis of AH

Although several clinical scoring systems are available to predict AH, their main use is in highlighting patients most at risk of having severe AH, to facilitate the institution of early therapeutic interventions. Hyperbilirubinemia a key feature of AH compared with other causes of decompensated ALD. However, hyperbilirubinemia is also commonly associated with sepsis and systemic inflammatory response syndrome (a condition that requires two or more of the following abnormalities temperature >38.3°C or <36°C, heart rate >90 beats/min, respiratory rate >20 breaths/min or $PaCO_2$ <32 mmHg, WBC >12,000 cells/mm^3, <4000 cells/mm^3, or >10 percent immature (band) forms).[24] It is thus important to segregate these patients with AH, especially because the corticosteroid (CS)-related mortality rate will be high in these groups of patients. Many of the scoring systems available draw on criteria such as clotting time, which are prone to significant variations between laboratories. Additionally, scores such as the Model for End-Stage Liver Disease (MELD) score and the Glasgow Alcoholic Hepatitis Score (GAHS) also use measures of renal function, which in the context of advanced liver disease are unreliable and change with clinical status (eg, urea with fluid status, feeding, and gastrointestinal bleeding). A recent study looking into the relative importance of AH histologic score compared with discriminant function or MELD noted that histologic examination has a markedly higher predictive utility for defining 28-day mortality.[25] It has, thus, been argued that liver biopsy may allow more reliable interpretation of data from clinical trials of new interventions by

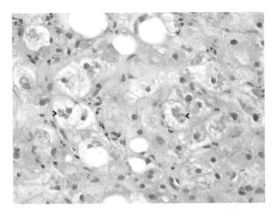

Fig. 1. AH with steatosis, neutrophilic infiltrate, and Mallory bodies within ballooned hepatocytes (*arrowhead*). As is typical in AH, the degree of macrovesiclar steatosis is not proportional to the degree of inflammation and degenerative changes. (Original magnification, ×400.) (*Courtesy of* Pamela B. Sylvestre, MD; University of Tennessee Health Science Center.)

accurately defining the "at-risk" severe-AH population with the most to gain from intervention, while also clearly identifying patients who have other causes of liver disease.

Histologic Findings

The classic histologic features of AH include steatosis, inflammation, ballooning, foamy degeneration, and necrosis, which are most prominent in the centrilobular region (**Fig. 1**).[26] Ballooned hepatocytes cause compression of the sinusoid and reversible portal hypertension. The inflammatory cell infiltrate, located primarily in the sinusoids and close to necrotic or degenerative hepatocytes consists of polymorphonuclear cells and mononuclear cells. Many patients with AH have fatty infiltration and Mallory bodies (also known as Mallory-Denk bodies, **Fig. 2**). Mallory bodies are intracytoplasmic

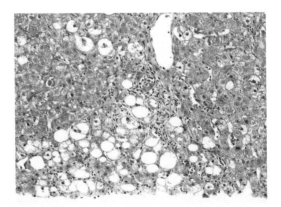

Fig. 2. Trichrome stained section demonstrating perisinusoidal arachnoid fibrosis (aka chicken wire fibrosis), a scarring pattern characteristic of steatohepatitis (both alcoholic and non-alcoholic steatohepatitis). (Original magnification, ×200.) (*Courtesy of* Pamela B. Sylvestre, MD; University of Tennessee Health Science Center.)

perinuclear aggregations of intermediate filaments found in ballooned hepatocytes and are eosinophilic on hematoxylin-eosin staining. Neither fatty infiltration nor Mallory bodies are specific for AH or are necessary for the diagnosis. Steatohepatitis with peri-portal ductular reaction and cholestasis is often seen in severe AH and is fairly specific for an alcoholic cause. Megamitochondria, seen on routine histologic examination in AH, may be associated with a milder form of AH, a lower incidence of cirrhosis, and fewer complications with a good long-term survival.[27] Furthermore, the degree of stea-tosis is not directly proportional to the degree of severity of AH.

Severity Assessment

Maddrey's discriminant function
The discriminant function index (DFI) was originally described by Maddrey and colleagues[28] in a placebo-controlled study to assess the benefit of CS therapy in 55 patients with AH. In their study they used a formula: 4.6 × prothrombin time (PT) (seconds) + serum bilirubin (mg/dL) to risk stratify patients who would most benefit from the CS therapy. They noted that patients with a DFI greater than 93 and treated with placebo had a 28-day survival of 25%, whereas those with a score of 93 or lower had 100% survival.[28] Subsequently this score was modified in 1989 [modified discrim-inant function [MDF]; Discriminant function = (4.6 × [PT – control PT]) + (serum bili-rubin)] using prolongation of PT in seconds (over control) instead of absolute value of PT.[29] It was noted that patients without treatment and with an MDF score of 32 or higher and/or the presence of encephalopathy had a 28-day survival of about 65%. A recent analysis confirmed this observation with untreated patients having 28-day survival of 68% among patients with an MDF of 32 or higher.[30] The American College of Gastroenterology recommends that patients with AH with an MDF score of 32 or higher be considered for CS therapy.[31]

The MELD
The MELD score is a statistical model predicting survival in patients with cirrhosis and is universally used to prioritize patients for liver transplantation.[32] The score is based on serum bilirubin and creatinine levels and international normalized ratio (INR). At least 3 studies suggested that the MELD score may also predict mortality in patients hospitalized for AH.[33–35] In one report, an MELD score of more than 11 performed as well as the discriminant function described earlier in predicting 30-day mortality.[33] In another study, the MELD score had similar predictive accuracy as the discriminant function in predicting 30- and 90-day mortality.[34] A MELD score of 21 had a sensitivity of 75% and specificity of 75% for predicting 90-day mortality. Moreover, serial moni-toring of MELD score with a change in score of 2 or more points in the first week of hospitalization has independently predicted in-hospital mortality.[35]

The advantage of the MELD score is the use of the INR instead of the PT, which is more comparable and uniform across the laboratories, because the calculation accounts for the sensitivity of the thromboplastin reagent used in the test.[36] American Association for Study of the Liver Diseases (AASLD) guidelines on the management of acute liver disease suggest that a cutoff MELD score of 18 be taken to predict severe AH and should be the criterion for initiating treatment.[37]

The GAHS
The GAHS is a multivariate model predicting mortality in AH.[38] It includes age, serum bilirubin (at days 1 and 6–9), blood urea nitrogen, PT, and peripheral white blood cell count. It was found to be a better predictor for mortality at 28 days than the discrim-inant function based on an initial validation study. The accuracy of the GAHS was confirmed by the validation study of 195 patients in this study. The GAHS was equally

accurate irrespective of the use of the INR or PT ratio or if the diagnosis of AH was biopsy-confirmed or on the basis of clinical assessment.[39]

A retrospective study from the United Kingdom specifically looked at the response to CS treatment with severe AH.[39] The study noted for patients with a GAHS of 9 or greater, the 28-day survival for untreated and CS-treated patients was 52% and 78% (P = .002), and the 84-day survival was 38% and 59% (P = .02), respectively. The study authors concluded that among patients with an MDF of 32 or greater, there was no appreciable benefit from treatment with CSs in patients with a GAHS less than 9. Patients with a GAHS of 9 or greater have an extremely poor prognosis if they are not treated with CSs or if such treatment is contraindicated.[39]

Child-Turcotte-Pugh score

Since the 1970s, the standard for assessing perioperative morbidity and mortality in patients with cirrhosis has been the Child-Turcotte-Pugh (CTP) scoring system, which is based on the patient's serum bilirubin and albumin levels, PT, and severity of encephalopathy and ascites.[40] This score categorizes the disease severity into 3 categories, stages A through C, with a total score of 5 to 6, 7 to 9, and greater than 9, respectively. The mortality rates in patients with cirrhosis with various stages are 10% to 15% for Child A status, 25% to 30% for Child B status, and 70% to 80% for Child C status at 1 year. CPT score is not traditionally used as a predictive model for AH but has been shown in studies to predict mortality at 3 to 6 months.[41]

Two of the most important studies, separated by 13 years, reported nearly identical results: mortality rates for patients undergoing major abdominal surgery were 10% for those with Child class A, 30% for those with Child class B, and 76% to 82% for those with Child class C cirrhosis.[42] In addition to predicting perioperative mortality, the Child class correlates with the frequency of postoperative complications, which include worsening encephalopathy, bleeding, liver failure, infection, hypoxia, renal failure, and intractable ascites.

Age-bilirubin-INR-creatinine score

This new scoring system for the prognostic stratification of patients with AH is called the age-bilirubin-INR-creatinine score. Age, serum bilirubin, serum creatinine, and INR independently predicted 90-day mortality.[43]

Based on the study cutoff values of 6.71 and 9.0, patients with low, intermediate, and high risk of death at 90 days (100%, 70%, and 25% of survival rate, respectively) were identified. Further studies are required to validate these results.

Lille model

In patients with severe AH who have been treated with glucocorticosteroids, a prognostic scoring system (the Lille model) has been proposed for predicting mortality.[44] The model, which combines 6 variables (age, renal insufficiency (creatinine >1.3 or creatinine clearance <40), albumin, PT, bilirubin, and evolution of bilirubin at day 7), performed better than the CTP score, discriminant function, or GAHS in predicting survival at 6 months. Survival at 6 months was lower for patients with a Lille score of 0.45 or higher compared with patients with a Lillie score of less than 0.45 (25% vs 85%, P< .0001). The authors concluded that CS be discontinued for patients with Lillie score of 0.45 or greater at 1 week. This is important in early identification of subjects with substantial risk of death according to the Lille model. This will improve management of patients suffering from severe AH and will help in the design of future studies for alternative treatment modalities.

Treatment

Abstinence

The most important and first step in the therapeutic intervention for patients with AH is abstinence.[45] Abstinence has been shown to improve the outcome and histologic features of hepatic injury, to reduce portal pressure, and to decrease progression to cirrhosis. It has also shown to improve survival at all stages in patients with ALD.[46–48] However, this may be less likely in female patients.[49–51] This improvement can be relatively rapid, and in 66% of patients abstaining from alcohol, significant improvement was observed in 3 months.

Disulfiram, one of the first agents to be used, was approved by the US Food and Drug Administration in 1983. Use of disulfiram is widespread but less clearly supported by the clinical trial evidence,[52] and based on its poor tolerability, its use has been largely supplanted by newer agents.

Acamprosate has shown potential utility in several studies. A recent systemic review that included 24 randomized controlled trials (RCTs) with 6915 participants concluded that acamprosate was an effective and safe treatment strategy for supporting continuous abstinence after detoxification in alcohol-dependent patients even though the sizes of treatment effects seem to be rather moderate in magnitude.[53] Despite the moderate efficacy, the authors favored this mode of treatment, in view of the relapsing nature of alcoholism and the limited therapeutic options currently available for its treatment.

Another drug with potential use is baclofen, particularly in patients with cirrhosis and liver failure from ALD.[54] In this study, patients with alcoholic decompensated cirrhosis were randomized to receive baclofen (n = 42) or placebo (n = 42). At 3 months, abstinence rates were better with the use of baclofen compared with placebo-treated patients (71% vs 29%; $P = .0001$) with longer cumulative abstinence duration (63 vs 31 days; $P = .001$). No side effects were reported with the use of baclofen in these patients with advanced cirrhosis.[54]

NONPHARMACOLOGIC THERAPY

Nutritional Therapy

Malnutrition is fairly common in patients with AH.[55] The nutritionist plays a valuable role in assessing the degree of malnutrition and guiding nutritional supplementation in malnourished alcoholic patients. An older study that looked the relationship of malnutrition to AH found a direct correlation with short-term (1-month) and long-term (1-year) mortality. Patients with mild malnutrition have a 14% mortality rate, compared with a 76% mortality rate in those with severe malnutrition at the end of 1 year from the time of diagnosis.[56] Older studies have attempted to show a benefit of nutritional supplementation.[57,58] A recent large meta-analysis concluded that there was a lack of compelling data to justify the routine use of parenteral nutrition, enteral nutrition, or oral nutritional supplements in patients with ALD.[59]

Despite these reservations, the AASLD practice guidelines recommends that all patients with AH or advanced ALD be assessed for nutritional deficiencies (protein-calorie malnutrition) and for vitamin and mineral deficiencies. Those with severe disease should be treated aggressively with enteral nutritional therapy. These guidelines suggest multiple feedings, emphasizing breakfast and a nighttime snack, with a regular oral diet at higher-than-usual dietary intake (1.2–1.5 g/kg for protein and 35–40 kcal/kg for energy).[52] The rationale is based on the observation that patients with cirrhosis use alternative fuel sources (such as fat) more rapidly during starvation compared with healthy volunteers.[60]

PHARMACOLOGIC THERAPY

The need to consider therapy is less urgent in patients with AH who have a low risk of complications as defined by an MDF score of <32, without hepatic encephalopathy, or a low MELD score (eg, MELD <18) or GAHS score of <8. This is particularly true in those whose liver score improves during hospitalization. This is shown by a decrease in total bilirubin. These patients will likely improve spontaneously with abstinence and supportive care alone. For those with more severe disease and therefore a more dismal prognosis, medical treatment should be considered.

Corticosteroids

The most extensively studied pharmacotherapy in AH is the use of CSs. Because autoimmunity is not a significant feature of this disease, the rationale behind the use of glucocorticosteroids is to block cytotoxic and inflammatory pathways.[61]

The use of CSs as specific therapy for AH has received a great deal of attention and selected studies are summarized in **Table 1**.[28,29,62–71] Unfortunately many of these early trials are small and poorly designed with limited statistical power. Others, although showing therapeutic effects to various degrees, differed in the inclusion/exclusion criteria, CS regimens, scoring systems, and spectrum of clinical disorders. Therefore, it is difficult to reach a consensus on the efficacy of CSs in the treatment of AH. In addition, the potential side effects of glucocorticosteroids are numerous,

Table 1
Randomized controlled trials to assess CS treatment in AH

Author (Year)	Sample Size CS	Placebo	Intervention	Survival Treated	Placebo	P
Maddrey et al,[28] 1978	24	31	Prednisolone 40 mg/d (30 d)	96%	81%	.05
Carithers et al,[29] 1989	35	31	Methyl prednisolone: 32 mg/d for 28 d, then 16 mg/d for 7 d, then 8 mg/d for 7 d	94%	65%	.006
Shumaker et al,[62] 1978	12	15	Prednisolone: 80 mg/d (4–7 d) tapered off over 4 wk	50%	53%	NS
Ramond et al,[63] 1992	32	29	Prednisolone: 40 mg/d (28 d)	87%	45%	.001
Helman et al,[64] 1971	20	17	Prednisolone: 40 mg/d (4 wk), then tapered over 2 wk	95%	65%	.01
Porter et al,[65] 1971	11	9	6 Methyl prednisolone 40 mg/d for 10 d	45%	23%	NS
Campra et al,[66] 1973	20	25	Prednisone 0.5 mg/k/d for 3wk then 0.25 mg/k/d for 3 wk	65%	64%	NS
Blitzer et al,[67] 1977	16	14	Prednisolone 40 mg for 14 d then tapering for 2 wk	65%	69%	NS
Depew et al,[68] 1980	15	13	Prednisolone 40 mg/d for 28 d then taper for 14 d	47%	46%	NS
Thedossi et al,[69] 1980	27	28	Methylprednisolone 1 g.d for 3d	37%	43%	NS
Lesesne et al,[70] 1978	7	7	Prednisolone 40 mg/d (30 d), tapered over 2 Wk	71%	0%	.001
Mendenhall et al,[71] 1984	90	173	Prednisone tapered over 28 d	77%	73%	NS

Abbreviations: CS, corticosteroids; NS, not significant.

including antianabolism, muscle breakdown (proteolysis), immunosuppression, increased susceptibility to infection, and increased risk of gastrointestinal bleeding.

The effect of glucocorticosteroid therapy in acute AH has been debated for more than 40 years. An earlier meta-analysis[72] suggested a beneficial role of CSs in patients with acute AH who have hepatic encephalopathy but without active gastrointestinal bleeding by reducing short-term mortality. A later analysis involving 12 controlled trials could not confirm these benefits.[73] By using individual patient data across clinical trials, an approach considered to be the "gold standard" for meta-analysis,[74] another study showed the survival benefit of CSs in the subgroup of patients with hepatic encephalopathy and/or those with an MDF of 32 or greater. All combined original data were retrieved from 3 large RCTs of prednisolone versus placebo. A total of 215 patients including 102 in the placebo arm and 113 in the CS arm were studied. The results confirmed that acute AH is a severe illness with high in-hospital mortality. The 1-month survival rate was 85% for patients in the treatment group and 65% in the placebo group ($P < .001$). Also, survival at 6 months was greater in patients receiving prednisolone than in those receiving placebo (65% vs 50%, $P < .01$). A more comprehensive Cochrane review of 15 trials in 2008 with a total of 721 randomized patients found 12 of the trials were at a risk of bias, and CSs significantly reduced mortality only in the subgroup of patients with MDF of 32 or greater or in those with encephalopathy. In all analyses, heterogeneity was significant and substantial.[75]

A study from France found an early an early change in bilirubin levels at 7 days (defined as bilirubin level at 7 days lower than that on the first day of treatment) predicted a significantly higher survival at 6 months [83% vs 24%, $P < .0001$].[76] It has been suggested that CS therapy be interrupted in nonresponders (ie, no decline in bilirubin level after 7 days of treatment).[77]

In yet another meta-analysis, patients from 5 RCTs evaluating CSs in patients with severe AH were classified into 3 groups using 2 new cutoffs of the Lille score: complete responders (Lille score ≤ 0.16; $\leq$35th percentile), partial responders (Lille score 0.16–0.56; 35th–70th percentile), and null responders (Lille score ≥ 0.56; $\geq$70th percentile).[74] It was concluded that CSs significantly improve the 28-day survival in complete responders and partial responders but not in null responders. This study proposed a new response-guided therapy based on the Lille model in patients with severe AH.[74]

Based on the most current evidence from multiple clinical trials, the following generalizations can be made. Patients with mild to moderate AH (defined as a Maddrey score of <32) without hepatic encephalopathy and with improvement in serum bilirubin or decline in the Maddrey score during the first week of hospitalization should be monitored closely. Such patients will likely not require nor benefit from specific medical interventions and are expected to recover with nutritional support and abstinence from alcohol.

Patients with severe disease (defined as a Maddrey score of $\geq$32 with or without hepatic encephalopathy) who do not have contraindications to glucocorticosteroids should be considered for a 4-week course of prednisolone (40 mg/d, typically stopped or followed by a taper during 2–4 weeks or depending on the clinical situation). Prednisolone is preferred to prednisone because the latter requires conversion to prednisolone (the active form) in the liver, a process that may be impaired in AH.

The guidelines point out that the efficacy of glucocorticosteroids has not been evaluated in patients with concomitant pancreatitis, gastrointestinal bleeding, renal failure, or active infection, which were exclusion criteria in many of the clinical trials. There is a threshold of severity, beyond which glucocorticosteroids may cause more harm than benefit. In one report, patients with a Maddrey score of greater than 54 who received glucocorticosteroids had higher mortality than those who had not received them.[52] However, more data are needed to establish a cutoff.

The effectiveness of nutritional therapy was compared with treatment with glucocorticosteroids in a controlled trial involving 71 patients with severe AH. These patients were randomly assigned to prednisolone (40 mg/d) or enteral tube feeding for 28 days followed by 1 year of follow-up.[78] Early mortality during treatment was similar in the 2 groups (25% vs 31%), although deaths occurred significantly earlier with enteral feeding (median 7 vs 23 days). The mortality in the long term was higher in the steroid group (37% vs 8%). Seven patients randomized to glucocorticosteroids died within the first 1.5 months of follow-up, most of whom had infections.

Combination therapies of CSs with pentoxyfylline[79] or CSs with N-acetylcysteine (NAC)[80] have not shown any additional benefit in improving survival in patients with severe AH.

Pentoxifylline

The observation that tumor necrosis factor (TNF) levels are increased in patients with AH provided a rationale for the study of pentoxifylline (PTX) in AH because of its anti-TNF action. The data available in literature vary with regard to its efficacy and are summarized in **Table 2**.[81–85] It may be an acceptable option in patients with severe disease, particularly those with a contraindication to glucocorticosteroids.

In a double-blind placebo-controlled RCT, PTX showed survival benefit at 1 month compared with placebo (76% vs 54%). This benefit was attributed mainly to the prevention of the hepatorenal syndrome (HRS) among patients treated with PTX compared with placebo (50% vs 92%, $P< .05$).[81] Although an anti-TNF agent, the TNF levels were not shown to be different among patients receiving PTX and those receiving placebo.[81]

A recent study that compared steroids to PTX showed superiority of PTX in the treatment of patients with AH with better survival rate at 3 month (85% vs 65%, $P = .04$).[86] This was again mainly to the result of the prevention of HRS with the use of PTX (6 of 34 patients receiving steroids developed HRS compared with 0 of 34 receiving PTX). However, the latest Cochrane systematic review of 5 RCTs (4 reported

Table 2
RCT to assess PTX for treatment of AH

Author	Sample Size		Intervention	Survival		P
	PTX	Placebo		Treated	Placebo	
Akriviadis et al,[81] 2000	49	52	Pentoxifylline 400 mg tid for 28 d	75%	54%	.037
McHutchison et al,[82] 1991	12	10	Pentoxifylline 400 mg tid for 10 d	91%	70%	NS
Lebrec et al,[83] 2007	bNR	NR	Pentoxifylline 400 mg tid	86%	84%	.07
Sidhu et al,[84] 2006	aNR	NR	Pentoxifylline 400 mg tid for 28 d	76%	60%	NS
Paladugu et al,[85] 2006	14	16	Pentoxifylline for 28 d	71%	56%	.09

Abbreviation: NR, not reported.
 a Fifty patients were enrolled.
 b This report is based on a subgroup analysis on 132 patients with AH. Survival was reported at 2 months. Survival at 6 months was also not significantly different (73% vs 69%, $P = .30$).

as abstracts) that included a total of 336 randomized participants could not find firm evidence in support of recommending PTX in the treatment of AH.[87]

In severe AH, about 40% of patients will obtain no benefit from CSs. Whether PTX is a salvage option for patients with nonresponse to CSs was studied recently; patients were identified as a nonresponder at 1 week (Lille score $\geq$0.45) and randomized to PTX or placebo.[88] A 2-step strategy was evaluated consisting of early withdrawal of CSs and a switch to PTX for 28 additional days in nonresponders identified using change in bilirubin level at 1 week (Lille score $\geq$0.45) and randomized to PTX or placebo. Nonresponders to CSs did not obtain any benefit from an early switch to PTX (36% vs 31%, $P>$ .05). Thus, the issue of the management of nonresponders remained unresolved.[88]

The guideline issued by the AASLD and the American College of Gastroenterology suggests pentoxifylline (400 mg orally 3 times daily for 4 weeks) as an alternative to glucocorticosteroids in patients with severe AH (Maddrey score $\geq$32), especially if there are contraindications to glucocorticosteroids.[52]

TNF-α Inhibitor

Infliximab, a monoclonal chimeric anti-TNF antibody, has also been studied. In the first clinical trial of infliximab, 20 patients with biopsy-proved AH and an MDF score between 32 and 55 were randomized to either 5 mg/kg infliximab plus 40 mg/d prednisone (n = 11) or prednisone alone.[89] No substantial difference in overall mortality was found, but substantial decreases in other prognostic markers, including cytokine levels and MDF scores, were seen in patients treated with combination therapy.

The use of etanercept (given 6 times over 3 weeks) was tested in 48 patients with moderate to severe AH (MELD score >15); unfortunately, no significant difference in 1-month mortality was seen in the treated patients compared with patients given placebo. However, an increase in mortality was seen at 6 months.[90]

Antioxidants

NAC

The combination of NAC, an antioxidant, with prednisolone has been studied. This study enrolled 174 patients who were randomly assigned to receive either predniso-lone 40 mg/d for 28 days along with intravenous NAC for 5 days or prednisolone 40 mg/d for 28 days alone. Combination therapy improved 1-month survival in patients with AH. However, the 6-month survival, which was the primary endpoint of the study, did not improve.[80]

Metadoxine

Metadoxine, a combination of 2 antioxidants, pyridoxine and pyrrolidone, is potentially a useful drug in the treatment of ALD. A controlled trial included 136 alcoholic patients diagnosed with fatty liver who were randomly assigned to metadoxine (1500 mg/d) or placebo for 3 months.[91] At the end of the study, there was significant improvement in liver function tests in both groups, although improvement was observed more rapidly in those randomized to metadoxine. The percentage of patients with persistent hepatic steatosis as assessed by ultrasound was also significantly lower in the meta-doxine group (28% vs 70%).[91] This benefit was observed in those who abstained from alcohol and patients who continued to drink, although the degree of improvement was less in the latter group. Further studies are required to better explain the significance of these observations on other clinical endpoints.

Miscellaneous Agents

Propylthiouracil

Propylthiouracil (PTU) has also been evaluated for the treatment of acute AH in at least 2 controlled trials, which produced discordant results.[92,93] The principle behind the use of PTU was to decrease the hypermetabolic state induced by alcohol. Explanations for the differences between the studies include the time at which PTU therapy was started and the heterogeneity in baseline thyroid function among patients, because neither study measured baseline T3 levels, which may influence the responsiveness to PTU.[94] A Cochrane review showed no benefit of PTU versus placebo on total or liver-related mortality. At present, PTU therapy should not be used routinely in patients with acute AH.

Colchicine

The rationale for its study was based on its many effects on hepatic fibrogenesis, including the inhibition of collagen production, the enhancement of collagenase activity, and the interference with collagen transcellular trafficking. In addition, colchicine also has favorable effects on cytokine production associated with fibroblast proliferation.

An RCT showed a survival benefit of oral colchicine.[95] However, subsequent controlled trials showed mixed results,[96] and a meta-analysis of 15 randomized trials with 1714 patients with varying degrees of ALD showed no benefit of colchicine on liver tests, histological examination, or overall mortality and liver-related mortality.[96]

Polyunsaturated lecithins

Polyunsaturated lecithin is extracted from soybeans and is a constituent of cell membranes. Its mechanism of action is unknown; one probable mechanism is an alteration in collagenase activity.[97] Polyunsaturated lecithin seems to improve histology and reduce activation of hepatic stellate cells in baboons with alcoholic liver injury.[98] A large multicenter trial in humans is now under way. An attractive aspect of this medication is its excellent side effect profile, because the compound is a normal cellular constituent.

Anabolic steroids

Androgens have also been used in an attempt to improve nutritional status. A large multicenter Veterans Administration trial of oxandrolone showed some benefit in long-term survival in one subgroup of treated patients.[71] However, these results have not been confirmed by others. Furthermore, a recent systematic review could not demonstrate any significant beneficial effects of anabolic-androgenic steroids on any clinically important outcomes (mortality, liver-related mortality, liver complications, and histology) of patients with AH and/or cirrhosis.[99] Thus, interest for this regimen has diminished.

Hepatic Regeneration Therapy

There are several growth factors that have been identified as influencing hepatocyte regeneration. The best studied in humans are insulin and glucagon, which have been evaluated in several controlled trials in patients with AH.[100,101] A treatment benefit has not been consistently demonstrated, and complications (including hypoglycemic deaths) have occurred.

Another regenerative agent, malotilate, was evaluated in a controlled trial that included 407 patients with ALD who were randomized to malotilate (750 mg or 1500 mg/d) or placebo.[102] The results suggested a possible survival benefit only in patients who were randomized to the lower dose of the drug. Although hepatic regeneration therapy seems promising, treatment should be limited to controlled clinical trials.

FUTURE TARGETS

In addition to medical treatment directed at the underlying pathophysiologic abnormalities, several studies have tested other aggressive interventions in patients with AH, such as a molecular adsorbent recirculating system.[103–105] Although the results of early studies were optimistic, with better than predicted outcomes in treated patients, a further case series was less promising.[106] Case reports have also described the outcome of patients with severe AH treated with leukocytopharesis after failing to improve substantially on steroids.[107,108] These reports are promising, but recommendations regarding their appropriate use must await results of comparative studies of outcomes in these patients.

Liver Transplantation in AH

Acute AH is a distinct clinical entity among patients with chronic alcohol abuse. Patients who have severe AH are at increased risk of dying in about 20% to 25% cases despite specific treatment with CSs and/or pentoxifylline. Undoubtedly, a need for an additional more effective treatment option is needed.

Liver transplantation (LT) is a definitive treatment option for patients with end-stage liver disease who have a greater than 10% risk of dying within 1 year but requires 6-month abstinence. Patients with severe AH who do not respond to CSs or pentoxifylline have a mortality of 50% to 75% at 6 months.[109] Multiple issues need to be addressed if these subjects are to be eligible for LT. These issues are related to ethical concerns of transplanting patients who are actively drinking alcohol and the high risk of recidivism after LT that affects the graft and patient survival. The rate of recidivism after LT varies according to different authors. In a review of 22 studies on ALD, relapse ranged from 3% to 49%, with graft dysfunction and death ranging from 0% to 27% and 0% to 6.5%, respectively.[110] Therefore, it is essential to accurately identify patients before LT who are likely to relapse to harmful drinking after receiving the transplant. McCallum and Masterton[110] identified multiple factors consistently associated with recidivism; such as younger age, associated polysubstance abuse, lack of social support, family history of alcohol abuse in a first-degree relative, poor response to previous rehabilitation programs, and noncompliance. A careful selection of a subset of the patients with acute severe AH thus might benefit from LT.

Available data on the outcome of patients with AH after orthotopic LT (OLT) are limited and restricted to retrospective analyses. In one such study,[111] among a series of 246 patients with ALD, 110 underwent OLT. About 7.2% (8 cases) had histologic evidence of AH on the explants. Comparison of these 8 cases with the remaining 102 cases without histologic AH in the explants showed similar patient survival post-OLT recidivism. Unfortunately, their retrospective study design precludes any meaningful analyses.[111]

In a small prospective study by the French group, 26 patients with severe AH nonresponsive to steroids (defined as $\geq$0.45 Lille score) were studied to assess the role of LT.[112] Each patient was matched to a control patient (who did not undergo LT and continued to receive medical management) for age, sexr, MDF, and Lille score. Patients received LT within an average of 9 days from the day they were labeled as nonresponsive. The cumulative 6-month survival rate ($\pm$SE) was higher among patients who received early transplantation than among those who did not (77% $\pm$ 8% vs 23% $\pm$ 8%, $P <$ .001). At the end of 1 year, patient survival in the transplanted group was higher compared with those not receiving LT (83% vs 44%, $P =$ .009). Among the nontransplanted patients, 50% to 90% deaths occurred within first 2 months. This benefit of early transplantation was maintained through 2 years of follow-up (hazard ratio, 6.08; $P =$ .004).[112]

Current data clearly show that LT is a potential treatment option for the group of patients with severe AH who continue to deteriorate despite intensive medical treatment. Further, 6 months of abstinence does not affect recidivism after OLT, although more data are needed to make a firmer conclusion. However, to preselect these patients who would derive the most benefit, we need to evolve the best criteria to identify candidates with the least risk of recidivism to harmful drinking for the optimal utilization of available organs in the setting of AH in the same way as is being done for other causes of acute liver failure.

SUMMARY

The diagnosis of AH is based on the appropriate alcohol intake history and is supported with clinical features such as fever, jaundice, ascites, elevated white blood cells, generally AST less than 500 IU/mL, and elevated AST:ALT ratio (usually >2:1). Although a liver biopsy may help confirm the diagnosis, it is generally not recommended. The biopsy may demonstrate hepatocyte ballooning, Mallory hyaline, neutrophilic infiltration, and perisinusoidal fibrosis. Although the spectrum of severity ranges from mild to severe, mortality for severe AH is quite high, in the range of 30% to 50% during a 28-day period. Assessment of disease severity can be made using MFD, MELD score, GAHS, and the Lillie model. Malnutrition is rampant among alcoholics, nutritional supplementation in integral in the management, and an enteral feeding tube should be considered if patients are too ill to eat voluntarily. Although results are variable, the most widely accepted pharmacologic intervention in AH is prednisolone 40 mg/d for 28 days. It should not, however, be used in patients with recent upper gastrointestinal bleeding, elevated creatinine, or uncontrolled infection. PTX 400 mg 3 times daily for 28 days is an alternate treatment option. Many other treatments (eg, antioxidants, anti–TNF-α treatment) have not proved to be beneficial and thus are not recommended. Early studies have shown some promise for aggressive interventions such as molecular adsorbent recirculating system, but more studies are needed. LT in acute AH is contentious because of the 6-month abstinence rule, ethical concerns, risk of recidivism, and potential for poor post-transplant graft and patient survival.

ACKNOWLEDGMENTS

We would like to express our sincere thanks to Dr Pamela Silvestre, Department of Pathology, University of Tennessee Health Sciences Center, for her input in improving the article and providing the relevant figures on the histopathology of AH.

REFERENCES

1. Savolainen VT, Liesto K, Männikkö A, et al. Alcohol consumption and alcoholic liver disease: evidence of a threshold level of effects of ethanol. Alcohol Clin Exp Res 1993;17:1112–7.
2. Lelbach WK. Cirrhosis in the alcoholic and its relation to the volume of alcohol abuse. Ann N Y Acad Sci 1975;252:85–105.
3. Grant BF, Dufour MC, Harford TC. Epidemiology of alcoholic liver disease. Semin Liver Dis 1988;8:12–25.
4. Lu XL, Luo JY, Tao M, et al. Risk factors for alcoholic liver disease in China. World J Gastroenterol 2004;10:2423–6.
5. Maddrey WC. Alcoholic hepatitis: clinicopathologic features and therapy. Semin Liver Dis 1998;8:91–102.

6. Levitsky J, Mailliard ME. Diagnosis and therapy of alcoholic liver disease. Semin Liver Dis 2004;24:233–47.
7. Uchida T, Kao H, Quispe-Sjogren M, et al. Alcoholic foamy degeneration–a pattern of acute alcoholic injury of the liver. Gastroenterology 1983;84:683–92.
8. Nanji AA, French SW, Mendenhall CL. Serum aspartate aminotransferase to alanine aminotransferase ratio in human and experimental alcoholic liver disease: relationship to histologic changes. Enzyme 1989;41:112–5.
9. Cohen JA, Kaplan MM. The SGOT/SGPT ratio–an indicator of alcoholic liver disease. Dig Dis Sci 1979;24:835–8.
10. Niemela O. Biomarkers in alcoholism. Clin Chim Acta 2007;377:39–49.
11. Nyblom H, Berggren U, Balldin J, et al. High AST/ALT ratio may indicate advanced alcoholic liver disease rather than heavy drinking. Alcohol 2004;39:336–9.
12. Yersin B, Nicolet JF, Dercrey H, et al. Screening for excessive alcohol drinking. Comparative value of carbohydrate- deficient transferrin, gamma-glutamyltransferase, and mean corpuscular volume. Arch Intern Med 1995;155:1907–11.
13. Conigrave KM, Degenhardt LJ, Whitfield JB, et al. CDT, GGT, and AST as markers of alcohol use: the WHO/ISBRA collaborative project. Alcohol Clin Exp Res 2002;26:332–9.
14. Sillanaukee P, Massot N, Jousilahti P, et al. Dose response of laboratory markers to alcohol consumption in a general population. Am J Epidemiol 2000;152:747–51.
15. Alte D, Luedemann J, Rose HJ, et al. Laboratory markers carbohydrate- deficient transferrin, gamma-glutamyl transferase, and mean corpuscular volume are not useful as screening tools for high-risk drinking in the general population: results from the Study of Health in Pomerania (SHIP). Alcohol Clin Exp Res 2004;28:931–40.
16. Reynaud M, Schellenberg F, Loisequx-Meunier MN, et al. Objective diagnosis of alcohol abuse: compared values of carbohydrate-deficient transferrin (CDT), gamma-glutamyl transferase (GGT), and mean corpuscular volume (MCV). Alcohol Clin Exp Res 2000;24:1414–9.
17. Poynard T, Zourabichvili O, Hilpert G, et al. Prognostic value of total serum bilirubin/gamma-glutamyl transpeptidase ratio in cirrhotic patients. Hepatology 1984;4:324–7.
18. Naveau S, Poynard T, Abella A, et al. Prognostic value of serum fibronectin concentration in alcoholic cirrhotic patients. Hepatology 1985;5:819–23.
19. Bortolotti F, De Paoli G, Tagliaro F. Carbohydrate-deficient transferrin (CDT) as a marker of alcohol abuse: a critical review of the literature 2001-2005. J Chromatogr B Analyt Technol Biomed Life Sci 2006;841:96–109.
20. De Feo TM, Fargion S, Duca L, et al. Carbohydrate-deficient transferrin, a sensitive marker of chronic alcohol abuse, is highly influenced by body iron. Hepatology 1999;29:658–63.
21. Schmitt UM, Stieber P, Jüngst D, et al. Carbohydrate-deficient transferrin is not a useful marker for the detection of chronic alcohol abuse. Eur J Clin Invest 1998;28:615–21.
22. Wurst FM, Alling C, Aradottir S, et al. Emerging biomarkers: new directions and clinical applications. Alcohol Clin Exp Res 2005;29:465–73.
23. Zimmer H, Schmitt G, Aderjan R. Preliminary immunochemical test for the determination of ethyl glucuronide in serum and urine: comparison of screening method results with gas chromatography-mass spectrometry. J Anal Toxicol 2002;26:11–6.

24. Katoonizadeh A, Laleman W, Verslype C, et al. Early features of acute-on-chronic alcoholic liver failure: a prospective cohort study. Gut 2010;59:1561–9.
25. Mookerjee RP, Lackner C, Stauber R, et al. The role of liver biopsy in the diagnosis and prognosis of patients with acute deterioration of alcoholic cirrhosis. J Hepatol 2011;55:1103–11.
26. Tannapfel A, Denk H, Dienes HP, et al. Histopathological diagnosis of non-alcoholic and alcoholic fatty liver disease. Virchows Arch 2011;458:511–23.
27. Chedid A, Mendenhall CL, Tosch T, et al. Significance of megamitochondria in alcoholic liver disease. Gastroenterology 1986;90:1858–64.
28. Maddrey WC, Boitnott JK, Bedine MS, et al. Corticosteroid therapy of alcoholic hepatitis. Gastroenterology 1978;75:193–9.
29. Carithers RL Jr, Herlong HF, Diehl AM, et al. Methylprednisolone therapy in patients with severe alcoholic hepatitis. A randomized multicenter trial. Ann Intern Med 1989;110:685–90.
30. Mathurin P, Mendenhall CL, Carithers RL Jr, et al. Corticosteroids improve short-term survival in patients with severe alcoholic hepatitis (AH): individual data analysis of the last three randomized placebo controlled double blind trials of corticosteroids in severe AH. J Hepatol 2002;36:480–7.
31. McCullough AJ, O'Connor JF. Alcoholic liver disease: proposed recommendations for the American College of Gastroenterology. Am J Gastroenterol 1998; 93:2022–36.
32. Kamath PS, Wiesner RH, Malinchoc M, et al. A model to predict survival in patients with end-stage liver disease. Hepatology 2001;33:464–70.
33. Sheth M, Riggs M, Patel T. Utility of the Mayo End-Stage Liver Disease (MELD) score in assessing prognosis of patients with alcoholic hepatitis. BMC Gastroenterol 2002;2:2.
34. Dunn W, Jamil LH, Brown LS, et al. MELD accurately predicts mortality in patients with alcoholic hepatitis. Hepatology 2005;41:353.
35. Srikureja W, Kyulo NL, Runyon BA, et al. MELD score is a better prognostic model than Child-Turcotte-Pugh score or Discriminant Function score in patients with alcoholic hepatitis. J Hepatol 2005;42:700.
36. Kamath PS, Kim WR. Is the change in MELD score a better indicator of mortality than baseline MELD score? Liver Transpl 2003;9:19–21.
37. O'Shea RS, Dasarathy S, McCullough AJ. Practice Guideline Committee of the American Association for the Study of Liver Diseases; Practice Parameters Committee of the American College of Gastroenterology. Alcoholic liver disease. Hepatology 2010;51:307–28.
38. Forrest EH, Evans CD, Stewart S, et al. Analysis of factors predictive of mortality in alcoholic hepatitis and derivation and validation of the Glasgow alcoholic hepatitis score. Gut 2005;54:1174–9.
39. Forrest EH, Morris AJ, Stewart S, et al. The Glasgow alcoholic hepatitis score identifies patients who may benefit from corticosteroids. Gut 2007;56: 1743.
40. Friedman LS. The risk of surgery in patients with liver disease. Hepatology 1999; 29:1617–23.
41. Jeong JY, Sohn JH, Son BK, et al. Comparison of model for end-stage liver disease score with discriminant function and child-Turcotte-Pugh scores for predicting short-term mortality in Korean patients with alcoholic hepatitis. Korean J Gastroenterol 2007;49:93–9 [in Korean].
42. Garrison RN, Cryer HM, Howard DA, et al. Clarification of risk factors for abdominal operations in patients with hepatic cirrhosis. Ann Surg 1984;199:648–55.

43. Dominguez M, Rincón D, Abraldes JG, et al. A new scoring system for prognostic stratification of patients with alcoholic hepatitis. Am J Gastroenterol 2008;103:2747–56.
44. Louvet A, Naveau S, Abdelnour M, et al. The Lille model: a new tool for therapeutic strategy in patients with severe alcoholic hepatitis treated with steroids. Hepatology 2007;45:1348–54.
45. Pessione F, Ramond MJ, Peters L, et al. Five-year survival predictive factors in patients with excessive alcohol intake and cirrhosis. Effect of alcoholic hepatitis, smoking and abstinence. Liver Int 2003;23:45–53.
46. Borowsky SA, Strome S, Lott E. Continued heavy drinking and survival in alcoholic cirrhotics. Gastroenterology 1981;80:1405–9.
47. Brunt PW, Kew MC, Scheuer PJ, et al. Studies in alcoholic liver disease in Britain. I. Clinical and pathological patterns related to natural history. Gut 1974;15:52–8.
48. Luca A, Garcia-Pagan JC, Bosch J, et al. Effects of ethanol consumption on hepatic hemodynamics in patients with alcoholic cirrhosis. Gastroenterology 1997;112:1284–9.
49. Pares A, Caballeria J, Bruguera M, et al. Histological course of alcoholic hepatitis. Influence of abstinence, sex and extent of hepatic damage. J Hepatol 1986; 2:33–42.
50. Powell WJ Jr, Klatskin G. Duration of survival in patients with Laennec's cirrhosis. Influence of alcohol withdrawal, and possible effects of recent changes in general management of the disease. Am J Med 1968;44:406–20.
51. Garbutt JC, West SL, Carey TS, et al. Pharmacological treatment of alcohol dependence: a review of the evidence. JAMA 1999;281:1318–25.
52. Alcoholic Liver Disease: Robert S, O'Shea, et al. The Practice Guideline Committee of the American Association for the Study of Liver Diseases and the Practice Parameters Committee of the American College of Gastroenterology.
53. Rösner S, Hackl-Herrwerth A, Leucht S, et al. Acamprosate for alcohol dependence. Cochrane Database Syst Rev 2010;(9):CD004332.
54. Leggio L, Ferrulli A, Zambon A, et al. Baclofen promotes alcohol abstinence in alcohol dependent cirrhotic patients with hepatitis C virus (HCV) infection. J Addict Behav 2012;37:561–4.
55. DiCecco SR, Francisco-Ziller N. Nutrition in alcoholic liver disease. Nutr Clin Pract 2006;21:245–54.
56. Mendenhall CL, Anderson S, Weesner RE, et al. Protein-calorie malnutrition associated with alcoholic hepatitis. Veterans Administration Cooperative Study Group on Alcoholic Hepatitis. Am J Med 1984;76:211.
57. Cabre E, Gonzalez-Huix F, Abad-Lacruz A, et al. Effect of total enteral nutrition on the short-term outcome of severely malnourished cirrhotics. A randomized controlled trial. Gastroenterology 1990;98:715.
58. Kearns PJ, Young H, Garcia G, et al. Accelerated improvement of alcoholic liver disease with enteral nutrition. Gastroenterology 1992;102:200.
59. Koretz RL, Avenell A, Lipman TO. Nutritional support for liver disease. Cochrane Database Syst Rev 2012;(5):CD008344.
60. Swart GR, Zillikens MC, van Vuure JK, et al. Effect of a late evening meal on nitrogen balance in patients with cirrhosis of the liver. BMJ 1989;299:1202.
61. Tan HH, Virmani S, Martin P. Controversies in the management of alcoholic liver disease. Mt Sinai J Med 2009;76(5):484–98.
62. Shumaker JB, Resnick RH, Galambos JT, et al. A controlled trial of 6-methylprednisolone in acute alcoholic hepatitis. With a note on published results in encephalopathic patients. Am J Gastroenterol 1978;69:443–9.

63. Ramond MJ, Poynard T, Rueff B, et al. A randomized trial of prednisolone in patients with severe alcoholic hepatitis. N Engl J Med 1992;326:507–12.

64. Helman RA, Temko MH, Nye SW, et al. Alcoholic hepatitis. Natural history and evaluation of prednisolone therapy. Ann Intern Med 1971;74:311–21.

65. Porter HP, Simon FR, Pope CE 2nd, et al. Corticosteroid therapy in severe alcoholic hepatitis. A double-blind drug trial. N Engl J Med 1971;284:1350–5.

66. Campra JL, Hamlin EM Jr, Kirshbaum RJ, et al. Prednisone therapy of acute alcoholic hepatitis. Report of a controlled trial. Ann Intern Med 1973;79: 625–31.

67. Blitzer BL, Mutchnick MG, Joshi PH, et al. Adrenocorticosteroid therapy in alcoholic hepatitis. A prospective, double-blind randomized study. Am J Dig Dis 1977;22: 477–84.

68. Depew W, Boyer T, Omata M, et al. Double-blind controlled trial of prednisolone therapy in patients with severe acute alcoholic hepatitis and spontaneous encephalopathy. Gastroenterology 1980;78:524–9.

69. Theodossi A, Eddleston AL, Williams R. Controlled trial of methylprednisolone therapy in severe acute alcoholic hepatitis. Gut 1982;23:75–9.

70. Lesesne HR, Bozymski EM, Fallon HJ. Treatment of alcoholic hepatitis with encephalopathy. Comparison of prednisolone with caloric supplements. Gastroenterology 1978;74:169–73.

71. Mendenhall CL, Anderson S, Garcia-Pont P, et al. Short-term and long-term survival in patients with alcoholic hepatitis treated with oxandrolone and prednisolone. N Engl J Med 1984;311:1464–70.

72. Imperiale TF, McCullough AJ. Do corticosteroids reduce mortality from alcoholic hepatitis? A meta-analysis of the randomized trials. Ann Intern Med 1990;113: 299–307.

73. Christensen E, Gluud C. Glucocorticoids are ineffective in alcoholic hepatitis: a meta-analysis adjusting for confounding variables. Gut 1995;37:113–8.

74. Mathurin P, O'Grady J, Carithers RL, et al. Corticosteroids improve short-term survival in patients with severe alcoholic hepatitis: meta-analysis of individual patient data. Gut 2011;60:255–60.

75. Rambaldi A, Saconato HH, Christensen E, et al. Systematic review: glucocorticosteroids for alcoholic hepatitis–a Cochrane Hepato-Biliary Group systematic review with meta-analyses and trial sequential analyses of randomized clinical trials. Aliment Pharmacol Ther 2008;27:1167–78.

76. Morris JM, Forrest EH. Bilirubin response to corticosteroids in severe alcoholic hepatitis. Eur J Gastroenterol Hepatol 2005;17:759–62.

77. Mathurin P, Abdelnour M, Ramond MJ, et al. Early change in bilirubin levels is an important prognostic factor in severe alcoholic hepatitis treated with prednisolone. Hepatology 2003;38:1363–9.

78. Cabré E, Rodríguez-Iglesias P, Caballería J, et al. Short- and long-term outcome of severe alcohol-induced hepatitis treated with steroids or enteral nutrition: a multicenter randomized trial. Hepatology 2000;32:36–42.

79. Sidhu SS, Goyal O, Singla P, et al. Corticosteroid Plus Pentoxifylline Is Not Better than Corticosteroid Alone for Improving Survival in Severe Alcoholic Hepatitis (COPE Trial). Dig Dis Sci 2012;57:1664–71.

80. Nguyen-Khac E, Thevenot T, Piquet MA, et al. Glucocorticoids plus N-acetylcysteine in severe alcoholic hepatitis. N Engl J Med 2011;365:1781–9.

81. Akriviadis E, Botla R, Briggs W, et al. Pentoxifylline improves short-term survival in severe acute alcoholic hepatitis: a double-blind, placebo-controlled trial. Gastroenterology 2000;119:1637–48.

82. McHutchison JG, Runyon BA, Draguesku JO, et al. Pentoxifylline may prevent renal impairment in severe alcoholic hepatitis. Hepatology 1991;14:96A.
83. Lebrec D, Dominique T, Oberti F, et al. Pentoxifylline for the treatment of patients with advanced cirrhosis. A randomized placebo controlled double blind trial. Hepatology 2007;46:A249–50.
84. Sidhu S, Singla M, Bhatia KL. Pentoxifylline reduces disease severity and prevents renal impairment in severe acute alcoholic hepatitis: a double blind, placebo controlled trial. Hepatology 2006;44(Suppl 1):373A–4A.
85. Paladugu H, Sawant P, Dalvi L, et al. Role of pentoxifylline in treatment of severe acute alcoholic hepatitis - a randomized controlled trial. J Gastroenterol Hepatol 2006;21:A459.
86. De BK, Gangopadhyay S, Dutta D, et al. Pentoxifylline versus prednisolone for severe alcoholic hepatitis: a randomized controlled trial. World J Gastroenterol 2009;15:1613–9.
87. Whitfield K, Rambaldi A, Wetterslev J, et al. Pentoxifylline for alcoholic hepatitis. Cochrane Database Syst Rev 2009;(4):CD007339.
88. Louvet A, Diaz E, Dharancy S, et al. Early switch to pentoxifylline in patients with severe alcoholic hepatitis is inefficient in non-responders to corticosteroids. J Hepatol 2008;48:465–70.
89. Spahr L, Rubbia-Brandt L, Frossard JL, et al. Combination of steroids with infliximab or placebo in severe alcoholic hepatitis: a randomized controlled pilot study. J Hepatol 2002;37:448–55.
90. Boetticher NC, Peine CJ, Kwo P, et al. A randomized, double-blinded, placebo-controlled multicenter trial of Etanercept in the treatment of alcoholic hepatitis. Gastroenterology 2008;135:1953–60.
91. Caballería J, Parés A, Brú C, et al. Metadoxine accelerates fatty liver recovery in alcoholic patients: results of a randomized double-blind, placebo-control trial. Spanish Group for the Study of Alcoholic Fatty Liver. J Hepatol 1998;28:54–60.
92. Orrego H, Kalant H, Israel Y, et al. Effect of short-term therapy with propylthiouracil in patients with alcoholic liver disease. Gastroenterology 1979;76:105–15.
93. Hallé P, Paré P, Kaptein E, et al. Double-blind, controlled trial of propylthiouracil in patients with severe acute alcoholic hepatitis. Gastroenterology 1982;82:925–31.
94. Israel Y, Walfish PG, Orrego H, et al. Thyroid hormones in alcoholic liver disease. Effect of treatment with 6-n-propylthiouracil. Gastroenterology 1979;76:116–22.
95. Kershenobich D, Vargas F, Garcia-Tsao G, et al. Colchicine in the treatment of cirrhosis of the liver. N Engl J Med 1988;318:1709–13.
96. Rambaldi A, Gluud C. Colchicine for alcoholic and non-alcoholic liver fibrosis and cirrhosis. Cochrane Database Syst Rev 2005;(2):CD002148.
97. Li J, Kim CI, Leo MA, et al. Polyunsaturated lecithin prevents acetaldehyde-mediated hepatic collagen accumulation by stimulating collagenase activity in cultured lipocytes. Hepatology 1992;15:373–81.
98. Lieber CS, Robins SJ, Li J, et al. Phosphatidylcholine protects against fibrosis and cirrhosis in the baboon. Gastroenterology 1994;106:152–9.
99. Rambaldi A, Gluud C. Anabolic-androgenic steroids for alcoholic liver disease. Cochrane Database Syst Rev 2006;(4):CD003045.
100. Trinchet JC, Balkau B, Poupon RE, et al. Treatment of severe alcoholic hepatitis by infusion of insulin and glucagon: a multicenter sequential trial. Hepatology 1992;15:76–81.
101. Bird G, Lau JY, Koskinas J, et al. Insulin and glucagon infusion in acute alcoholic hepatitis: a prospective randomized controlled trial. Hepatology 1991;14:1097–101.

102. Keiding S, Badsberg JH, Becker U, et al. The prognosis of patients with alcoholic liver disease. An international randomized, placebo-controlled trial on the effect of malotilate on survival. J Hepatol 1994;20:454–60.
103. Parés A, Deulofeu R, Cisneros L, et al. Albumin dialysis improves hepatic encephalopathy and decreases circulating phenolic aromatic amino acids in patients with alcoholic hepatitis and severe liver failure. Crit Care 2009;13:R8.
104. Laleman W, Wilmer A, Evenepoel P, et al. Effect of the molecular adsorbent recirculating system and Prometheus devices on systemic haemodynamics and vasoactive agents in patients with acute-on-chronic alcoholic liver failure. Crit Care 2006;10:R108.
105. Jalan R, Sen S, Steiner C, et al. Extracorporeal liver support with molecular adsorbents recirculating system in patients with severe acute alcoholic hepatitis. J Hepatol 2003;38:24–31.
106. Wolff B, Machill K, Schumacher D, et al. MARS dialysis in decompensated alcoholic liver disease: a single-center experience. Liver Transpl 2007;13:1189–92.
107. Tsuji Y, Kumashiro R, Ishii K, et al. Severe alcoholic hepatitis successfully treated by leukocytapheresis: a case report. Alcohol Clin Exp Res 2003;27:26S–31S.
108. Okubo K, Yoshizawa K, Okiyama W, et al. Severe alcoholic hepatitis with extremely high neutrophil count successfully treated by granulocytapheresis. Intern Med 2006;45:155–8.
109. Dureja P, Lucey MR. The place of liver transplantation in the treatment of severe alcoholic hepatitis. J Hepatol 2010;52:759–64.
110. McCallum S, Masterton G. Liver transplantation for alcoholic liver disease: a systematic review of psychosocial selection criteria. Alcohol Alcohol 2006;41:358–63.
111. Castel H, Moreno C, Antonini T, et al. Early transplantation improves survival of non-responders to steroids in severe alcoholic hepatitis: a challenge to the 6 month rule of abstinence. Hepatology 2009;50(Suppl 4):307A.
112. Mathurin P, Moreno C, Samuel D, et al. Early liver transplantation for severe alcoholic hepatitis. N Engl J Med 2011;365:1790–800.

Management of Alcohol Abuse

Anthony P. Albanese, MD*

KEYWORDS

- Alcohol abuse • Alcohol dependence • Alcohol use disorder • Addiction treatment
- Recovery • Detoxification • Rehabilitation • Alcoholism

KEY POINTS

- The diagnosis and treatment of alcohol use disorders are the first and most important steps in the treatment of alcoholic liver disease.
- Alcohol is the most common substance use disorder in the United States.
- The societal costs of alcohol abuse when considering lost earnings, medical and legal consequences, property destruction, and treatment is estimated to be more than $185 billion.
- This article provides clinicians with a basic understanding of the tools available to diagnose and treat this cunning and baffling brain and multisystem disease.

DEFINITION

The idea of drinking alcoholic beverages to alter mood is not new. The ninth chapter of the biblical book of Genesis tells a story of Noah, the most righteous man on earth, getting drunk.[1] Although techniques to brew, ferment, and distill alcoholic beverages have changed somewhat over the years, the basic essence has not. Alcohol is consumed worldwide by people of many different cultual and ethnic backgrounds. The attempt to legislate abstinence in the United States, "the noble experiment" of prohibition, started in 1919 and failed in 1933. Each group has some sense of boundary over which further drinking is considered excessive. Because these boundaries vary with society, coming up with universally acceptable definitions of alcohol misuse and abuse is difficult. Variation even exists on the size of a standard drink, although most would consider this to be approximately 14 g of absolute (95%) ethyl alcohol.[2,3] Many organizations have developed definitions of alcohol misuse, abuse, dependency, and alcoholism. Alcohol misuse generally implies one or more episodes of overuse or incorrect use. To ingest alcohol through the eye (an "eye-shot") instead of by mouth might be an example of incorrect use.

Disclosures: The author is on the speaker's bureau for Genentech and Merck.
No conflict of interest.
Hepatology and Chemical Dependency, VA Northern California Healthcare System, University of California Davis School of Medicine, Sacramento, CA, USA
* Sacramento VA Medical Center, 10535 Hospital Way SMAT/111, Mather, CA 95655.
E-mail address: Anthony.Albanese@va.gov

Clin Liver Dis 16 (2012) 737–762
http://dx.doi.org/10.1016/j.cld.2012.08.006
1089-3261/12/$ – see front matter Published by Elsevier Inc.

An example of misuse might be a mild/moderate alcohol user with no previous consequences being cited for driving under the influence (DUI) after drinking more heavily at a wedding or graduation party and then driving. The definitions of abuse vary slightly, but most involve the 3 C's: craving, compulsion, and continued use despite negative consequences. The definitions of alcohol dependence and alcoholism usually include the physiologic phenomena of tolerance and/or withdrawal symptoms. The *Diagnostic and Statistical Manual of Mental Disorders*, Fourth Edition, Text Revision (DSM IV-TR) has distinct divisions between the diagnoses of alcohol abuse and dependence. Both definitions begin with the phrase, "Maladaptive pattern of alcohol use leading to clinically significant impairment or distress...."[4] The abuse diagnosis requires that 1 of 4 criteria be met, whereas the dependence diagnosis requires fulfilling 3 of 7. The DSM, Fifth Edition (DSM V; scheduled to be published in 2013) does not use this "either/or" paradigm, but will combine both diagnoses into an Alcohol Use Disorder category, with 2 to 3 of 11 fulfilled criteria being considered moderate disease, and 4 or more classified as severe disease.[5] The new definition is not yet finalized, but would likely be "A maladaptive pattern of substance use leading to clinically significant impairment or distress, as manifested by 2 (or more) of the following, occurring within a 12-month period:

1. Recurrent substance use resulting in a failure to fulfill major role obligations at work, school, or home.
2. Recurrent substance use in situations in which it is physically hazardous.
3. Continued substance used despite having persistent or recurrent social or interpersonal problems caused or exacerbated by the effects of the substance.
4. Tolerance as defined by either a need for markedly increased amounts of the substance to achieve intoxication or desired effect OR markedly diminished effect with continued use of the same amount of the substance.
5. Withdrawal, as manifested by either the characteristic withdrawal syndrome for the substance OR the same substance is taken to relieve or avoid withdrawal symptoms.
6. The substance is often taken in larger amounts or over a longer period than was intended.
7. There is a persistent desire or unsuccessful efforts to cut down or control substance use.
8. A great deal of time is spent in activities necessary to obtain the substance, use the substance, or recover from its effects.
9. Important social, occupational, or recreational activities are given up or reduced because of substance use.
10. The substance use is continued despite knowledge of having a persistent or recurrent physical or psychological problem that is likely to have been caused or exacerbated by the substance.
11. Craving or strong desire or urge to use a specific substance."[5]

PREVALENCE

Large studies, such as the National Survey on Drug Use and Health (NSDUH), National Longitudinal Alcohol Epidemiologic Survey, and National Epidemiologic Survey on Alcohol and Related Conditions, estimate the overall prevalence of alcohol use disorders at 6% to 8.5% in the United States.[6–8] The NSDUH 2009 study shows that the incidence of alcohol abuse and dependence diagnoses is highest in people whose first alcohol use was before the age of 14 years, with decreasing incidence as the age of first drink increases. The lowest incidence in this study occurs with first use after the age of 21 years. Alcohol is the most common substance use disorder in the United States. The societal costs of alcohol abuse, when considering lost earnings, medical and legal consequences, property destruction, and treatment, is estimated to be more than $185 billion.[9,10]

The terms "alcoholic" and "alcoholism" refer to alcohol dependence. They were popularized in the 1930s with the publication of "The Big Book" of Alcoholics Anonymous (AA). Today these terms are sometimes considered to be insulting or stigmatizing. The natural history of alcohol dependence can be separated into 2 phenotypes, which often vary by age of onset and personality traits.[11,12] The first type, type 1 (or A), is noted in approximately 75% of men with alcohol dependence. Drinking patterns are usually similar to those of peers until age reaches the early to mid 20s when alcohol use escalates. The first major alcohol-related life problems emerge between the late 20s and early 40s. Consequences of dependency mount during the 50s, with attempts to control drinking, exacerbations, and remissions. Often treatment or recovery support is sought during this phase of illness. Traits include a low degree of novelty seeking and fighting, and a high degree of guilt, harm avoidance, and reward dependence. Type 2 (or B) is a much smaller subset that begins alcohol use during preteen or early teenage years, with a rapidly escalating course. This type is characterized by a high degree of novelty seeking, and often other drug use. Traits include a low degree of guilt, fear, and harm avoidance. Medical, legal, and social consequences often escalate by the late teens or early 20s. The Cooperative Study on the Genetics of Alcoholism sought to determine whether certain genetic patterns could be identified in families with alcohol-dependent members. The study showed genetic similarities in the alcohol-dependent individuals on chromosomes 1 and 5 at a level that warrants further study.[13,14]

DIAGNOSIS

Alcohol abuse is diagnosed by obtaining a thorough, honest history. The history should include

1. Age of first use, first intoxication, and first regular use
2. Use patterns of parents, grandparents, siblings, spouse, and friends
3. Consequences of use, including blackouts, arguments, lost work, health and legal issues
4. Heaviest use, current pattern of use, longest abstinence, and number of quit attempts

Several reliable screening tools are available, ranging from simple to complex, which can help the interviewer incorporate and standardize this part of the history. A commonly used screening tool is the CAGE questionnaire. If 2 questions are answered positively, the survey has a reported 60% to 90% sensitivity and 40% to 95% specificity.[15] One problem is that the questionnaire can miss binge drinkers. The CAGE is not copyrighted and represents 4 questions asked during the history:

- Have you ever felt you should Cut down on your drinking?
- Have people Annoyed you by criticizing your drinking?
- Have you ever felt bad or Guilty about your drinking?
- Have you ever taken a drink first thing in the morning (Eye-opener) to steady your nerves or get rid of a hangover?

Another screening tool is the Alcohol Use Disorder Identification Test (AUDIT). It is a 10-item questionnaire in which each item scores 0 to 4 points (maximum score = 40), with a score of 8 or more indicating potential problems. The AUDIT has a sensitivity of 57% to 95% and specificity of 78% to 96% for hazardous or harmful drinking, and a sensitivity of 61% to 96% and specificity of 85% to 96% for alcohol abuse or dependence.[16] The AUDIT is copyrighted by the World Health Organization, with the test and module available for free. The AUDIT-Consumption (AUDIT-C) is a shorter version asking 3 questions. It is used as the screening test in Veterans Administration Medical Centers across the United States and has been shown to have good reliability.[17,18] The Michigan Alcohol Screening Test (MAST) is a 25-question test that can be either self-administered or given through interview. It is a reliable, widely used screen that is useful in assessing alcohol-related problems longitudinally.[19] The Brief (BMAST),[20] Short (SMAST),[21] and Malmo[22] Modifications (MmMAST) are shorter versions that retain good sensitivity and specificity. Screening tests for specific populations include the Geriatric MAST[23] and the Problem-Oriented Screening Instrument for Teenagers (POSIT). These tests are not copyrighted and are free.

Unfortunately, the addictive illness (which sometimes accompanies alcohol abuse) often involves elements of denial, rationalization, and lack of complete candor. For these reasons, biologic confirmation through physical and laboratory examination is important to confirm the history when possible. The physical examination can give many clues to alcohol abuse, but the findings are often nonspecific. The odor of alcohol on breath can be helpful, but is not necessarily a reliable indicator of ethanol consumption. The odor reflects impurities and other flavorings of the beverage rather than the alcohol itself.

A partial list of body systems potentially affected by alcohol abuse includes[24]

1. Central nervous system (CNS): "great mimicker" of psychiatric disorders; causes decreased sleep latency, blackouts, peripheral neuropathy, Wernicke-Korsakoff syndrome, cerebellar degeneration, Marchiafava-Bignami disease (corpus callosum demyelination/necrosis), and dementia.
2. Gastrointestinal: causes esophagitis, gastritis, enteritis, increased gastric acid production, lowers lower esophageal sphincter tone; promotes absorption of iron; interferes with absorption of some B vitamins; toxic to pancreas; associated with esophageal, gastric, pancreatic, hepatocellular, and colon cancer; leads to fatty liver and cirrhosis.
3. Hematopoietic: causes pancytopenia, toxic granulocytosis, and elevated mean corpuscular volume (MCV).
4. Cardiovascular: increases high-density lipoprotein; 1 to 2 drinks per day may decrease the risk of cardiac death; decreases myocardial contractility and peripheral vasodilatation; decreases blood pressure in low dose; increases blood pressure long-term in high doses; causes cardiomyopathy, arrhythmias, and "holiday heart."
5. Genitourinary: modest doses increase sex drive but decrease erectile capacity, testicular atrophy with shrinkage of the seminiferous tubules; causes amenorrhea, decreased ovarian size, infertility, and spontaneous abortions.
6. Other: causes fetal alcohol syndrome, alcoholic myopathy, osteonecrosis with increased fractures and avascular necrosis of the femoral heads, and modest reversible decreases in T3 and T4.

Laboratory analysis can also provide clues of heavy alcohol consumption. Elevations in MCV, aspartate aminotransferase (AST), alanine aminotransferase (ALT), alkaline phosphatase, gamma glutamyl transpeptidase (GGT), AST/ALT ratio, iron saturation, ferritin, and carbohydrate-deficient transferrin (CDT) may be noted. Specificity can be increased by combining markers such as GGT, MCV, and CDT, but many of these laboratory values can be elevated because of liver disease from other causes. They should not be mistaken for proof of alcohol use. Neither should a positive urine drug screen for alcohol be considered proof of alcohol use. Sugar in the urine of diabetics being fermented into alcohol by yeast contaminating the sample has been reported.

ETHANOL PHARMACOLOGY

To understand how laboratory analysis can be a benefit in diagnosing an alcohol use disorder, it is important to briefly review ethanol metabolism. Ethanol ($C_2H_5O_2$) is a colorless, volatile, flammable, water-soluble liquid that can be produced naturally through the fermentation of certain carbohydrates, or synthetically through the hydration of ethylene. It has a burning taste and is rapidly absorbed into the bloodstream through the mucous membranes (including the mouth), stomach, small intestine, and colon. Absorption could be impaired or delayed by the presence of food in the stomach. Because of its high water solubility, alcohol can distribute from the bloodstream into all tissues.

Alcohol acts on a variety of brain receptors that facilitate or inhibit the permeability of ions (Cl^-, Na^+, K^+, or Ca^{++}) through their respective channels. Alcohol is a γ-aminobutyric acid (GABA) and serotonin agonist, facilitating passage of chloride through the GABA "a" channel (GABAa), and facilitating passage of sodium through the serotonin type 3 (5-HT3) channel.[11] Variations in the serotonin transporter–linked polymorphic region (5'-HTTLPR) have been noted to be associated with susceptibility to alcohol intoxication and alcohol dependence.[25] Subjects with homozygous long allele (LL) in this transporter region (vs short [S] allele) have been associated with reduced intoxication and a higher risk of developing alcohol dependence.[26]

Alcohol is also a glutamate antagonist, inhibiting passage of sodium and calcium through N-methyl D-aspartate (NMDA) and non-NMDA channels. These actions lead to stimulation of dopamine production in the ventral tegmental area and nucleus accumbens producing a pleasurable "brain reward."[27,28] There is also evidence that alcohol may act on opioid receptors, further stimulating the dopamine reward system, enhancing its self-reinforcing properties. Some evidence shows that the effect of alcohol on the μ-opioid receptor is variable,[29] and that genetic differences in the μ-opioid receptor (OPRM1 118G vs 118A) may result in a more pronounced reward.[30,31] In addition to its ability to produce a brain reward, alcohol may also act as a stress reliever.[32] The role of alcohol as an inhibitor of the stress-related neuropeptide corticotropin-releasing factor has also been explored.[33] Alcohol is metabolized at a rate of around 120 mg/kg/h (linear zero-order kinetics) in naïve users, but this can be higher in regular heavy drinkers. Metabolism occurs via gastric and (primarily) hepatic alcohol dehydrogenases, along with microsomal ethanol oxidizing systems (MEOS-CYP2E1). The major metabolic pathway accounts for between 90% and 98% of alcohol metabolism.[34] Three genes encode hepatic alcohol dehydrogenase, with alpha, beta, and gamma subunits; the sigma subunit is primarily found in gastric mucosa. Alcohol metabolism is different between men and women because of lower weight, total body water content, and fluctuations in gonadal hormone levels.[35] An Italian study in 1990 showed decreased gastric alcohol dehydrogenase activity and first-pass metabolism in women, potentially leading to higher blood alcohol levels per unit weight than in men.[36] The remainder of ingested alcohol is either excreted or processed through minor metabolic pathways. These pathways include conjugation with glucuronic acid and sulfate to form ethyl glucuronide or ethyl sulfate.[37] Both metabolites can be found in serum, urine, and hair sample analysis.

After drinking ethanol, these metabolites are excreted in the urine for longer periods than alcohol itself, leading to a broader detection window. Ethyl glucuronide and ethyl sulfate are direct measures of alcohol consumption, not indirect markers of potential use. Ethyl glucuronide, unlike ethyl sulfate, can be produced in vitro after specimen collection or be hydrolyzed by urinary bacteria, potentially causing false-positives or false-negatives.[38] Another direct biomarker (only formed in the presence of ethanol) is phosphatidyl ethanol, a membrane phospholipid found in the erythrocyte fraction of blood.[39] These direct biomarkers have been shown to correlate well with blood alcohol concentrations in subjects with alcohol abuse–related consequences.[40]

DETERMINING LEVEL OF TREATMENT

Diagnosing alcohol use disorders may be important for many reasons. Before its classification as "a chronic brain disease" by the National Institute for Drug Abuse (NIDA), addiction was considered a biopsychosocial-spiritual illness. The cumbersome aspects of the latter definition were accepted because it implies that addiction affects all areas of a person's life. Health care professionals are often most concerned about the well-being of patients rather than the legal, social, or moral implications of the diagnosis. Confirmatory physical findings and laboratory results can help break through the denial, rationalization, and lack of candor that frequently accompany addiction.

Years ago, treatment of an alcohol or other substance use disorder implied that the subject might be whisked away to a distant 28-day recovery program to undergo rigorous lessons in submission and humility. Twenty-eight day treatment centers have been popularized, and spoofed in literature and movies. Use of the 28-day residential program for all levels of severity and all substance use disorders was based on rationale but not necessarily evidence. The 28-day treatment program certainly has a place in the treatment of substance use disorders today, but this level of care is now more frequently selected based on established criteria determining need.

Currently treatment options are evaluated and considered based on severity of illness, presence (or absence) of co-occurring disorders, social support, and willingness of the patient to engage. Many care providers, insurance companies, and societies have formulated criteria, but those published by the American Society of Addiction Medicine (ASAM) are considered the standard. Included in the ASAM Patient Placement Criteria (now version PPC-2R) are care recommendations for adults and adolescents.[41] This article focuses on the adult table. The ASAM Patient Placement Criteria uses a numerical system to differentiate levels of care, with level IV, which indicates hospital admission to either a medical or psychiatric unit, as the highest level (**Table 1**). In level IV, patients are medically managed in an environment that has nursing care and medical services available 24 hours a day. The cost of hospital services can be thousands to tens of thousands of dollars per day, depending on level of care, tests, and procedures performed. The next lower level (III.7) permits the use of critical pathways and order sets that allow the physician to order and monitor treatment without having to manage the patient as intensely. Although facilities that provide care at the III.7 level have 24-hour nursing care, these are frequently not full hospitals that have laboratory, radiology, and on-call medical personnel readily available at all hours. Level III.7 services are less expensive than those available at the hospital, but prices vary greatly depending on clientele and funding source.

Level III.5 is medium- to high-intensity "clinically managed" treatment. Care is often provided by licensed psychologists, social workers, or therapists, with medical services available on an as-needed basis. The programs providing a higher intensity of service often have providers with a broad range of technical expertise practicing in a comfortable treatment setting or therapeutic community. Level III.3 is a medium-intensity level of residential treatment, often without the amenities or range of services available at the higher level. Level III.1 is considered low-intensity residential treatment. This treatment level is most often used as a step-down or transitional stage for patients that need structure and a safe living environment to maintain gains made at a higher service level. Patients often begin working or going to school again while in this treatment level, and process work-related stressors with their recovering peers and therapists. Sometimes level III.1 treatment facilities provide banking services to help patients budget and use their money wisely.

Level II.5, the "day treatment program," is the most structured therapy in an outpatient setting. Level II.5 programs provide the treatment of a medium- to high-intensity residential program during the day, with the patient going home at night. Time spent in treatment at this level is usually more than 20 hours per week. Level II.1 (the next lower step) is also known as the intensive outpatient program (IOP). IOPs have several groups or individual sessions per treatment day (some have more, some have less). The intentional flexibility of level II.1 allows treatment to be provided in the evenings and/or weekends in addition to the usual daytime weekday hours. Time spent in treatment at this level is usually 9 to 19 hours per week.

Level I is outpatient-based treatment, with the frequency of office visits being decided by the provider and the patient. Patients with co-occurring psychiatric disorders or behavioral issues that might interfere with the group dynamic may respond better to individual therapy in an office visit setting.

Time spent in treatment at this level is usually less than 9 hours per week. Level 0.5 (single office-based intervention) is the lowest treatment level. This level of intervention is designed to address patients who may not meet the criteria for a substance abuse or dependence diagnosis but are noted to be at risk. Patients may be referred to recovery groups for support but are not scheduled for follow-up sessions to address alcohol or other substance misuse. Opioid maintenance treatment (OMT) with methadone or buprenorphine is a separate heading. OMT can be very structured, with daily visits, regular drug screens, and counseling sessions. It could also be unstructured, with monthly office visits for prescription renewals and no therapy requirements.

Which treatment level to use is decided based on the patient's performance on a 6-dimensional assessment. Dimension 1 is alcohol intoxication and/or severe alcohol/other drug withdrawal symptoms. Patients with severe withdrawal symptoms necessitating 24-hour medical care require hospitalization. Patients with less severe symptoms can be considered for less intensive and less costly treatment options. Dimension 2 is biomedical conditions and complications. Patients with traumatic injuries or uncontrolled medical issues (eg, malignant hypertension, diabetic ketoacidosis or hyperosmolar nonketotic hyperglycemia, decompensated cirrhosis) generally require treatment in the level 4 setting. Dimension 3 is emotional, behavioral, or cognitive conditions and complications. Patients with co-occurring psychiatric, behavioral, or cognitive disorders that impair perception of reality, or those at significant risk of harming themselves or others, require additional treatment in a setting that allows concomitant treatment of both processes. This care is often provided in a hospital-based locked psychiatric ward or medical ward with one-on-one observation.

Dimension 4 is treatment readiness to change. The keyword that summarizes this dimension to the author is *insight*. The question providers must ask is about the patient's motivation to change. Is the request for treatment more related to the avoidance of external consequences or to an internal desire to change? However, dimension 4 responses do not qualify patients for level 4 services. It makes sense that the hospital is not the correct level of care to impart insight. In the absence of dimension 1, 2, or 3 factors, this issue is best addressed in a lower, less costly level of care.

Table 1
Adult admission criteria: crosswalk of levels 0.5 through IV

Criteria Dimensions	Levels of Service									
	Level 0.5 Early Intervention	OMT Opioid Maintenance Therapy	Level I Outpatient Services	Level II.1 Intensive Outpatient	Level II.5 Partial Hospitalization	Level III.1 Clinically-Managed Low Intensity Residential Services	Level III.3 Clinically-Managed Medium Intensity Residential Services	Level III.5 Clinically-Managed Medium/High Intensity Residential Services	Level III.7 Medically-Monitored Intensive Inpatient Services	Level IV Medically-Monitored Intensive Inpatient Services
Dimension 1: Alcohol Intoxication and/or Withdrawal Potential	No withdrawal risk	Withdrawal prevented by OMT	Minimal risk of severe withdrawal	Minimal risk of severe withdrawal	Minimal risk of severe withdrawal	No withdrawal risk	Moderate withdrawal risk (not severe)	Moderate withdrawal risk (not severe)	Moderate risk of severe withdrawal	Severe withdrawal risk
Dimension 2: Biomedical Conditions and Complications	None or stable	None or stable	None or stable	None or stable	None or stable	None or stable	None or stable	Stable; may need medical monitoring	Medical monitoring required	Needs 24 hour medical care
Dimension 3: Emotional/Behavioral Conditions and Complications	None or stable	None or manageable in outpatient structure	None or stable	Mild severity; needs monitoring	Mild to moderate severity; needs monitoring	None or minimal	Mild to moderate severity	Unable to control impulses	Moderate severity	Severe problems need 24 hour Psychiatric care

Dimension 4: Readiness to Change (insight)	Has insight into use affecting goals	Requires structure therapy to progress	Cooperative, but needs motivation and monitoring	Moderate resistance structure required	Significant resistance; more structure needed	Needs structure to maintain therapeutic gains	Little insight; needs motivating strategies	No insight may not believe treatment is necessary	High resistance and poor impulse control	Not applicable for this level of care
Dimension 5: Relapse/ Continued Use Potential (automaticity)	Need skills to change current use	High relapse risk without OMT	Able to maintain abstinence	Higher automaticity; needs monitoring and support	Significant automaticity; needs more monitoring and support	Understands relapse, but still needs structure	Higher automaticity requiring 24 hour monitoring	Inadequate skills to prevent immediate relapse	Unable to control use with dangerous consequence	Not applicable for this level of care
Dimension 6: Recovery Environment	Good social support	Supportive recovery environment	Supportive recovery environment	Less supportive structure needed to cope	Environment unsupportive; higher structure improves patient coping	Dangerous environment; structure permits success in recovery	Dangerous environment; structure permits success in recovery	Dangerous environment; structure permits success in recovery	Dangerous recovery environment; structure permits success in recovery	Not applicable for this level of care

Adapted from Mee-Lee D, Shulman GD, Fishman M, et al, editors. ASAM patient placement criteria for the treatment of substance-related disorders, second Edition-revised (ASAM PPC-2R). Chevy Chase (MD): American Society of Addiction Medicine, Inc; 2001. p. 27–33; with permission.

Dimension 5 is relapse, continued use, or continued problem potential. The keyword that summarizes this dimension to the author is *automaticity*. The patient may be able to sit in a counseling or group session, understand, and verbally ascend to willingness to change, but may be unable to resist alcohol use when confronted with cues or stressors associated with drinking in the past. Inability to resist impulse is not a reason for hospitalization but may, in some cases (depending on severity), preclude the use of outpatient treatment settings.

Dimension 6 is recovery environment. This dimension is closely related to dimension 5 in that a lonely or unsupportive environment can exert pressure on the patient to return to the same escape mechanism (alcohol, other drugs, or behaviors) used before the treatment intervention. The benefits of a supportive recovery environment cannot be overstated, because a dangerous environment that encourages relapse can rapidly undermine gains made in treatment. Sometimes a safe environment can be built through attending sobriety meetings and/or developing a network of sober accountability partners and friends. Other times more drastic measures are necessary, such as removing the patient from a destructive home or exposure to negative influences from friends or family members.

CASE EXAMPLE
Initial Presentation

A 63-year-old man voluntarily presents to the emergency room tremulous and agitated with a blood alcohol level of 320 mg/dL. He is noted to have a blood pressure of 210/120 mm Hg and his pulse is 120 beats per minute (bpm). He complains of nausea with vomiting, headache, and a prickly sensation on his arms and legs. He is unkempt, disheveled, and malodorous. Fundoscopic, heart, lung, and abdominal examinations are normal. The complete blood cell count and chemistry panel are normal and a urine toxicology screen is pending. Addiction consultation is called to assist with appropriate treatment and disposition. What level of treatment does this patient require?

Treatment recommendations

Patient requires level 4 treatment. Because of his elevated pulse and blood pressure along with vomiting, he is unsuitable for a lower level of care. He may be placed on a protocol or symptom-triggered detoxification regimen, given fluids, thiamine, anti-nauseants, and antihypertensives as needed.

Background

The next day, the patient is feeling much better, though he still feels tremulous and anxious. He continues to have headaches and the prickly skin sensation, but nausea is improved and he had no vomiting overnight. The blood pressure is now 140/80 mm Hg, and his pulse is 96 bpm. The patient is now ready to tell his story. He has been using alcohol since his teenage years and has never had previous addiction treatment. He married his college sweetheart after graduation. During his 20s he would binge drink weekends while watching sports with his friends. During is 30s he discovered wine tasting, and would share a bottle of wine every evening while still binge drinking on weekends with friends. During his 40s and 50s his work promotions allowed business lunches with alcohol use. He began meeting clients and coworkers after work for drinks before coming home and drinking wine before, during, and after dinner. He would go out with "bar buddies" but lost interest in any previously enjoyable activities (movies, evening walks, sex) after arriving home for the evening. He began having arguments with his wife about his heavy drinking and boring lifestyle. He retired from work at the age of 62 years and stayed home most days, starting his drinking with mimosas in the morning and continuing use all day. Fights with his wife escalated. Approximately 3 weeks before the admission, he physically assaulted his wife during an argument. She called the police, who removed him from his home. She changed the locks, secured the doors and windows, and installed an alarm system. She is charging him with domestic violence, has requested a restraining order, and has not spoken to him since. He has been living with his bar buddies, drinking nonstop. He knows he needs to change but does not know how. He is very angry with his wife. What is the next treatment step for him?

Diagnosis and treatment plan

He has type 1 alcohol dependence as manifested by multiple negative consequences (fights with spouse, including a legal intervention for domestic violence), tolerance, and withdrawal symptoms. He wants to get away from his consequences, but his internal motivation to change is questionable (angry at wife). His automaticity is unknown, but his recovery environment is dangerous. The plan is to complete detoxification and address any remaining medical issues, then transition him into a residential treatment facility (3.3 or 3.5), depending on what is available through his insurance provider.

Follow-Up

Patient returns after 1 month in a medium-intensity residential treatment facility (level 3.3). He has enjoyed attending the groups and recovery activities. He reports no desire to drink alcohol anymore and does not feel tempted when he passes the grocery store or the bar. He understands that he hurt his wife and that he needs to make amends. He has joined AA and has a sponsor. He is working on step 2. He asks to stay in treatment another month because he does not want to go back to live with his bar buddies. The program has contacted his wife, who is amenable to the possibility of a reconciliation, but "not yet." What is the next treatment step for him?

Assessment and Recommendations

He has developed insight and does not report problems with automaticity. His major issue is dimension 6—the dangerous recovery environment. He could transition to the lower-cost 3.1 level of treatment. Now that he understands his role in damaging his marriage, it may be possible to explore involving the wife in her own recovery program. As they both recover, potential for outpatient couples therapy and reunion exists.

TYPES OF TREATMENT

Many treatment strategies have been attempted to treat people with alcohol use disorders, ranging from quick 1-hour sessions or 1-weekend seminars to lifelong therapies. Proper treatment depends on proper diagnosis, and understanding that there is a spectrum of drinking disorders. The NIDA concept of addiction as a chronic brain disease is important once the diagnosis of dependence is established. Patients not exhibiting criteria for addiction frequently respond to brief counseling and motivational interviewing/enhancement to facilitate self-change. As consequences mount in frequency and severity, the strategy should be adjusted. This section discusses treatment tools, including behavioral therapies, pharmacologic therapies, complementary and alternative therapies, and support groups.

DETOXIFICATION

Patients that present in alcohol withdrawal often require pharmaceutically assisted detoxification. Withdrawal symptoms can begin hours to days after cessation of heavy prolonged alcohol use. The symptoms should not be from another medical or psychiatric disorder, and should cause clinically significant impairment of function. Two of the following 8 criteria listed in the DSM IV-TR should be noted[4]:

1. Autonomic hyperactivity
2. Increased hand tremor
3. Insomnia
4. Nausea or vomiting
5. Transient visual, tactile, or auditory hallucinations or illusions
6. Psychomotor agitation
7. Anxiety
8. Grand mal seizures

Symptoms result from an unmasking of the chronic suppression of excitatory neurotransmitters (predominantly glutamate) by GABA.[42,43] Delirium tremens (DTs) is defined by systemic autonomic instability in addition to the hallucinosis and CNS hyperactivity. Withdrawal seizures are usually generalized tonic-clonic, and occur most often between 12 and 48 hours after cessation of alcohol use, the same time frame as acute alcoholic hallucinosis. The DTs usually begin between 48 and 96 hours after cessation of alcohol use, and have a mortality rate of up to 5%. Common electrolyte abnormalities include hypokalemia, hypomagnesemia, and hypophosphatemia, which can lead to rhabdomyolysis, cardiac arrhythmias, and further systemic decompensation. Uncomplicated DTs may last up to 7 days, and frequently require treatment in the intensive care unit.

Treatment of alcohol withdrawal is predominantly supportive, with use of sedatives to prevent seizures and alleviate CNS hyperactivity. Benzodiazepines and barbiturates have both been used successfully in the treatment of acute, severe alcohol withdrawal. Both are GABAa agonists, and increase the flow of the chloride ion through the channel, causing inhibition of excitatory biogenic amines.[44] Barbiturates cause the channel to stay open (increasing potential for overdose), whereas benzodiazepines allow the channel to open and close at a more rapid rate. Because of the improved safety profile, benzodiazepines are the most commonly used sedative to manage alcohol withdrawal. Barbiturates (phenobarbital) or propofol can be added to benzodiazepines to treat refractory DTs.

In 1997, a working group from ASAM published an evidence-based practice guideline on the pharmacologic management of alcohol withdrawal.[45] This publication was a meta-analysis reviewing 134 articles, including 65 prospective controlled trials involving 42 medications. Outcomes reviewed included severity of withdrawal syndrome, DTs, withdrawal seizures, completion of withdrawal, entry into a rehabilitation program, and cost. Benzodiazepines (chlordiazepoxide, diazepam, lorazepam, oxazepam) were considered equally efficacious in reducing seizures and DTs, and were recommended for moderate to severe withdrawal. Thiamine administration on admission was also recommended, as was use of individualized treatment regimens.

The choice of benzodiazepine is often based on the experience of the provider and unique characteristics of the patient. Diazepam and chlordiazepoxide are long-acting benzodiazepines that are metabolized in the liver to other active compounds. Diazepam is usually given in 5- to 10-mg doses, whereas chlordiazepoxide is usually given in 25- to 50-mg doses. These agents may take several weeks to be completely cleared from the body after a 3- to 5-day course (3–6 doses per day), and provide a smooth, gradual self-taper.

Lorazepam and oxazepam are short/intermediate-acting benzodiazepines that do not have active metabolites and may be a safer alternative in patients who are elderly or have decompensated liver disease or respiratory compromise. Lorazepam is usually given in 1- to 2-mg doses, whereas oxazepam is given in 15- to 30-mg doses. They may also be given 3 to 6 times per day, but late-onset withdrawal symptoms and seizures may occur.[46] Clonazepam (0.5–1 mg per dose) is a long-acting benzodiazepine also metabolized in the liver but without active metabolites. Benzodiazepines may be given proactively in front-loaded or fixed-dose protocols, or reactively to treat patient symptoms.

Carbamazepine and divalproex have both been used successful to treat less severe alcohol withdrawal symptoms, and may be considered in milder withdrawal situations with outpatient protocols.[47–50] Although protocols vary significantly, nonbenzodiazepine detoxification may start at around 200 mg for carbamazepine or 250 mg for divalproex, given 3 to 4 times per day or for the first day or 2 then tapered off over a period of 7 to 10 days. Doses may need to be lower in elderly patients.

Several quantifying instruments have been developed and used to better assess risk of morbidity and mortality from alcohol withdrawal. The most well-known, and commonly used is the Clinical Institute Withdrawal Assessment of Alcohol Scale, Revised (CIWA-Ar).[51] This scale has well-documented validity and reliability. The CIWA-Ar has 10 sign/symptoms categories, 9 of which are scored from 0 to 7 and the tenth from 0 to 4, for a total possible 67 points. A score of less than 8 to 10 points indicates mild withdrawal, whereas a score of 15 or higher indicates severe symptoms.[46] Some have chosen to use a mild (0–8), moderate (9–15), severe (>15) scale, and base decisions regarding whether to use medications, outpatient detoxification, or inpatient treatment on the score. Others use a mild (<10) versus significant (≥10) scale to determine whether to use pharmaceutically assisted detoxification. The 10 parameters measured by the CIWA-AR are as follows:

1. Nausea/vomiting: 0–7
2. Tremor: 0–7
3. Paroxysmal sweats: 0–7
4. Tactile disturbances: 0–7
5. Auditory disturbances: 0–7
6. Visual disturbances: 0–7
7. Anxiety: 0–7
8. Agitation: 0–7
9. Headache, fullness in head: 0–7
10. Orientation and clouding of sensorium: 0–4

The CIWA-Ar can be administered by a trained provider in approximately 2 minutes. No points are given for abnormal pulse or blood pressure. The CIWA-Ar has been used to measure symptoms to determine the need for medication using symptom-triggered detoxification protocols. Patients receiving symptom-triggered protocols have been shown to use less medication and have a shorter treatment period than patients on fixed-dose protocols.[52,53] One issue with using short-acting benzodiazepines in symptom-triggered detoxification protocols is that they require patient assessment to be performed regularly and sometimes frequently. Sometimes this is difficult to accomplish on a general medical ward, leading to protocol errors.[54] The staff must be able and willing to use assessment tools in a correct, timely manner.

STAGES OF CHANGE AND MOTIVATIONAL INTERVIEWING

Detoxification (separation of the patient from alcohol) may be considered the beginning of substance abuse treatment, but the terms are not synonymous. Time in detoxification can be used to determine the next appropriate level of treatment, the type of treatment, and whether anticraving pharmacologic therapy will be used. The treatment provider should work with the patient to optimize motivation to change, which can be done through techniques of motivational interviewing. Use of open-ended questions, affirmations, and reflective questioning will allow the interviewer to determine the patient's insight and readiness to change. The "stages of change" provide a framework with which to better define this process (**Table 2**).[55,56] The first stage is precontemplation. This stage may be categorized by rationalization and denial of the severity of consequences. Patients in this stage may feel that the effort of changing is not justified by the reward. The second stage is contemplation. Patients in this stage are becoming more aware of the benefits of changing their behavior, and understanding the severity of the consequences of avoiding change. The third stage of change is preparation, in which the patient realizes that change may not be easy but is still necessary. The patient makes mental and physical adjustments necessary to make the change. The fourth stage is action, in which the individual makes observable changes necessary to reduce or eliminate consequences. The fifth stage is maintenance, which may be categorized as relapse prevention. The patient learns the stresses and triggers of temptation for returning to old behavior, and uses new behaviors (learned in the action step) to prevent relapse. The sixth and final stage of change is termination. This is the theoretical stage in which a temptation or chance to relapse is no longer present. Sometimes patients with severe physical, social, or legal consequences of alcohol dependence believe that they have reached this stage of change after detoxification, without having worked through the preceding stages.

During a motivational interview, the provider gives information that may relate to the physical or social consequences of alcohol abuse. The provider may also dispel preconceived ideas about addiction treatment, making the idea of changing behavior less frightening to the patient. By helping the patient understand the severity of the consequences and lower the fear related to change, the provider can facilitate movement toward action. The provider then affirms the patient's "change talk," being careful not to belittle the ideas, motivation, or plans. An open, honest, nonjudgmental relationship is the building block for further conversation if the first attempt at behavioral change is unsuccessful.

Table 2
Summarized Stages of Change

Stages of Change	
Stage	Description
Precontemplation	Rationalization of issue. Denial of the severity of consequences. Feeling that change is not justified by the reward.
Contemplation	Awareness of the potential benefits for behavioral change. Understanding of possible consequences.
Preparation	Realization of the necessity of change. Mental and physical adjustments.
Action	Observable changes to reduce consequences.
Maintenance	Relapse prevention. Develops skills to identify stresses and triggers. Implement new behaviors to prevent relapse.
Termination	There is no longer a threat of relapse. Confidence in coping without relapse.

BEHAVIORAL THERAPIES

Once the patient is ready to move toward action, the various therapeutic options must be considered. Several models are primarily used for the treatment of alcohol (and other substance) abuse.[57] Many treatment programs offer group therapy sessions as part of their treatment model. Recovery groups can be educational, support-related, therapeutic, or focused on skill development. Many programs combine different types of groups. Educational recovery groups may use lecture or videos in addition to discussion to improve the understanding of addiction, process of recovery, and prevention of relapse. Support-related 12-step or secular facilitation groups encourage participation in outside support groups to develop a network, including sponsors and accountability partners. The most widely established support groups are Alcoholics/Narcotics Anonymous, but other support groups, such as Celebrate Recovery, Life Ring, or SMART Recovery, also encourage the development of a community-based support system. Therapy groups may use motivational enhancement therapy (MET)[58] to help patients resolve ambivalence about changing behaviors, increasing their commitment to recovery. They may also be insight-oriented, with a goal of raising insight and self-awareness of stressors and relapse triggers. Skills groups may use cognitive behavioral therapy (CBT)[59] or dialectic behavioral therapy to reverse maladaptive thoughts and beliefs that support substance use or other problem-solving and stress management techniques. Other therapies, such as individual counseling, family therapy, and contingency management (giving intermittent small rewards for achieving objective recovery goals), are often used in addition to groups by many recovery programs.

Project MATCH (Matching Alcoholism Treatment to Client Heterogeneity) was a multicenter clinical trial designed to discover whether matching patient characteristics to treatment options would improve outcomes. The study included 1726 alcohol-dependent patients (2 parallel groups of either directly admitted outpatients or those stepping down from inpatient or day-treatment program) who were randomly assigned to 12-step facilitation (TSF), CBT, or MET for a treatment period of 12 weeks. One-year follow-up interviews were performed with more than 90% of patients. Significant and sustained improvements in drinking outcomes were achieved from baseline by patients in all 3 treatment groups, with little difference in outcome by type of treatment. In the outpatient study arm, those with lower psychiatric severity showed better results with TSF than those using CBT.[60] A secondary analysis showed that patients with a high anger score treated with MET had better posttreatment outcomes than those treated with CBT, and patients with high alcohol dependence had better results with TSF than those using CBT. Patients with low alcohol dependence had better results with CBT.[61] A 3-year follow-up (for 952 patients) was subsequently performed, revealing that the patients with a high anger score continued to do better after MET. With regard to overall outcomes, the reductions in drinking observed after 1 year were sustained in the third year. Although few differences were seen among the 3 cohorts, the research group noted a possible slight advantage in those receiving TSF.[62]

PHARMACOLOGIC THERAPIES APPROVED BY THE U.S. FOOD AND DRUG ADMINISTRATION

Although several models of therapy-based substance abuse treatment have provided evidence of effectiveness,[63] considerable room for improvement still exists. Several pharmacologic therapies for alcohol abuse have shown benefit in reducing hazardous drinking, and should be considered. The U.S. Food and Drug Administration (FDA) has approved 4 medications for the treatment of alcohol dependence: disulfiram, acamprosate, oral naltrexone, and injectable long-acting naltrexone. A thorough literature review can be found in "TIP 49: Incorporating Alcohol Pharmacotherapies Into Medical Practice: A Review of the Literature" from the U.S. Department of Health and Human Services.[64] Disulfiram is an anticraving drug approved nearly 60 years ago that inhibits the conversion of acetaldehyde to acetate by aldehyde dehydrogenase. This agent can cause nausea, vomiting, flushing, and headache with alcohol intake. A black box warning states that it should not be given to patients whom have ingested alcohol within the preceding 12 hours. The dose range is 125 to 500 mg/d, but it has been used in higher doses at less frequent intervals. Recent literature reviews have shown only modest short-term reductions in alcohol use.[65] One study showed significantly better abstinence with observed dosing during the initial phase (12 weeks), but results were similar to those with naltrexone and acamprosate during the second phase (52 weeks) of treatment.[66] Patients who agree to supervised disulfiram use have better abstinence rates and improved outcomes.[67]

Acamprosate was approved by the FDA in 2004, but has been used in Europe since the 1980s. The exact mechanism of acamprosate is unclear, but it is structurally similar to GABA and thought to modulate the effects of glutamate at the NMDA receptor in the brain. It has been studied in doses from 1332 to 3000 mg/d, but the usual dose is 666 mg (2 tablets) 3 times daily (1998 mg/d). Acamprosate has no black box warnings and no pharmacokinetic differences based on gender or degree of alcohol dependency. No dosage adjustments are needed with mild to moderate hepatic impairment or mild renal disease. Dose adjustment is necessary in moderate renal disease (creatinine clearance of 30–50 mL/min), and acamprosate is contraindicated in severe renal disease (<30 mL/min). The 3 European studies that served as pivotal trials[68–70] all underwent FDA reanalysis, which showed improved outcomes in complete abstinence, time to first drink, and percent days abstinent.[71] Several good multicenter studies in the United States have shown variable improvement in outcomes.[72,73] Despite this, the meta-analyses performed on the many worldwide trials show a significant reduction in drinking frequency.[74,75] Acamprosate has been shown to reduce the risk of returning to any drinking and to improve duration of abstinence. It is considered to be a moderately effective medication in the treatment of alcohol dependence.[76,77]

Oral naltrexone was approved by the FDA in 1994 as an anticraving medication for treatment of alcohol dependence. Naltrexone is a μ-opioid receptor (OPRM1) antagonist, thought to work through blocking the brain reward contribution from the opioid system. This effect may be most prominent in a subset of patients with certain genetic polymorphisms (Asp40 allele).[31] A black box warning states not to use naltrexone in patients with acute hepatitis or hepatic failure. Caution should be used in patients with severe liver or renal disease, but no dosage adjustment is recommended. Patients who use naltrexone should not be using opioids for the treatment of chronic pain, and should carry a card informing medical providers they are taking an opioid receptor blocking agent.

Seminal articles by Volpicelli and colleagues[78] and O'Malley and colleagues[79] published in 1992 showed a significant decrease in relapse drinking with naltrexone. The interesting paradigm shift of using "less heavy drinking days" as a measure of success was advanced by these studies. Many clinicians at that time felt that the only measure of treatment success was complete abstinence and did not acknowledge the clinical significance of these study results. Naltrexone has been administered at doses of 25 to 100 mg/d, with the usual dose being 50 mg/d. Oral naltrexone has been extensively studied in the past 2 decades, with most studies showing increased efficacy over placebo, although some have not.[64]

The COMBINE study[72] was a National Institute on Alcohol Abuse and Alcoholism–sponsored multicenter, randomized, controlled study that evaluated the efficacy of medications (oral naltrexone and acamprosate), behavioral therapies, and their combinations for the treatment of alcohol dependence. The study included 1383 patients from 11 academic sites. Subjects were randomized to either 100 mg of oral naltrexone, 3 g of acamprosate, both, or neither. Behavioral therapies consisted of either combined behavioral intervention or medical management, both, or neither. Medication placebo groups were included. The study was conducted for 16 weeks, with reevaluation 1 year after treatment. The investigators concluded that "within the context of medical management, naltrexone yielded outcomes similar to those obtained from specialist behavioral treatment." They found no evidence of increased efficacy for acamprosate alone or in combination with naltrexone, and found that placebo plus medical management was more effective than specialist combined behavioral intervention alone. The 1-year posttreatment phase published in 2008 assessed drinking behavior and clinical status at weeks 26, 52, and 68. Patients treated with medical management and either combined behavioral intervention, naltrexone, or both experienced sustained benefit.[80]

A critical factor in the efficacy of naltrexone in the treatment of alcohol dependence is patient compliance.[81] Unfortunately, medication adherence is generally not good, with a retrospective database review showing that more than 85% of patients did not refill their naltrexone prescription at some point within 6 months after starting treatment.[82] To assist patients in overcoming motivational difficulties with adherence, long-acting implantable and injectable forms of naltrexone were developed. In April 2006, the FDA approved extended-release naltrexone (XR-NTX)[83] for the treatment of alcohol dependence and prevention of relapse to opioid dependence. This (polylactide-co-glycolide) microsphere formulation is administered intramuscularly and releases naltrexone for 1 month after injections. Comparing the 380 mg dose with placebo, one study showed a 25% decrease in heavy drinking days over a 6-month period.[84] Medication adherence is a problem with XR-NTX, as with the other approved alcohol dependence medications.[85] One study found that "persistence days on medication" were significantly higher than with the other 3 FDA-approved medications.[86] This study also showed that, despite the higher up-front cost for XR-NTX (approximately $1100 per month), the number of emergency department visits and hospital days saved (because of relapse prevention) make it a cost-effective option. An open-label pilot study examining the use of XR-NTX in repeat DUI offenders showed significantly fewer drinks per day and more abstinent days over the 3-month period.[87]

OTHER PHARMACOLOGIC THERAPIES

The issues of poor adherence and moderate efficacy with the current FDA-approved medications have prompted the search for other options.[88] Topiramate, baclofen, ondansetron, sertraline, nalmefene, and aripiprazole are among the medications currently under investigation. Topiramate is thought to work as a GABA agonist and glutamate antagonist.[89] Topiramate was shown in a randomized controlled trial to have a lower percentage than placebo (by 16%) of heavy drinking days by participants (N = 371).[90] In this study, participants randomized to topiramate were titrated from a starting dose of 25 mg/d up to 300 mg/d over a 6- to 8-week period. Adverse effects involving paresthesia, taste perversion, and anorexia were problematic. Baclofen is a GABAb agonist currently under investigation. A recent, retrospective, open-label study assessed the proportions of high-risk drinkers who were either abstinent or drinking at low levels 1 year after starting high-dose baclofen therapy (129 ± 71 mg/d).[91] The authors were able to follow-up on 132 of 181 patients. Of these patients, 80% were either abstinent or drinking at low levels.

Ondansetron is an antagonist of the 5-HT3 receptor, and was approved for the treatment of nausea and vomiting. One study randomized 283 alcohol-dependent patients according to serotonin transporter (5-HTT) genotype (LL, LS, SS), with additional genotyping for another transporter polymorphism (TT/TG/GG). Participants received either ondansetron 4 μg/kg twice daily or placebo for 11 weeks plus CBT.[92] The investigators noted that individuals with the LL genotype had a lower mean number of drinks per day and a higher percentage of days abstinent than those receiving placebo, with the greatest effect seen in individuals with the LL/TT genotypes.

Sertraline, a selective serotonin reuptake inhibitor approved for the treatment of depression, anxiety, and other psychiatric disorders, has also been evaluated for potential efficacy in alcohol use disorders. One study evaluated the effect of sertraline on alcohol-dependent patients, separating them by phenotype (late onset/low vulnerability [LOA] vs early onset/high vulnerability [EOA]) and serotonin transporter (5-HTT) genotype (LL, LS, SS).[93] The patients (N = 134) were randomized to receive up to 200 mg of sertraline or placebo daily during the 12-week study. The medication effect varied significantly by phenotype and genotype, with the LOA/LL patients reporting fewer drinking and heavy drinking days. The study participants were followed up for 6 months posttreatment, with continued significantly beneficial effects seen in the LOA/LL group only.[94]

The opioid antagonist nalmefene was assessed in a randomized double-blind study in Finland.[95] Subjects (N = 242) took 10 to 40 mg of nalmefene or placebo for the 28-week study, with minimal psychosocial intervention. The study was extended another 24 weeks for 57 subjects in the nalmefene arm, who were randomized to either continue nalmefene or receive placebo. The study showed significantly decreased drinking for those receiving nalmefene over placebo in both phases.

Aripiprazole is an atypical antipsychotic medication also approved for the treatment of bipolar disorder. It is a partial agonist of the dopamine 2 and serotonin 1A receptors, and an antagonist of the serotonin 2A receptor. In one study, alcohol-dependent subjects not seeking treatment were randomized to either aripiprazole or placebo, with the dose titrated to 15 mg over a 14-day period.[96] Functional MRI was performed during exposure to alcohol-related cues. Brain activity was higher in the right ventral striatum of individuals receiving placebo and blunted in those receiving aripiprazole. Patients treated with aripiprazole also had significantly less heavy drinking during the 14-day period.

COMPLEMENTARY AND ALTERNATIVE MEDICINE

Submitting to treatment for an alcohol use disorder can be difficult for patients. When making the decision to take the first, most difficult step toward treatment, people have a natural tendency to wonder if perhaps an easier or better option exists. Complementary and alternative medicines (CAMs) for addiction treatment are available worldwide and have been gaining popularity in the United States. Identifying and describing the wide variety of available CAMs would be a difficult process. Even the definition of CAM is challenging in this paradigm, because behavior therapies, 12-step support groups, and stress relieving/relaxation techniques are a part of established nonalternative recovery programs. The National Center for Complementary and Alternative Medicine was established in 1998 and is one of 27 centers that constitute the National Institutes of Health. It divides CAM into 5 subsets[97]:

1. Alternative medical systems (acupuncture, homeopathy, naturopathy, traditional healers)

2. Biologically based therapies (chelation; nonvitamin, nonmineral, and natural products; diets)
3. Manipulative and body-based therapies (chiropractic/osteopathic, massage, movement)
4. Mind–body therapies (biofeedback, relaxation, hypnosis)
5. Energy-healing therapy

Studies using biofeedback[98] and electroacupuncture[99,100] indicate that these therapies may be helpful. A paucity of randomized, placebo/sham controlled studies are available using these therapies. Lack of evidence however, is different from lack of efficacy. Many testimonials of success have been shared by individuals who overcame their struggles with alcohol using CAM. Furthermore, companies with proprietary formulations or therapies have introduced CAM products directly to consumers using testimony as a marketing tool. The potential benefit of these therapies is difficult to report because they often have not undergone the rigorous scrutiny required for presentation or publication in scientific meetings or journals.

SUPPORT GROUPS

A review article about alcohol abuse would be remiss to not mention the very important role of support groups in recovery history and process. The largest and most well-established group is Alcoholics Anonymous (AA), the idea of which was birthed in Akron Ohio in 1935 by cofounders Bill Wilson and (Dr) Bob Smith. The first "Big Book" of AA was published in 1939 and included the 12 steps with which AA, and many subsequent groups, would be identified. The 12 steps illuminate a spiritual (not religious) recovery path taken by millions of people worldwide. Currently more than 2 million people attend more than 115,000 AA recovery groups around the world. "Friends of Bill W," a pseudonym for AA, find fellowship on cruise ships, in airplanes, and at many other spontaneous and interesting places. In the chapter "How it Works" of AA, the steps are listed[101]:

1. We admitted we were powerless over alcohol—that our lives had become unmanageable.
2. Came to believe that a Power greater than ourselves could restore us to sanity.
3. Made a decision to turn our will and our lives over to the care of God *as we understood Him.*
4. Made a searching and fearless moral inventory of ourselves.
5. Admitted to God, to ourselves, and to another human being the exact nature of our wrongs.
6. Were entirely ready to have God remove all these defects of character.
7. Humbly asked Him to remove our shortcomings.
8. Made a list of all persons we had harmed, and became willing to make amends to them all.
9. Made direct amends to such people wherever possible, except when to do so would injure them or others.
10. Continued to take personal inventory and when we were wrong promptly admitted it.
11. Sought through prayer and meditation to improve our conscious contact with God *as we understood Him*, praying only for knowledge of His will for us and the power to carry that out.
12. Having had a spiritual awakening as the result of these steps, we tried to carry this message to alcoholics, and to practice these principles in all our affairs.

Many other groups have used the steps in this spiritual recovery pathway to overcome other chemical and behavioral addictions, such as Narcotics Anonymous, Gamblers Anonymous, Overeaters Anonymous, Co-Dependents Anonymous, and Sex and Love Addicts Anonymous. Several other recovery groups in addition to these should be mentioned.

Celebrate Recovery was founded by John Baker in 1991, and is intended to bring the 12-step recovery process to people admitting they need support to overcome "habits, hurts, and hang-ups." It was designed to be broad enough to allow participants with behavioral issues (eg, anger, gambling, past abuse, codependency, sex addiction, overeating) to benefit from the 12-step recovery process along with those with alcohol or other chemical dependencies. Celebrate Recovery is growing rapidly and, with approximately 20,000 groups meeting in the United States and 20 other countries, is now second to the Anonymous groups in size. Celebrate Recovery has a program for teens (The Landing), and a "pre-covery" program (Celebration Station) for children from 5 to 12 years of age.[102] Participants start the meeting together in a large group for a testimonial or step study, then separate into smaller gender- and issue-specific groups for individual sharing.

The spiritual nature of the 12-step programs has raised questions about the legality of court-mandated attendance. Several circuit court decisions have upheld the assertion that mandated 12-step meeting attendance is a violation of the Establishment Clause in the First Amendment to the U.S. Constitution.[103] Several secular organizations have regular insight-oriented meetings, including LifeRing, SMART recovery, Women for Sobriety, Secular Organizations for Sobriety, and Moderation Management. These programs combine to offer approximately 2000 meetings in the United States and other countries.

SUMMARY

The diagnosis and treatment of alcohol use disorders are the first and most important steps in the treatment of alcoholic liver disease. This article provides clinicians with a basic understanding of the tools available to diagnose and treat this cunning and baffling brain and multisystem disease.

REFERENCES

1. Genesis 9:20–1 (RSV).
2. National Institute on Alcohol Abuse and Alcoholism (NIAAA). The physicians' guide to helping patients with alcohol problems (revised). Bethesda, MD: NIAAA; 2004. NIH Publication No. 04-3769.
3. Alcohol and public health. Frequently asked questions. Centers for Disease Control and Prevention Web site. Available at: http://www.cdc.gov/alcohol/faqs.htm.
4. Diagnostic and Statistical Manual of Mental Disorders. Fourth edition. Text revision. Washington (DC): American Psychiatric Association; 2000. p. 191–295.
5. Substance abuse and addictive disorders. American Psychiatric Association Web site. Available at: http://www.dsm5.org/proposedrevision/Pages/Substance UseandAddictiveDisorders.aspx.
6. Results from the 2010 National Survey on Drug Use and Health: summary of national findings. Available at: http://oas.samhsa.gov/NSDUH/2k10NSDUH/2k10Results.htm.
7. U.S. alcohol epidemiologic data reference manual. National Institutes of Health, National Institute on Alcohol Abuse and Alcoholism Web site. Available at: http://pubs.niaaa.nih.gov/publications/manual.htm.

8. Grant BF, Stinson FS, Dawson DA, et al. Prevalence and co-occurrence of substance use disorders and independent mood and anxiety disorders: results from the National Epidemiological Survey on Alcohol and Related Conditions. Arch Gen Psychiatry 2004;61:807–16.

9. Harwood H. Report from Lewin Group for NIAAA 2000 NIH Pub No. 98-4327 from Harwood HJ, Fountain D, Livermore G. Economic cost of alcohol and drug abuse in the United States, 1992: a report. Addiction 1999;94:631–5.

10. Bouchery EE, Harwood J, Sacks JJ, et al. Economic costs of excessive alcohol consumption in the U.S., 2006. Am J Prev Med 2011;41(5):546–7.

11. Woodward JJ. The pharmacology of alcohol. In: Gram AW, Schultz TK, Mayo-Smith MF, et al, editors. ASAM principles of addiction medicine. 3rd edition. Chevy Chase (MD): American Society of Addiction Medicine Inc; 2003. p. 101–18.

12. Cloninger CR. Neurogenetic adaptive mechanisms in alcoholism. Science 1987; 236:410–6.

13. Dick DM, Nurnberger J Jr, Edenberg HJ, et al. Suggestive linkage on chromosome 1 for quantitative alcohol-related phenotype. Alcohol Clin Exp Res 2002; 26(10):1453–60.

14. Dick DM, Plunkett J, Wetherill LF, et al. Association between GABRA1 and drinking behaviors in the collaborative study on the genetics of alcoholism sample. Alcohol Clin Exp Res 2006;30(7):1101–10.

15. Beresford TP, Blow FC, Hill E, et al. Comparison of CAGE questionnaire and computer-assisted laboratory profiles in screening for covert alcoholism. Lancet 1990;336:482–5.

16. Fiellin DA, Reid MC, O'Connor PG. Outpatient management of patients with alcohol problems. Ann Intern Med 2000;133:815–27.

17. Bradley KA, Bush KR, Epler AJ, et al. Two brief alcohol screening tests from the alcohol use disorders Identification test (AUDIT). Arch Intern Med 2003;163: 821–9.

18. Bradley K, Williams EC, Achtmeyer CE, et al. Implementation of evidence-based alcohol screening in the Veterans Health Administration. Am J Manag Care 2006;12:597–606.

19. Selzer ML. The Michigan Alcoholism Screening Test: the quest for a new diagnostic instrument. Am J Psychiatry 1971;127:1653–8.

20. Pokorny AD, Miller BA, Kaplan HB. The brief MAST: a Shortened version of the Michigan alcoholism screening test. Am J Psychiatry 1972;129:342–5.

21. Harburg E, Gunn R, Gleiberman L, et al. Using the short Michigan alcoholism screening test to study social drinkers: Tecumseh, Michigan. J Stud Alcohol 1988;49(6):522–31.

22. Tell D, Nilsson PM. Early ageing in middle-aged men is associated with adverse social factors and increased mortality risk: the Malmo Preventive Project. Scand J Public Health 2006;34(4):346–52.

23. Naegle MA. Screening for alcohol use and misuse in older adults: using the short Michigan alcoholism screening test—geriatric version. Am J Nurs 2008; 108(11):50–8.

24. Schuckit MA. Alcohol and alcoholism. In: Longo DL, Fauci AS, Kasper DL, et al, editors. Harrison's principles of internal Medicine. 18th edition. New York: McGraw-Hill; 2012.

25. Barr CS, Newman TK, Becker ML, et al. Serotonin transporter gene variation is associated with alcohol sensitivity in rhesus macaques exposed to early-life stress. Alcohol Clin Exp Res 2003;27:812–7.

26. Laucht M, Treutlein J, Schmid B, et al. Impact of psychosocial adversity on alcohol intake in you adults: moderation by the LL genotype of the serotonin transporter polymorphism. Biol Psychiatry 2009;66:102–9.

27. Koob GF, Sanna PP, Bloom FE. Neuroscience of addiction. Neuron 1998;21:467–76.

28. Koob GF, Roberts AJ, Schulteis G, et al. Neurocircuitry targets in ethanol reward and dependence. Alcohol Clin Exp Res 1998;22:3–9.

29. Boileau I, Assaad JM, Pihl RO, et al. Alcohol promotes dopamine release in the human nucleus accumbens. Synapse 2003;49:226–31.

30. Ray LA, Hutchinson KE. A polymorphism of the mu-opioid receptor gene (OPRM1) and sensitivity to the effects of alcohol in humans. Alcohol Clin Exp Res 2004;28:1789–95.

31. Anton RF, Oroszi G, O'Malley S. An evaluation of mu-opioid receptor (OPRM-1) as a predictor of naltrexone response in the treatment of alcohol dependence: results from the Combined Pharmacotherapies and Behavioral Interventions for Alcohol Dependence (COMBINE) study. Arch Gen Psychiatry 2008;65(2):135–44.

32. Heilig M, Goldman D, Berrettini W, et al. Pharmacogenetic approaches to the treatment of alcohol addiction. Nature 2011;12:670–84.

33. Liu X, Weiss F. Additive effect of stress and drug cues on reinstatement of ethanol seeking: exacerbation by history of dependence and role of concurrent activation of corticotrophin-releasing factor and opioid mechanisms. J Neurosci 2002;22:7856–61.

34. Schuckit MA. Ethanol and methanol. In: Brunton LL, Chabner BA, Knollmann BC, editors. Goodman & Gilman's the pharmacological basis of therapeutics. 12th edition. New York: McGraw-Hill; 2011.

35. National Institute for Alcohol Abuse and Alcoholism Alcohol Alerts # 10 & #46 #10 Alcohol and Women. Available at: http://pubs.niaaa.nih.gov/publications/aa10.htm. Are women more vulnerable to alcohol's effects? Available at: http://pubs.niaaa.nih.gov/publications/aa46.htm. Accessed April 30, 2012.

36. Frezza M, di Padova C, Pozzato G, et al. High blood alcohol levels in women. The role of decreased gastric alcohol dehydrogenase activity and first-pass metabolism. N Engl J Med 1990;322(2):95.

37. Wurst FM. Ethyl sulphate: a direct ethanol metabolite reflecting recent alcohol consumption. Addiction 2006;101(2):204–11.

38. Helander A, Böttcher M, Fehr C, et al. Detection times for urinary ethyl glucuronide and ethyl sulfate in heavy drinkers during alcohol detoxification. Alcohol Alcohol 2009;44(1):55–61.

39. Varga A, Hansson P, Lundqvist C, et al. Phosphatidylethanol in blood as a marker of ethanol consumption in healthy volunteers: Comparison with other markers. Alcohol Clin Exp Res 1998;22:1832–7.

40. Marques P, Tippetts S, Allen J, et al. Estimating driver risk using alcohol biomarkers, interlock BAC tests, and psychometric assessments: initial descriptives. Addiction 2010;105(2):226–39.

41. Mee-Lee D, Shulman GD, Fishman M, et al, editors. ASAM patient placement criteria for the treatment of substance-related disorders, second Edition-revised (ASAM PPC-2R). Chevy Chase (MD): American Society of Addiction Medicine, Inc; 2001. p. 27–33.

42. Morrow AL, Suzdak PD, Karanian JW. Chronic ethanol administration alters gamma-aminobutyric acid, pentobarbital, and ethano-mediated 36Cl$^-$ uptake in cerebral cortical synaptoneurosomes. J Pharmacol Exp Ther 1988;246:158.

43. Tsai G, Gastfriend DR, Coyle JT. The glutamatergic basis of human alcoholism. Am J Psychiatry 1995;153:332.

44. Korpi ER, Grunder G, Luddens H. Drug interactions at the GABA(A) preceptors. Prog Neurobiol 2002;67(2):113–59.

45. Mayo-Smith MF. Pharmacological management of alcohol withdrawal: a meta-analysis and evidence -based practice guideline. JAMA 1997;278:144–51.

46. Miller NS, Kipnis SS. Detoxification and substance abuse treatment: a treatment improvement protocol TIP 45. DHHS Publication No SMA08–4131. Rockville (MD): U.S. Department of Health and Human Services; 2006.

47. Malcom R, Myrick H, Brady KT, et al. Update on anticonvulsants for the treatment of alcohol withdrawal. Am J Addict 2001;10(Suppl):16–23.

48. Reoux JP, Saxon AJ, Malte CA, et al. Divalproex Sodium in alcohol withdrawal: a randomized double-blind placebo-controlled clinical trial. Alcohol Clin Exp Res 2001;25(9):1324–9.

49. Eyer F, Schreckenberg M, Hecht D, et al. Carbamazepine and valproate as adjuncts in the treatment of alcohol withdrawal syndrome: a retrospective cohort study. Alcohol Alcohol 2011;46(2):177–84.

50. Barrons R, Roberts N. The role of carbamazepine and oxcarbazepine in alcohol withdrawal syndrome. J Clin Pharm Ther 2010;35(2):153–67.

51. Sullivan JT, Sykora K, Schneiderman J, et al. Assessment of alcohol withdrawal: the revised clinical institute withdrawal instrument for alcohol scale (CIWA-Ar). Br J Addict 1989;84:1353–7.

52. Saitz R, Mayo-Smith MF, Roberts MS, et al. Individualized treatment for alcohol withdrawal. A randomized double-blind controlled trial. JAMA 1994;272:519.

53. Daeppen JB, Gache P, Landry U, et al. Symptom-triggered vs. fixed-schedule doses of benzodiazepine for alcohol withdrawal: a randomized treatment trial. Arch Intern Med 2002;162:1117.

54. Weaver MF, Hoffman HJ, Johnson RE, et al. Alcohol withdrawal pharmacotherapy for inpatients with medical comorbidity. J Addict Dis 2006;25(2):17–24.

55. Prochaska JO, DiClemente CC, Norcross JC. In search of how people change: applications to the addictive behaviors. Am Psychol 1992;47:1102–14.

56. Prochaska JO. In: Ries RK, Fiellin DA, Miller SC, et al, editors. Principles of addiction Medicine. 4th edition. Chevy Chase (MD): American Society of Addiction Medicine, Inc; 2009. p. 745–61.

57. Leamon MH, Wright TM, Myrick H. Substance related disorders. In: Hales RE, Yudofsky SC, Gabbard GO, editors. The American psychiatric publishing textbook of psychiatry. Arlington (VA): American Psychiatric Publishing Inc; 2008. p. 365–406.

58. Miller WR, Zweben A, Di Clemente CC, et al. Motivational enhancement therapy Manual. Rockville (MD): U.S. Dept of Health and Human Services; 1994.

59. Kadden R, Carroll KM, Donavan D, et al. Cognitive behavioral coping skills therapy manual. Rockville (MD): U.S. Dept of Health and Human Services; 1994.

60. Project MATCH Research Group. Matching alcoholism treatments to client heterogeneity: project MATCH post treatment drinking outcomes. J Stud Alcohol 1997;58:7–29.

61. Project MATCH Research Group. Project MATCH secondary a priori hypotheses. Addiction 1997;92(12):1671–98.

62. Project MATCH Research Group. Matching alcoholism treatments to client heterogeneity: project MATCH three year drinking outcomes. Alcohol Clin Exp Res 1998;22(6):1300–11.

63. Helping patients who drink too much: a clinician's guide. National Institutes of Health; National Institute on Alcohol Abuse and Alcoholism Web site. Updated 2005 edition. Available at: http://pubs.niaaa.nih.gov/publications/Practitioner/CliniciansGuide2005/clinicians_guide.htm.

64. Incorporating alcohol pharmacotherapies into medical practice: a review of the literature. Rockville (MD): U.S. Department of Health and Human Services; 2009.

65. Jorgensen CH, Pedersen B, Tonnesen H. The efficacy of disulfiram for the treatment of alcohol use disorder. Alcohol Clin Exp Res 2011;35(10):1749–58.

66. Laaksonen E, Koski-Jannes A, Salspuro M, et al. A randomized, mulitcentre, open-labeled, comparative trial of disulfiram, naltrexone, and acamprosate in the treatment of alcohol dependence. Alcohol Alcohol 2008;43(1):53–61.

67. Chick J, Gough K, Falkowski W, et al. Disulfiram treatment of alcoholism. Br J Psychiatry 1992;161:84–9.

68. Pelc I, Verbanck P, Le Bon O, et al. Efficacy and safety of acamprosate in the treatment of detoxified alcohol-dependent patients: a 90- day placebo-controlled dose-finding study. Br J Psychiatry 1997;171:73–7.

69. Sass H, Soyka M, Mann K, et al. Relapse prevention by acamprosate: results from a placebo-controlled study on alcohol dependence. Arch Gen Psychiatry 1996;53:673–80.

70. Paille FM, Guelfi JD, Perkins AC, et al. Double-blind randomized multicentre trial of acamprosate in maintaining abstinence from alcohol. Alcohol Alcohol 1995; 30:239–47.

71. Kranzler HR, Gage A. Acamprosate efficacy in alcohol-dependent patients: summary of results from three pivotal trials. Am J Addict 2008;17(1):70–6.

72. Anton RF, O'Malley SS, Ciraulo DA, et al. Combined pharmacotherapies and behavioral interventions for alcohol dependence: the COMBINE study: a randomized controlled trial. JAMA 2006;295:2003–17.

73. Mason BJ, Goodman AM, Chabac S, et al. Effect of oral acamprosate on abstinence in patients with alcohol dependence in a double-blind, placebo-controlled trial: the role of patient motivation. Jpn Psychol Res 2006;40:383–93.

74. Mason BJ. Treatment of alcohol-dependent outpatients with acamprosate: a clinical review. J Clin Psychiatry 2001;62(Suppl 10):42–8.

75. Mann K, Lehert P, Morgan MY. The efficacy of acamprosate in the maintenance of abstinence in alcohol-dependent individuals: results of a meta-analysis. Alcohol Clin Exp Res 2004;28:51–63.

76. Garbutt JC, West SL, Carey TS. Pharmacological treatment of alcohol dependence: a review of the evidence. JAMA 1999;281(14):1318–25.

77. Witkiewitz K, Saville K, Hamreus K. Acamprosate for treatment of alcohol dependence: mechanisms, efficacy, and clinical utility. Ther Clin Risk Manag 2012;8:45–53.

78. Volpicelli JR, Alterman AI, Hayashida M, et al. Naltrexone in the treatment of alcohol dependence. Arch Gen Psychiatry 1992;49:876–80.

79. O'Malley SS, Jaffe AJ, Chang G, et al. Naltrexone and coping skills therapy for alcohol dependence: a controlled study. Arch Gen Psychiatry 1992;49:881–7.

80. Donovan DM, Anton RF, Miller WR, et al. Combined pharmacotherapies and behavioral interventions for alcohol dependence (The COMBINE Study): examination of posttreatment drinking outcomes. J Stud Alcohol Drugs 2008;69(1):5–13.

81. Volpicelli JR, Rhines KC, Rhines JS, et al. Naltrexone and alcohol dependence: the role of subject compliance. Arch Gen Psychiatry 1997;54:737–42.

82. Kranzler HR, Stephenson JJ, Montejano L, et al. Persistence with oral naltrexone for alcohol treatment: implications for health-care utilization. Addiction 2008; 103(11):1801–8.

83. Vivitrol (naltrexone for extended-release injectable suspension) prescribing information. Waltham (MA): Alkermes, Inc; 2010.
84. Garbutt JC, Kranzler HR, O'Malley SS, et al. Efficacy and tolerability of long-acting injectable naltrexone for alcohol dependence: a randomized controlled trial. JAMA 2005;293:1617–25.
85. Bryson WC, McConnell J, Korthuis PT, et al. Extended-release naltrexone for alcohol dependence: persistence and healthcare costs and utilization. Am J Manag Care 2011;17(Suppl 8):S213–221.
86. Baser O, Chalk M, Rawson R, et al. Alcohol dependence treatments: comprehensive healthcare costs, utilization outcomes, and pharmacotherapy persistence. Am J Manag Care 2011;17(Suppl 8):S222–234.
87. Lapham SC, McMillan GP. Open-label pilot study of extended-release naltrexone to reduce drinking and driving among repeat offenders. J Addict Med 2011;5(3):163–9.
88. Edwards S, Kenna GA, Swift RM, et al. Current and promising pharmacotherapies and novel research target areas in the treatment of alcohol dependence: a review. Curr Pharm Des 2011;17(14):1323–32.
89. Johnson BA. Recent advances in the development of treatments for alcohol and cocaine dependence: focus on topiramate and other modulators of GABA or glutamate function. CNS Drugs 2005;19(10):873–96.
90. Johnson BA, Rosenthal N, Capece JA, et al. Topiramate for treating alcohol dependence: a randomized controlled trial. JAMA 2007;298:1641–51.
91. Rigal L, Anexandre-Dubroeucq C, de Beaurepaire R, et al. Abstinence and "low-risk" consumption 1 year after the initiation of high-dose baclofen: a retrospective study among "high-risk" drinkers. Alcohol Alcohol 2012;47(4):439–42.
92. Johnson BA, Ait-Daoud N, Seneviratne C, et al. Pharmacogenetic approach at the serotonin transporter gene as a method of reducing the severity of alcohol drinking. Am J Psychiatry 2011;168(3):265–75.
93. Kranzler HR, Armeli S, Tennen H, et al. A double-blind, randomized trial of sertraline for alcohol dependence: moderation by age of onset [corrected] and 5-hydroxytryptamine transporter-linked promoter region genotype. J Clin Psychopharmacol 2011;31(1):22–30.
94. Kranzler HR, Armeli S, Tennen H. Post-treatment outcomes in a double-blind, randomized trial of sertraline for alcohol dependence. Alcohol Clin Exp Res 2012;36(4):739–44.
95. Karhuvaara S, Simojoki K, Virta A, et al. Targeted nalmefene with simple medical management in the treatment of heavy drinkers: a randomized double-blind placebo controlled multicenter study. Alcohol Clin Exp Res 2007;31(7):1179–87.
96. Myrick H, Li X, Randall PK, et al. The effect of aripiprazole on cue-induced brain activation and drinking parameters in alcoholics. J Clin Psychopharmacol 2010;30(4):365–72.
97. Nahin RL, Barnes MA, Stussman BJ, et al. Costs of complementary and alternative Medicine (CAM) and frequency of visits to CAM Practitioners: United States, 2007. Natl Health Stat Report 2009;30(18):1–15.
98. Sokhadze TM, Cannon RL, Trudeau DL. EEG Biofeedback as a treatment for substance use disorders: review, rating of efficacy, and recommendations for further research. Appl Psychophysiol Biofeedback 2008;33(1):1–28.
99. Li J, Zou Y, Ye JH. Low frequency electroacupuncture selectively decreases voluntarily ethanol intake in rats. Brain Res Bull 2001;86(5–6):428–34.

100. Overstreet DH, Cui CL, Ma YY, et al. Electroacupuncture reduces voluntary alcohol intake in alcohol-preferring rats via an opiate-sensitive mechanism. Neurochem Res 2008;33(10):2166–70.
101. Wilson B. Alcoholics anonymous. 3rd edition. New York: Alcoholics Anonymous World Services, Inc; 1976. p. 59–60.
102. Baker J. Celebrate Recovery summit material. Saddleback (CA): Saddleback Church; 2012.
103. Peele S. Resisting 12-step coercion: how to fight forced participation in AA, NA, or 12-step treatment. 2001. Available at: http://www.morerevealed.com/library/resist.

Long-term Management of Alcoholic Liver Disease

Garmen A. Woo, MD*, Christopher O'Brien, MD, AGAF, FRCMI

KEYWORDS

• Alcoholic liver disease • CAGE • AUDIT-C • Long-term management • Nutrition

KEY POINTS

- Alcoholic liver disease is a major cause of end-stage liver disease worldwide.
- Prevalence of alcoholic liver disease is strongly correlated to the cumulative lifetime consumption of alcohol. Genetic and environmental factors, such as gender, genetic polymorphisms, obesity, and viral hepatitis, also affect the development of cirrhosis from alcohol use.
- Early detection of alcoholism with screening tools and abstinence is important for both prevention and management of alcoholic liver disease. Abstinence is best achieved with concomitant psychological and pharmacological therapies.
- Treatment of alcoholic liver disease includes discontinuation of alcohol consumption, nutritional support, and management of the sequelae of cirrhosis. Liver transplantation should be considered in those patients with decompensated cirrhosis as early as possible.

Chronic consumption of alcohol in large amounts remains the hallmark for hepatic damage and subsequent development of alcoholic liver disease.[1] The spectrum of this disease ranges from fatty liver to hepatic inflammation, necrosis, and progressive fibrosis, and is a major cause of morbidity and mortality worldwide.[2] Alcohol accelerates the progression of other liver diseases, such as hepatitis C virus, hepatocellular carcinoma, and hemochromatosis. Alcoholic liver disease is also a major cause of end-stage liver disease that requires transplantation in most developed countries.[3]

The cumulative lifetime alcohol consumption is strongly associated with the prevalence of alcoholic liver disease.[1] The type of beverage and pattern of drinking also affects the risk for developing alcoholic liver disease.[1] Yet, it remains unclear why, despite reaching the required 'threshold' for alcohol intake, only 10% to 35% of heavy, long-term alcohol drinkers will develop alcoholic hepatitis and only 8% to 20% will develop cirrhosis.[4,5] Both environment and genetic factors have been explored.

Supporting funds: None.

Disclosures: The authors have nothing to disclose.

Center for Liver Diseases, Miller School of Medicine, University of Miami, 1500 Northwest 12th Avenue, Suite #1101, Miami, FL 33136, USA

* Corresponding author.

E-mail address: gwoo@med.miami.edu

Clin Liver Dis 16 (2012) 763–781

http://dx.doi.org/10.1016/j.cld.2012.08.007

1089-3261/12/$ – see front matter © 2012 Elsevier Inc. All rights reserved.

liver.theclinics.com

Environmental risk factors, such as the dose and pattern of alcohol intake, and dietary and lifestyle factors are noted to be important in determining disease risk.[6,7] Coexisting external factors, such as obesity and hepatitis C infection, combined with daily alcohol use increase the likelihood of developing associated liver disease by as high as 100-fold.[8]

Host factors predisposing to the development of alcoholic liver disease are not as well known. There are several studies demonstrating that women develop liver disease after exposure to lower quantities of alcohol and over shorter periods.[3,9,10] This gender difference may be attributable to several factors, such as differences in gastric alcohol dehydrogenase (ADH) levels and a higher proportion of body fat in women.[11] The rates of development of cirrhosis and mortality are also found to be higher in African American and Hispanic individuals compared with their White counterparts; but this may be more attributable to the longer and heavier drinking patterns seen in African American and Hispanic individuals.[12,13] There may be a genetic predisposition in the development of alcoholic liver disease. Polymorphisms of genes encoding for ADH and cytochrome P-450 enzymes have been associated with higher occurrences of liver disease.[14] In a study by Marcos and colleagues,[15] carriers of genotype TT and GT from the −330T>G interleukin (IL)-2 gene polymorphism were significantly higher in alcoholic individuals with cirrhosis compared with alcoholic individuals without liver disease. In addition, the presence of a deletion allele in NFKB1 polymorphism may be associated with a higher risk of developing alcoholic liver disease.[16] Further studies in this area are needed.

OVERVIEW OF MANAGEMENT
Detection

Alcoholism is essentially another medical disease; yet, there is a large stigma associated with having an alcohol-related diagnosis. Although there is a need to intervene early to prevent liver disease, fewer than 13% of those with an alcohol problem actually get diagnosed and even fewer than 6% of these diagnosed patients receive medical treatment.[17] Based on a national survey, few people are questioned about alcohol use when they visit a general practitioner and when an alcohol problem is identified, most do not receive appropriate follow-up.[18] Screening for alcohol problems by physicians in the primary care setting with various tools, including paper-and-pencil questionnaires, should be performed regularly to promote detection as well as to initiate brief counseling and use of medical treatment when appropriate.[19]

Screening tools

The US Preventive Services Task Force recommends screening for alcohol misuse in all adults.[20] A variety of screening tools are available; but the 2 most commonly used are the CAGE questionnaire and the Alcohol Use Disorder Identification Test (AUDIT).

CAGE is the mnemonic for the 4 questions listed in **Box 1**. One positive response to any of these questions suggests the need for further evaluation; whereas, positive responses to 2 or more suggest the possibility of alcohol misuse.[21,22] Although the brevity of the CAGE questionnaire makes it easy to incorporate into routine practice, it does not distinguish between current and past alcohol use and is insensitive in detecting heavy drinking, especially in women.[23,24]

AUDIT uses 10 questions to assess the quantity of alcohol consumed and the individual's experience with using alcohol.[25] Responses to these questions generate an additive score that correlates with risk for alcohol dependence. Although the AUDIT is not affected by gender or ethnic bias, its major limitation is the length of the questionnaire.[26] A modified version, the AUDIT-C, comprises only 3 questions (**Box 2**). Its relative sensitivity and specificity is 0.86 and 0.81, respectively, and has been

---

Box 1
The CAGE questionnaire

1. Have you ever felt the need to Cut down on drinking?

2. Have you ever felt Annoyed by criticism of your drinking?

3. Have you ever had Guilty feelings about your drinking?

4. Do you ever take a morning Eye opener (a drink first thing in the morning to steady your nerves or get rid of a hangover)?

Scoring: Each response is scores as 0 or 1, with a higher score indicative of alcohol-related problems, and a total of ≥ 2 being clinically significant.

---

validated as a screening tool in the outpatient setting and in the white, African American, and Hispanic populations.[27,28]

Abstinence

The American Association for the Study of Liver Diseases (AASLD) Practice Guidelines for alcoholic liver disease emphasize abstinence, as this is pertinent to the treatment and overall long-term survival.[3,4,15] The success rate in achieving abstinence varies considerably, from 30% to 90%.[6] The most important factor associated with cessation of alcohol consumption and long-term abstinence is the patient's awareness of alcohol toxicity and its associated consequences.[6,29] Other factors, such as patient's honest attitude, cessation of alcohol use at knowledge of liver disease, family recognition and adequate social support, lack of illicit drug use, and appropriate psychiatric evaluation, also help predict successful outcome.[6,29] Incorporation of behavior modification and support groups, such as Alcoholics Anonymous, increases the likelihood of sustained sobriety and is recommended for patients who have difficulty in abstaining.[30] On the other hand, awareness of alcohol dependence, previous alcohol abuse

---

Box 2
Alcohol use disorder identification test (AUDIT)-C

1. How often did you have a drink containing alcohol in the past year?
   Never — 0 points
   Monthly or less — 1 points
   Two to four times a month — 2 points
   Two to three times per week — 3 points
   Four or more times per week — 4 points
2. How many drinks did you have on a typical day when you were drinking in the past year?
   1 or 2 — 0 points
   3 or 4 — 1 points
   5 or 6 — 2 points
   7 to 9 — 3 points
   10 or more — 4 points
3. How often did you have 5 or more drinks on one occasion in the past year?
   Never — 0 points
   Less than monthly — 1 points
   Monthly — 2 points
   Weekly — 3 points
   Daily or almost daily — 4 points

The AUDIT-C is scored on a scale of 0–12. Scores of 0 reflect no alcohol use. Scores of 4 or more in men is considered positive. Scores of 3 or more in women is considered positive.

treatments, and consumption of alcohol-free beer did not significantly predict maintenance of abstinence.[29] If abstinence is achieved, the clinical and histologic benefits
can be impressive, even if the patients have severe liver disease.[31]

However, the reason most patients find it difficult to abstain is that alcoholism is
a disease itself. Alcoholism is a physical dependence that includes tolerance, impaired
control, and craving.[31] Therefore, addressing the underlying addiction to alcohol is the
most critical step in managing alcoholic liver disease.

Psychological treatment of dependency

Alcohol addiction is divided into abuse and dependence. Alcohol abuse is defined as
excessive drinking without harmful physical and social consequences, whereas alcohol
dependence is defined as continued drinking despite physical and social harms.[32]
Despite its psychological and social sequelae, alcohol dependence is essentially a brain
disorder.[33] Formal or intensive psychotherapy, such as inpatient and outpatient rehabilitation programs, have demonstrated effectiveness in assisting patients achieve and
maintain sobriety; yet motivating patients to follow this treatment regimen, monitoring
their compliance, and preventing relapse remain as major obstacles.[34] Interventions,
such as brief behavioral compliance enhancement treatment or medical management,
appear to be sufficient.[33] Studies indicate that heavy drinkers who receive brief interventions of less than 1 hour in length while incorporating motivational counseling techniques are more likely to have modified their drinking habits 6 to 12 months after the
intervention compared with the control group.[35] As such, referral to and communication
with an addiction specialist and actively participating in Alcoholics Anonymous should
be promoted and encouraged.[13] In addition, adjuvant pharmacotherapy provides
added benefit in achieving abstinence. Without a pharmacologic adjunct to psychosocial therapy, the clinical outcome is poor, with up to 70% of patients resuming drinking
within 1 year.[36,37] Therefore, the optimal treatment for alcohol dependence involves
psychosocial intervention and pharmacotherapy.

Pharmaceutical treatment of dependency

Disulfiram, naltrexone, and acamprosate have traditionally been used for the treatment of alcohol dependence.[17] These drugs have the ability to reduce alcohol craving
and consequently increase abstinence and prevent relapse. Disulfiram inhibits acetaldehyde dehydrogenase by blocking the metabolism of acetaldehyde.[38] This then
leads to the accumulation of acetaldehyde, which results in flushing, tachycardia,
hypotension, dyspnea, vomiting, vertigo, anxiety, and headache within 30 minutes
of alcohol ingestion.[39] However, disulfiram has no effect at reducing the urge or
propensity to drink, whereas naltrexone has been reported to do.[40] Naltrexone is an
opiate receptor antagonist and its antidrinking properties have been attributed to cor-
ticomesolimbic dopamine system modulation.[33,41] Acamprosate is a modulator of
glutamate neurotransmission at metabotropic-5 glutamate receptors and affects
the hypothalamic pituitary adrenal axis as well as beta-endorphin production.[33,42]
Naltrexone and acamprosate have been used to induce or maintain abstinence in
chronic heavy drinkers, yet neither of these medications has had consistent beneficial
effects nor has been studied in large numbers of patients.[31,33,43] In addition,
naltrexone has the potential to inflict hepatocellular injury and is relatively contraindicated in those with elevated hepatic enzymes.[29,31]

Newer medications, such as baclofen, topiramate, and ondansetron, are becoming
better alternatives in treating alcohol dependence. Baclofen is an agonist at the
presynaptic gamma aminobutyric acid b-receptor and appears to suppress the
cortico-mesolimbic dopamine system neurons.[31,33] In Addolorato and colleagues'[44]

randomized, double-blind controlled study, more than 70% of alcohol-dependent patients with liver cirrhosis achieved and maintained alcohol abstinence with baclofen compared with 29% with placebo. Baclofen may eventually surpass the other anti-craving drugs, especially among those with severe liver disease, as this drug is better tolerated and is excreted primarily through the kidneys.[33,44]

Topiramate, a sulfamate-substituted fructopyranose derivative, is presumed to decrease its antidrinking effects by the cortico-mesolimbic dopamine system.[33] Top-iramate has demonstrated efficacy in reducing heavy drinking, decreasing craving and withdrawal symptoms, and promoting abstinence in many clinical studies, including 2 large, randomized, placebo-controlled, clinical trials.[45–47] Similar to baclofen, topira-mate is generally well tolerated and is excreted mostly unchanged by the kidneys in the urine.[48] The common adverse events associated with topiramate use include paresthesia, taste perversion, anorexia, and difficulty with concentration.[33] Ondanse-tron, a 5-HT3 antagonist, also exerts its antidrinking effects through the cortico-mesolimbic dopamine system modulation.[33] In comparing ondansetron with placebo, Johnson and colleagues[49] found that the ondansetron recipients had fewer drinks per drinking day and higher percentage of days abstinent. Despite its therapeutic potential with milder adverse events, such as constipation, headaches, and sedation, unfortu-nately, ondansetron is not yet commercially available at the treatment dose necessary for alcohol dependence.[33,50]

REVIEW OF PROPOSED LIVER-SPECIFIC THERAPY

Aside from treating the addiction, various pharmacotherapies aimed at the underlying mechanisms of injury represent another approach in treating alcoholic liver disease.[13] The molecular pathogenesis of alcoholic liver disease and cirrhosis involves alcohol metabolism and secondary mechanisms, such as oxidative stress, endotoxins, cyto-kines, and immune regulators.[1]

Oxidative stress contributes to the development of alcoholic liver disease. Alcohol leads to generation of highly reactive oxygen species through various biochemical path-ways, which in turn, causes liver cell damage and necrosis.[1,51] The by-products of these pathways can also generate superoxide radicals to perpetuate further liver damage as well as lead to accumulation of intracellular lipids and promote steatosis.[1,51]

Alcohol exposure also impairs the host immune response. Excess alcohol intake increases the intestinal permeability to a variety of substances, such as bacterial endotoxins.[1] These endotoxins, when bounded, cause exaggerated transcription of proinflammatory cytokines, such as tumor necrosis factor (TNF) and IL-6 and synthe-size acute-phase proteins, such as transforming growth factor, all of which contribute to necro-inflammation, apoptosis, and fibrogenesis.[51] The metabolites of alcohol may also generate neo-antigens, thus, leading to an immune reaction with antibody production or T-cell activation, resulting in further tissue damage.[51] However, the exact role of the alcohol-induced immune-mediated abnormalities in the development of alcohol liver disease is not yet defined.[1,51]

Despite significant advances in the understanding of the pathogenesis of alcohol-related liver injury, there are no US Food and Drug Administration–approved treat-ments for chronic, alcoholic liver disease.[13]

Nutritional Therapy

Alcoholic liver disease has a profound effect on nutrient intake, nutrition status, and metabolism; thereby, contributing to the development of malnutrition.[52] The mecha-nisms for malnutrition are multifactorial, such as decreased caloric intake, malabsorption, and maldigestion. Alcohol-dependent patients often replace nutrient-dense foods with empty calories from alcohol. Inadequate oral hygiene leading to poor dentition also contributes to compromised nutrition intake.[52] In addition, owing to the nature of their liver disease, these patients often consume fewer calories or nutrients because of early satiety, anorexia, dietary restrictions, and fatigue.[52] Excess alcohol use leads to gastrointestinal tract dysfunction, such as altered gut integrity, pancreatic insufficiency, decreased bile excretion, and decrease in intestinal enzymes, resulting in decreased intestinal absorption and incomplete digestion of nutrients. Similarly, alcohol leads to hepatocyte dysfunction; thereby, decreasing the amount of functional liver mass and resulting in abnormal oxidation of fat and decreased processing and storage of nutrients.[53]

The severity of malnutrition correlates with the severity of liver disease. Advanced liver disease is associated with an increased catabolic state.[52] The inflammation present in alcoholic liver disease promotes a depletion of skeletal muscle and visceral proteins.[13] In addition, the diminished ability to store glycogen, impairments in amino acid uptake, and reduced liver protein synthesis contribute to protein calorie malnutrition often seen in alcoholic liver disease.[52,54] This hypermetabolic state, in combination with the reduced energy and protein intake seen in those with chronic liver disease, increases the occurrence of muscle loss.[52] The degree of protein calorie malnutrition worsens with the progression of the liver disease and frequently worsens in the hospital as a result of fasting for procedures and metabolic complications of liver disease, such as hepatic encephalopathy.[52] Malnutrition in those with advanced liver disease is also associated with worsening of the complications of liver disease, such as infection, encephalopathy, and ascites, and is negatively associated with overall patient survival.[54,55]

Nutrient and vitamin deficiencies are also a frequent complication of alcoholic liver disease. Micronutrient deficiencies of folate, vitamin B6, vitamin A, and thiamine are among the most commonly encountered. Mineral and element levels of selenium, zinc, copper, and magnesium are often altered in alcoholic liver disease.[56]

Nutrition therapy can improve response to treatment, alleviate symptoms, and improve overall quality and quantity of life.[52,57] The goals of nutrition therapy should include providing adequate calories, protein, and nutrients to support hepatocyte regeneration within the existing metabolic alterations of liver disease.[52] Hirsch and colleagues[58] showed that by adding oral supplements of up to 1000 kcal and 35 g of protein per day to the diet, individuals with chronic liver disease could improve their nutritional status and cellular immunity as well as reduce bacterial overgrowth. A study conducted by Mendenhall and colleagues[55] also demonstrated that adequate caloric intake in patients with alcoholic liver disease improves liver function and survival rates. As important as the adequacy of calories and protein consumed is, Swart and colleagues[59] showed that the frequency with which food is consumed is equally as important. In their study, cirrhotic patients who consumed a late-night feeding had a reduction in catabolic rate compared with those who did not. Based on this, it is recommended that prolonged fasting of 4 to 6 hours be avoided and consumption of 4 to 6 small meals per day be encouraged in individuals with cirrhosis so as to minimize gluconeogenesis and to prevent and treat muscle wasting.[59–61] Those patients who are unable to take adequate nutrition through diet or nutrition supplementation, especially in the inpatient setting, may require enteral or parenteral nutrition for maintenance.[52] A consensus of 35 to 40 kcal per kg caloric intake and 1.0 to 1.5 g of protein per kg of dry or estimated lean weight is adequate and beneficial, but should be adjusted according to individual symptoms and comorbidities, such as diabetes and renal function.[61]

Antioxidants

The rationale for using antioxidants in alcoholic liver disease derives from evidence that oxidative stress is instrumental in the pathogenesis of alcoholic liver disease.[31] Phillips and colleagues[62] compared using corticosteroids versus an antioxidant cocktail, consisting of β-carotene, vitamins C and E, selenium, methionine, allopurinol, desferrioxamine, and N-acetylcysteine, in patients with severe alcohol steatohepatitis; and found that the antioxidants were inferior to the corticosteroids in terms of survival rates at 30 days. The survival advantage for the corticosteroid-treated patients, however, was lost at 1 year of follow-up.[62] Stewart and colleagues[63] also investigated the role of antioxidants in patients with severe alcohol steatohepatitis. The active group received an initial loading dose of N-acetylcysteine of 150 mg/kg followed by 100 mg/kg/d for 1 week, and vitamins A and E, biotin, selenium, zinc, manganese, copper, magnesium, folic acid, and coenzyme Q daily for 6 months. In this study, antioxidant therapy showed no benefit alone and in combination with corticosteroids.[63] Despite the theoretical mechanism of antioxidants in treating the underlying pathophysiologic abnormalities, there are no convincing data to support its current use in alcoholic liver disease.[61]

Pentoxifylline

Pentoxifylline (PTX) is a nonselective phosphodiesterase inhibitor that has been shown to decrease the production of cytokines, such as TNF and IL-5, IL-6, and IL-12.[64] Several randomized trials treating those with severe alcoholic hepatitis with PTX has shown to be associated with a reduction in mortality compared with placebo.[65,66] In one study, the in-hospital mortality in PTX-treated patients was 40% lower than that in the placebo group.[67] Importantly, almost all of the improvement in survival in the treated group was a result of a substantial lower risk of developing hepatorenal syndrome, which was responsible for 50% of the deaths in the treatment arm compared with 91% in the placebo arm.[39,67] As a result, the advantage of administrating PTX to increase survival in those with severe alcoholic hepatitis is thought to be related to the prevention of hepatorenal syndrome.[39] Further trials are needed to determine whether PTX should become a standard treatment for patients with alcoholic hepatitis.[64]

Propylthiouracil

Propylthiouracil (PTU), is normally used to inhibit thyroid hormone production, but may also be useful in preventing oxidative stress to the liver. Chronic alcohol use produces a hypermetabolic state with increased oxygen consumption, which may lead to relative hypoxia of the liver. PTU has been postulated to attenuate this hypermetabolic state, to function as an antioxidant, and to improve portal blood flow.[68] Orrego and colleagues[69] studied the use of PTU in over 300 patients with various types of liver disease, including alcoholic liver disease, and found that mortality was reduced by nearly 50% in patients receiving PTU. However, a Cochran review evaluating PTU therapy for alcohol liver disease, combining 6 trials with 710 patients, yielded no significant effects of PTU versus placebo on mortality, liver-related mortality, complications of liver disease, or liver histology.[70] As a result of the lack of confirmatory studies, PTU has not yet been adopted as a treatment for alcoholic liver cirrhosis.[64]

Colchicine

Colchicine has been suggested as a treatment for alcohol liver disease because of its antifibrotic effects in vitro. However, a meta-analysis of several randomized, controlled trials with colchicine therapy found no benefit with regard to mortality or liver histology in cirrhosis.[71,72] Other large studies conducted also confirm that colchicine therapy in alcoholic cirrhosis has no beneficial effect on overall mortality or liver-related mortality.[73–75] Thus, despite the biochemical rationale, colchicine does not appear to be effective in treating alcoholic liver disease.[68]

S-adenosylmethionine

S-adenosylmethionine (SAMe) is a precursor for glutathione and thus may be protective against alcohol-induced liver injury.[31,76] SAMe or AdoMet is converted and activated by the liver from the amino acid, methionine. With alcohol consumption, SAMe is depleted owing to decreased hepatic methionine adenosyltransferase activity, the enzyme responsible for conversion of methionine to SAMe.[68] In addition, the depletion of SAMe also affects the metabolism of other amino acids, such as glutathione, which can protect both the hepatocytes and gastric mucosa from alcohol damage.[56] In one randomized study by Mato and colleagues,[77] supplementation with SAMe for 2 years in patients with alcoholic liver cirrhosis had decreased liver mortality (16% vs 30%) compared with the placebo-treated group. However, in a database review of several randomized trials with a combined sample of 434 patients with alcoholic liver disease, SAMe did not show any significant benefit on mortality or complication rates.[78] Other studies suggest that SAMe is hepatoprotective as it downregulates production of cytotoxic, proinflammatory cytokines, such as TNF, in vitro and in animal models.[79] Overall, more research is still needed to evaluate the role of SAMe in treating alcoholic liver disease.[52,68]

Glutathione Prodrugs

Glutathione (GSH) prodrugs, such as N-acetylcysteine, have been widely used in many forms of hepatotoxicity with beneficial results.[80] Maintaining adequate hepatocyte glutathione levels has been documented to prevent liver injury; therefore, GSH prodrugs can directly protect the hepatocytes as well as inhibit the production of proinflammatory cytokines, such as TNF and IL-8.[68] Pena and colleagues[81] demonstrated that procysteine, another GSH prodrug, can increase whole-blood GSH as well as inhibit TNF and IL-8 production when administered intravenously to stable alcoholic cirrhosis. However, large randomized studies using GSH prodrugs with regard to overall mortality are still lacking in patients with alcoholic liver disease.[68]

Silymarin/Milk Thistle

Silymarin, an extract of milk thistle, is an over-the-counter herbal remedy commonly used by patients with chronic hepatitis C. Because its proposed mechanism of action includes scavenging free radicals and reducing liver fibrogenesis, there has been interest in its use in patients with alcoholic liver disease.[82] Milk thistle is well tolerated with minimal adverse events; unfortunately, a systematic meta-analysis of all the randomized clinical studies found no significant beneficial effect of milk thistle on overall mortality, liver-related deaths, or biochemical liver tests.[82,83] As a result, there is no evidence to support the use of milk thistle in those with alcoholic liver disease.

Probiotics

Probiotics are currently in use for treating hepatic encephalopathy; yet, they could also preserve normal barrier function, thereby preventing bacterial permeability seen in alcoholic liver disease.[84,85] However, the potential beneficial effects of probiotics in alcoholic liver disease have only been investigated in animal models and in small pilot studies.[39] Forsyth and colleagues[86] used rat models to study the effects of the probiotic, lactobacillus GG (LGG), in alcoholic liver disease. In this study, LGG significantly reduced alcohol-induced gut hyperpermeability and intestinal markers of oxidative stress in alcohol-fed rats. The mechanisms for probiotics' beneficial effects on barrier function are not known, but it is suggested that probiotics indirectly inhibit the production of pathogenic bacteria as well as preserve a normal gut flora.[86] More studies, including large randomized trials, need to be carried out to determine the relevance of probiotics in clinical practice.[85]

Anabolic-Androgenic Steroids

Severe muscle wasting seen in alcoholic liver disease is mediated by both nutritional deficiencies and decreased functional levels of anabolic and androgenic steroids.[87] As such, use of anabolic-androgenic steroids to increase fat-free mass, muscle mass, and strength may be beneficial.[88] However, a Cochrane database reviewing the randomized clinical trials of 499 patients with alcoholic liver disease and cirrhosis demonstrated no significant effects of anabolic-androgenic steroids on mortality, liver-related mortality, complications of liver disease, and liver histology.[89] Furthermore, anabolic-androgenic steroids did not significantly affect a number of other outcome measures, including sexual function, and were associated with a slight increase in the occurrence of serious adverse events.[89] A review of all clinical trials using anabolic-androgenic steroids in the treatment of chronic diseases, including alcoholic liver disease, yielded similar results.[88] Although the beneficial effects of anabolic steroids in chronic disorders are promising, the relevant end points, such as quality of life, improved physical functioning, and survival, were not significant.[88] Thus, the lack of any observed benefit decreases the enthusiasm for using these hormones in patients with alcoholic liver disease.[89]

ASSESSING SURGICAL RISKS IN ALCOHOLIC CIRRHOSIS

The Child-Turcotte-Pugh (CTP) scoring system is based on the patient's serum bilirubin and albumin levels, prothrombin time, and severity of encephalopathy and ascites.[90] Two studies using the CTP scoring system reported similar results in terms of predicting perioperative mortality: 10% for those with Child class A, 30% for those with Child class B, and 76% to 82% for those with Child class C cirrhosis.[91,92] Emergency surgery is associated with a higher mortality rate compared with nonemergent surgery: 22% versus 10% for patients in Child class A; 38% versus 30% for those in Child class B; and 100% versus 82% for those in Child class C.[92]

The Model for End-Stage Liver Disease (MELD) score can also be used to predict perioperative mortality. The largest retrospective study of the MELD score as a predictor of perioperative mortality, conducted by Teh and colleagues,[93] evaluated 772 patients with cirrhosis who underwent abdominal, orthopedic, or cardiovascular surgery. In this selected cohort, patients with a MELD score of 7 or less had a mortality rate of about 6%; patients with a MELD score of 8 to 11 had a mortality rate of about 10%; and patients with a MELD score of 12 to 15 had a mortality rate of about 25%.

In addition to the CTP and MELD score, the American Society of Anesthesiologists (ASA) classification and the patient's age were shown to contribute to postoperative mortality risk.[93] An ASA class of IV added the equivalent of 5.5 MELD points to the mortality rate, whereas an ASA class of V was associated with a 100% mortality rate.[93] As a result of this study, the Web site, www.mayoclinic.org/meld/mayomodel9.html, can be used to calculate the 7-day, 30-day, 90-day, 1-year, and 5-year surgical mortality risk based on a patient's age, ASA class, international normalized ratio, and serum bilirubin and creatinine levels.[93]

PREVENTION OF COMPLICATIONS/DECOMPENSATED LIVER DISEASE

Once cirrhosis develops, patients are at risk for developing complications such as variceal bleeding, ascites with spontaneous bacterial peritonitis, hepatic encephalopathy, and hepatocellular carcinoma. Based on a multicenter study, the incidence rates for developing ascites, hepatic encephalopathy, and variceal bleeding in cirrhotic patients are 49%, 24%, and 22%, respectively.[94] The development of these complications has a significant impact on the prognosis of patients with alcoholic cirrhosis. Powell and Klatskin[95] showed that the 5-year survival in patients with overt hepatic decompensation, drinkers versus abstainers, is 34% and 60%, whereas patients with compensated cirrhosis, drinkers versus abstainers, had a 5-year survival of 68% and 89%, respectively. Therefore, clinical management of these complications is critical for the long-term survival of these patients.[68]

Gastroesophageal Varices

Gastroesophageal varices, as a result of portal hypertension, are present in approximately 50% of patients with cirrhosis. Therefore, it is recommended that patients with cirrhosis undergo endoscopic screening for varices at the time of diagnosis.[96] In those patients with compensated cirrhosis, the main objective for screening is to prevent variceal hemorrhage as well to prevent future events that could lead to decompensation. If no varices are seen on the initial screening endoscopy, the esophagogastroduodenoscopy (EGD) should be repeated in 2 to 3 years.[96] If small varices are seen, then the EGD should be repeated in 1 to 2 years.[96]

In those patients with decompensated cirrhosis, the EGD should be repeated at yearly intervals, as acute variceal hemorrhage occurs frequently.[96] The use of nonselective β-blockers can reduce the rates of variceal rebleeding to 43% in patients with medium or large varices.[97] Shunting therapy with either a radiological (transjugular intrahepatic portosystemic shunt) or surgical approach to markedly reduce portal pressures should be reserved for those patients who fail to respond to endoscopic or pharmacologic therapy.[98,99]

Ascites and Spontaneous Bacterial Peritonitis

Ascites is the most common complication of cirrhosis. It affects approximately 50% of patients with compensated cirrhosis.[100] Ascites caused by alcohol-induced liver injury can be dramatically reversed with abstinence and pharmacotherapy.[101] One study demonstrates that patients with Childs C cirrhosis attributable to alcohol and who stop drinking have a 75% 3-year survival, whereas those who continue to drink die within 3 years.[102]

Physicians should also be vigilant for spontaneous bacterial peritonitis (SBP).[103] It affects 10% to 30% of patients with ascites with a high recurrence rate of up to 70% within the first year. SBP also carries a poor long-term prognosis, with mortality reaching 50% to 70% at year 1.[101,102] Therefore, patients with cirrhosis and ascites presenting with fever, abdominal pain, or unexplained encephalopathy should undergo a diagnostic paracentesis and receive empiric antibiotic treatment until the diagnosis is made.

Hepatic Encephalopathy

Hepatic encephalopathy (HE), a reversible neuropsychiatric and functional syndrome, occurs in 50% to 70% of patients with cirrhosis.[104] HE usually manifests with progressive deterioration of the neurologic functions, ranging from altered mental status to deep coma.[105] This often results in an elevated serum ammonia level, which is detected in 60% to 80% of affected patients.[106,107] Current treatment includes lactulose and Rifaximin, which aimed to reduce or to inhibit production of intestinal ammonia or minimize its absorption from the gastrointestinal tract.[108] However, other factors that can precipitate HE include constipation, infection, gastrointestinal bleeding, certain medications, electrolyte imbalances, and medication noncompliance.[109]

Hepatorenal Syndrome

Hepatorenal syndrome (HRS) is a reversible form of renal failure that occurs with cirrhosis.[110] Patients with cirrhosis develop progressive circulatory dysfunction, which results in renal fluid retention and ascites. This extreme form of hemodynamic alteration also culminates in renal vasoconstriction, resulting in type 2 HRS.[111] Type 2 HRS is characterized by slowly progressive renal failure with refractory ascites; whereas, Type 1 HRS is characterized by rapid development of renal failure and deterioration in the function of the other organs in the setting of a precipitating event.[112,113] The overall prognosis for HRS is poor and dismal without liver transplantation.[111]

Hepatocellular Carcinoma

Patients with cirrhosis should be screened for hepatocellular carcinoma (HCC).[103,114] Alcohol intake increases the individual's risk for development of HCC.[52] In one study, alcoholic liver disease accounted for 32% of all HCCs.[115] In another, alcoholic liver disease was the risk factor for HCC in 35% of its subjects.[116] These studies confirm that alcoholic cirrhosis is a significant risk factor for HCC; thereby, warranting surveillance. The screening tests used to diagnose HCC include radiology, such as ultrasound or computed tomography scan and alpha-fetoprotein (AFP) serology. The ideal surveillance interval is not known but a surveillance interval of 6 to 12 months has been proposed based on tumor doubling times.[114] A randomized controlled trial of 6-month surveillance interval with AFP and ultrasound showed a survival benefit compared with no surveillance.[117] A retrospective study reported that survival is no different in patients screened at 6-month versus 12-month intervals, however.[118]

EFFECT OF ALCOHOLIC LIVER DISEASE ON BONE DISEASE

Hepatic osteodystrophy (HO) is the generic term defining the group of alterations in bone mineral metabolism found in patients with chronic liver disease. The origin of HO is multifactorial and its etiology and severity vary in accordance with the underlying liver disease. Its exact prevalence is unknown, but different studies estimate that it could affect 20% to 50% of patients. The reported mean prevalence of osteoporosis ranges from 13% to 60% in chronic cholestasis to 20% in chronic viral hepatitis and 55% in viral cirrhosis. Alcoholic liver disease is not always related to osteopenia; nonetheless, screening for osteopenia and osteoporosis is recommended in those with advanced chronic liver disease, regardless of its etiology.[119]

Bone loss and fractures are in part caused by direct and indirect effects of ethanol on bone remodeling but also to the peculiar lifestyle of the alcoholic individual (ie, prone to falls, traffic accidents, and violence).[120] Gonzalez-Reimers and colleagues[120] analyzed many factors, such as ethanol consumption, liver function impairment, bone densitometry, hormone alterations, nutritional status, and environmental factors related with job, social status, and eating habits, in relation to bone fractures seen in those engaged in heavy alcohol use. In this study, more than 50% of the patients had bone fractures and low vitamin D levels and deranged nutritional status were the main associated factors. Although bone mineral density values were lower among those with fractures, these differences were not statistically significant.[120]

LIVER TRANSPLANTATION

Alcoholic liver disease is a common indication for liver transplantation (LT) worldwide and is associated with good posttransplant outcomes. One recent large study showed that survival rates following LT in patients with alcohol are similar to the rates for patients with other causes of cirrhosis (89% vs 84% at 3 years, and 84% vs 81% at 5 years).[121] There remains ambivalence about the role of transplantation in patients suffering from alcoholic liver disease, based partly on concerns that this is a self-inflicted disease, risk for alcohol relapse posttransplant, and functional outcome post-transplant in an era of donor organ shortage and priority setting.[122]

Some type of alcoholic relapse after transplantation (often called recidivism) occurs in approximately 20% to 30% of patients despite formal psychological assessments before listing.[29] In 1997, a consensus conference of the AASLD and the American Society of Transplantation concluded that "there is a strong consensus for requiring that most alcoholic patients should be abstinent from alcohol for at least 6 months before they can be listed for liver transplantation."[123] In the literature on alcoholism, 6 months appears too short to determine meaningful abstinence and that sobriety is robust after 5 years.[124]

Altamirano and colleagues[29] studied the factors that influence both cessation in alcohol consumption and sustained alcohol abstinence in patients with alcoholic liver disease evaluated for LT. In this study, the risk factors that identify those patients with a high likelihood for alcohol relapse posttransplantation include preexisting psychotic disorders, unremitting multidrug abuse including tobacco consumption, and lack of insight of alcohol as the cause of their disease at initial assessment. Other negative prognostic factors include repeated and unsuccessful attempts at rehabilitation and lack of strong social support.[123] Other studies also confirmed that noncompliance and personality disorder contributed significantly in predicting alcohol relapse, whereas duration of sobriety before evaluation, being listed for LT, and presence of hepatitis C virus (HCV) or other psychiatric diagnoses did not significantly predict recidivism. Conversely, favorable factors in predicting abstinence include self-acknowledgment of their addiction, family recognition of the problem, and the presence of a strong social network, such as a spouse, a job, and a home.[29] Vaillant also identified 4 prognostic elements that are indicative of social integration: substitute activities, a source of improved self-esteem or hope, a rehabilitation relationship, and a perception by the drinker of the negative consequences of alcoholic relapse.[124]

Although alcohol recidivism occurs, it does not appear to affect graft and patient survival or compliance.[122] Moreover, the outcomes for patients who undergo transplantation for alcohol liver disease are at least as good as those for patients with most other diagnoses and are better than those for patients with HCV.[123] The causes of death after transplantation differ between recipients with alcoholic liver disease and recipients without alcoholic liver disease. A retrospective analysis of the European Liver Transplant Registry by Burra and colleagues[125] showed that cardiovascular causes and de novo malignancies were significantly overrepresented in patients who had undergone transplantation for alcoholic liver disease versus recipients without alcoholic liver disease. Similarly, Watt and colleagues[126] showed that in a prospective cohort of 780 primary graft recipients, alcoholic liver disease was significantly associated with the risk of cardiovascular death 1 year after LT.

REFERENCES

1. Seth D, Haber PS, Syn WK, et al. Pathogenesis of alcohol-induced liver disease: classical concepts and recent advances. J Gastroenterol Hepatol 2011;26(7): 1089–105.
2. Gao B, Bataller R. Alcoholic liver disease: pathogenesis and new therapeutic targets. Gastroenterology 2011;141(5):1572–85.
3. Altamirano J, Bataller R. Alcoholic liver disease: pathogenesis and new targets for therapy. Nat Rev Gastroenterol Hepatol 2011;8(9):491–501.
4. Day CP. Who gets alcoholic liver disease: nature or nurture? J R Coll Physicians Lond 2000;34(6):557–62.
5. Espinoza P, Ducot B, Pelletier G, et al. Interobserver agreement in the physical diagnosis of alcoholic liver disease. Dig Dis Sci 1987;32(3):244–7.
6. Day CP. Genes or environment to determine alcoholic liver disease and non-alcoholic fatty liver disease. Liver Int 2006;26(9):1021–8.
7. Wilfred de Alwis NM, Day CP. Genetics of alcoholic liver disease and nonalco-holic fatty liver disease. Semin Liver Dis 2007;27(1):44–54.
8. Mueller S, Millonig G, Seitz HK. Alcoholic liver disease and hepatitis C: a frequently underestimated combination. World J Gastroenterol 2009;15(28): 3462–71.
9. Becker U, Deis A, Sorensen TI, et al. Prediction of risk of liver disease by alcohol intake, sex and age: a prospective population study. Hepatology 1996;23(5): 1025–9.
10. Fuch CS, Stampfer MJ, Colditz GA, et al. Alcohol consumption and mortality among women. N Engl J Med 1995;332(19):1245–50.
11. Mas VR, Fassnacht R, Archer KJ, et al. Molecular mechanisms involved in the interaction effects of alcohol and hepatitis C virus in liver cirrhosis. Mol Med 2010;16(7–8):287–97.
12. Siu L, Foont J, Wands JR. Hepatitis C virus and alcohol. Semin Liver Dis 2009; 29(2):188–99.
13. Frazier TH, Stocker AM, Kershner NA, et al. Treatment of alcoholic liver disease. Ther Adv Gastroenterol 2011;4(1):63–81.
14. Basra S, Anand BS. Definition, epidemiology and magnitude of alcoholic hepa-titis. World J Hepatol 2011;3(5):108–13.
15. Marcos M, Pastor I, González-Sarmiento R, et al. A new genetic variant involved in genetic susceptibility to alcoholic liver cirrhosis: –330T>G polymorphism of the interleukin-2 gene. Eur J Gastroenterol Hepatol 2008;20(9):855–9.
16. Marcos M, Pastor I, González-Sarmiento R, et al. A functional polymorphism of the NFKB1 gene increases the risk for alcoholic liver cirrhosis in patients with alcohol dependence. Alcohol Clin Exp Res 2009;33(11):1857–62.
17. To SE, Vega CP. Alcoholism and pathways to recovery: new survey results on views and treatment options. MedGenMed 2006;8(1):2.
18. D'Amico EJ, Paddock SM, Burnam A, et al. Identification of and guidance for problem drinking by general medical providers: results from a national survey. Med Care 2005;43(3):229–36.
19. Grucza RA, Przybeck TR, Cloninger CR. Screening for alcohol problems: an epidemiological perspective and implications for primary care. Mo Med 2008; 105(1):67–71.
20. U.S. Preventive Services Task Force. Screening and behavioral counseling inter-ventions in primary care to reduce alcohol misuse: recommendation statement. Ann Intern Med 2004;140(7):554–6.

21. Bush B, Shaw S, Cleary P, et al. Screening for alcohol abuse using the CAGE questionnaire. Am J Med 1987;82(2):231–5.

22. Ewing JA. Detecting alcoholism. The CAGE questionnaire. JAMA 1984;252(14): 1905–7.

23. Bradley KA, Bush KR, McDonell MB, et al. Screening for problem drinking: comparison of CAGE and AUDIT. Ambulatory Care Quality Improvement Project (ACQUIP). Alcohol use disorders identification test. J Gen Intern Med 1998; 13(6):379–88.

24. Bradley KA, Boyd-Wickizer J, Powell SH, et al. Alcohol screening questionnaires in women: a critical review. JAMA 1998;280(2):166–71.

25. Saunders JB, Aasland OG, Babor TF, et al. Development of the alcohol use disorders identification test (AUDIT): WHO collaborative project on early detection of persons with harmful alcohol consumption—II. Addiction 1993;88(6):791–804.

26. Steinbauer JR, Cantor SB, Holzer CE 3rd, et al. Ethnic and sex bias in primary care screening tests for alcohol use disorders. Ann Intern Med 1998;129(5):353–62.

27. Kriston L, Holzel L, Weiser AK, et al. Meta-analysis: are 3 questions enough to detect unhealthy alcohol use? Ann Intern Med 2008;149(12):879–88.

28. Frank D, DeBenedetti AF, Volk RJ, et al. Effectiveness of the AUDIT-C as a screening test for alcohol misuse in three race/ethnic groups. J Gen Intern Med 2008;23(6):781–7.

29. Altamirano J, Bataller R, Cardenas A, et al. Predictive factors of abstinence in patients undergoing liver transplantation for alcoholic liver disease. Ann Hepatol 2012;11(2):213–21.

30. Babineaux MJ, Anand BS. General aspects of the treatment of alcoholic hepatitis. World J Hepatol 2011;3(5):125–9.

31. Tan HH, Virmani S, Martin P. Controversies in the management of alcoholic liver disease. Mt Sinai J Med 2009;76(5):484–98.

32. Lucey MR. Management of alcoholic liver disease. Clin Liver Dis 2009;13(2): 267–75.

33. Johnson BA. Medication treatment of different types of alcoholism. Am J Psychiatry 2010;167(6):630–9.

34. Miller WR, Walters ST, Bennett ME. How effective is alcoholism treatment in the United States? J Stud Alcohol 2001;62(2):211–20.

35. Kaner EF, Dickinson HO, Beyer F, et al. The effectiveness of brief alcohol interventions in primary care settings: a systemic review. Drug Alcohol Rev 2009; 28(3):301–23.

36. Swift RM. Drug therapy for alcohol dependence. N Engl J Med 1999;340(19): 1482–90.

37. Finney JW, Hahn AC, Moos RH. The effectiveness of inpatient and outpatient treatment for alcohol abuse: the need to focus on mediators and moderators of setting effects. Addiction 1996;91(12):1773–96.

38. Shen ML, Lipsky JJ, Naylor S. Role of disulfiram in the in vitro inhibition of rat liver mitochondrial aldehyde dehydrogenase. Biochem Pharmacol 2000;60(7): 947–53.

39. Kershenobich D, Corona DL, Kershenovich R, et al. Management of alcoholic liver disease: an update. Alcohol Clin Exp Res 2011;35(5):804–5.

40. Johnson BA. Update on neuropharmacological treatments for alcoholism: scientific basis and clinical findings. Biochem Pharmacol 2008;75(1):34–56.

41. Snyder JL, Bowers TG. The efficacy of acamprosate and naltrexone in the treatment of alcohol dependence: a relative benefits analysis of randomized controlled trials. Am J Drug Alcohol Abuse 2008;34(4):449–61.

42. Hammarberg A, Nylander I, Zhou Q, et al. The effect of acamprosate on alcohol craving and correlation with hypothalamic pituitary adrenal (HPA) axis hormones and beta-endorphin. Brain Res 2009;1305(Suppl):S2–6.
43. Bouza C, Angeles M, Munoz A, et al. Efficacy and safety of naltrexone and acamprosate in the treatment of alcohol dependence: a systemic review. Addiction 2004;99(7):811–28.
44. Addolorato G, Leggio L, Ferrulli A, et al. Effectiveness and safety of Baclofen for maintenance of alcohol abstinence in alcohol-dependent patients with liver cirrhosis; randomized, double-blind controlled study. Lancet 2007;370(9603):1915–22.
45. Kenna GA, Lomastro TL, Schiesl A, et al. Review of topiramate: an antiepileptic for the treatment of alcohol dependence. Curr Drug Abuse Rev 2009;2(2):135–42.
46. Johnson BA, Ait-Daoud N, Bowden CL, et al. Oral topiramate for treatment of alcohol dependence: a randomized controlled trial. Lancet 2003;361(9370):1677–85.
47. Johnson BA, Rosenthal N, Capece JA, et al. Topiramate for treating alcohol dependence: a randomized controlled trial. JAMA 2007;298(14):1641–51.
48. Shank RP, Gardocki JF, Streeter AJ, et al. An overview of the preclinical aspects of topiramate: pharmacology, pharmacokinetics, and mechanism of action. Epilepsia 2000;41(Suppl 1):S3–9.
49. Johnson BA, Ait-Daoud N, Seneviratne C, et al. Pharmacogenetic approach at the serotonin transporter gene as a method of reducing the severity of alcohol drinking. Am J Psychiatry 2011;168(3):265–75.
50. Edward S, Kenna GA, Swift RM, et al. Current and promising pharmacotherapies, and novel research target areas in the treatment of alcohol dependence: a review. Curr Pharm Des 2011;17(14):1323–32.
51. Gramenzi A, Caputo F, Biselli M, et al. Review article: alcoholic liver disease—pathophysiological aspects and risk factors. Aliment Pharmacol Ther 2006;24(8):1151–61.
52. DiCecco SR, Francisco-Ziller N. Nutrition in alcoholic liver disease. Nutr Clin Pract 2006;21(3):245–54.
53. Griffith CM, Schenker S. The role of nutritional therapy in alcoholic liver disease. Alcohol Res Health 2006;29(4):296–306.
54. Muller MJ, Lautz HU, Plogmann B, et al. Energy expenditure and substrate oxidation in patients with cirrhosis: the impact of cause, clinical staging and nutritional state. Hepatology 1992;15(5):782–94.
55. Mendenhall C, Roselle GA, Gartside P, et al. Relationship of protein calorie malnutrition to alcoholic liver disease: a reexamination of data from two Veterans Administration cooperative studies. Alcohol Clin Exp Res 1995;19(3):635–41.
56. Halsted CH. Nutrition and alcoholic liver disease. Semin Liver Dis 2004;24(3):289–304.
57. McClain CJ, Barve SS, Barve A, et al. Alcoholic liver disease and malnutrition. Alcohol Clin Exp Res 2011;35(5):815–20.
58. Hirsch S, de la Maza MP, Gattas V, et al. Nutritional support in alcoholic cirrhotic patients improves host defenses. J Am Coll Nutr 1999;18(5):434–41.
59. Swart GR, Zillikens MC, van Vuure JK, et al. Effect of late evening meal on nitrogen balance in patients with cirrhosis of the liver. BMJ 1989;200(6709):1202–3.
60. Verboeket-van de Venne WP, Westerp KR, van Hoek B, et al. Energy expenditure and substrate metabolism in patients with cirrhosis of the liver: effects of the pattern of food intake. Gut 1995;36(1):110–6.

61. O'Shea RS, Dasarathy S, McCullough AJ, et al. AASLD practice guidelines: alcoholic liver disease. Hepatology 2010;51(1):307–28.

62. Phillips M, Curtis H, Portmann B, et al. Antioxidants versus corticosteroids in the treatment of severe alcoholic hepatitis—a randomized clinical trial. J Hepatol 2006;44(4):784–90.

63. Stewart S, Prince M, Bassendine M, et al. A randomized trial of antioxidant therapy alone or with corticosteroids in acute alcoholic hepatitis. J Hepatol 2007;47(2):277–83.

64. Day CP. Treatment of alcoholic liver disease. Liver Transpl 2007;13(11 Suppl 2): S69–75.

65. Assimakoupoulos SF, Thomopoulos KC, Labropoulou-Karatza C. Pentoxifylline: a first line treatment option for severe alcoholic hepatitis and hepatorenal syndrome? World J Gastroenterol 2009;15(25):3194–5.

66. Akriviadis E, Botla R, Briggs W, et al. Pentoxifylline improves short-term survival in severe acute alcoholic hepatitis: a double-blind, placebo-controlled trial. Gastroenterology 2000;119(6):1637–48.

67. McCullough AJ, O'Shea RS, Dasarathy S. Diagnosis and management of alcoholic liver disease. J Dig Dis 2011;12(4):257–62.

68. Bergheim I, McClain CJ, Arteel GE. Treatment of alcoholic liver disease. Dig Dis 2005;23(3–4):275–84.

69. Orrego H, Blake JE, Blendis LM, et al. Long-term treatment of alcoholic liver disease with propylthiouracil. N Engl J Med 1987;317(23):1421–7.

70. Rambaldi A, Iaquinto G, Gluud C. Anabolic androgenic steroids for alcoholic liver disease: a Cochrane review. Am J Gastroenterol 2002;97(7): 1674–81.

71. Rambaldi A, Gluud C. Colchicine for alcoholic and nonalcoholic liver fibrosis and cirrhosis. Cochrane Database Syst Rev 2005;(2):CD002148.

72. Morgan TR, Weiss DG, Nemchausky B, et al. Colchicine treatment of alcoholic cirrhosis: a randomized, placebo-controlled clinical trial of patient survival. Gastroenterology 2005;128(4):882–90.

73. Kershenobich D, Vargas F, Garcia-Tsao G, et al. Colchicine in the treatment of cirrhosis of the liver. N Engl J Med 1988;318(26):1709–13.

74. Morgan TR, Nemchausky N, Schiff ER, et al. Colchicine does not prolong life in patients with advanced alcoholic cirrhosis: results of a prospective, randomized, placebo-controlled, multicenter VA trial [abstract]. Gastroenterology 2002;122:641.

75. Cortez-Pinto H, Alexandrino P, Camilo ME, et al. Lack of effect of colchicines in alcoholic cirrhosis: final results of a double blind randomized trial. Eur J Gastroenterol Hepatol 2002;14(4):377–81.

76. Lee TD, Sadda MR, Mendler MH, et al. Abnormal hepatic methionine and glutathione metabolism in patients with alcoholic hepatitis. Alcohol Clin Exp Res 2004;28(1):173–81.

77. Mato JM, Camara J, Fernandez de Paz J, et al. S-adenosylmethionine in alcoholic liver cirrhosis: a randomized, placebo-controlled, double-blind, multicenter clinical trial. J Hepatol 1999;30(6):1081–9.

78. Rambaldi A, Gluud C. S-Adenosyl-l-methionine for alcoholic liver diseases. Cochrane Database Syst Rev 2006;(2):CD002235.

79. McClain CJ, Hill DB, Song Z, et al. S-adenosylmethionine, cytokines, and alcoholic liver disease. Alcohol 2002;27(3):185–92.

80. Meister A. Glutathione metabolism and its selective modification. J Biol Chem 1988;263(33):17205–8.

81. Pena LR, Hill DB, McClain CJ. Treatment with glutathione precursor decreases cytokine activity. JPEN J Parenter Enteral Nutr 1999;23(1):1–6.
82. Rambaldi A, Jacobs BP, Gluud C. Milk thistle for alcoholic and/or hepatitis B or C virus liver diseases. Cochrane Database Syst Rev 2007;(4):CD003620.
83. Rambaldi A, Jacobs BP, Iaquinto G, et al. Milk thistle for alcoholic and/or hepatitis B or C liver diseases—a systematic cochrane hepato-biliary group review with meta-analyses of randomized clinical trials. Am J Gastroenterol 2005; 100(11):2583–91.
84. Kirpich IA, Solovieva NV, Leikhter SN, et al. Probiotics restore bowel flora and improve liver enzymes in human alcohol-induced liver injury: a pilot study. Alcohol 2008;42(8):675–82.
85. Lata J, Jurankova J, Kopacova M, et al. Probiotics in hepatology. World J Gastroenterol 2011;17(24):2890–6.
86. Forsyth CB, Farhadi A, Jakate SM, et al. Lactobacillus GG treatment ameliorates alcohol-induced intestinal oxidative stress, gut leakiness, and liver injury in a rat model of alcoholic steatohepatitis. Alcohol 2009;43(2):163–72.
87. Gluud C. Testosterone and alcoholic cirrhosis. Epidemiologic, pathophysiologic, and therapeutic studies in men. Dan Med Bull 1988;35(6):564–75.
88. Woerdeman J, de Ronde W. Therapeutic effects of anabolic androgenic steroids on chronic diseases associated with muscle wasting. Expert Opin Investig Drugs 2011;20(1):87–97.
89. Rambaldi A, Gluud C. Anabolic-androgenic steroids for alcoholic liver disease. Cochrane Database Syst Rev 2006;(4):CD003045.
90. Friedman LS. Surgery in the patient with liver disease. Trans Am Clin Climatol Assoc 2010;121:192–204.
91. Garrison RN, Cryer HM, Howard DA, et al. Clarification of risk factors for abdominal operations in patients with hepatitis cirrhosis. Ann Surg 1984;199(6):648–55.
92. Mansour A, Watson W, Shayani V, et al. Abdominal operations in patients with cirrhosis: still a major surgical challenge. Surgery 1997;122(4):730–5.
93. Teh SH, Nagorney DM, Stevens SR, et al. Risk factors for mortality after surgery in patients with cirrhosis. Gastroenterology 2007;132(4):1261–9.
94. Lucena MI, Andrade RJ, Tognoni G, et al. Multicenter hospital study on prescribing patterns for prophylaxis and treatment of complications of cirrhosis. Eur J Clin Pharmacol 2002;58(6):435–40.
95. Powell WJ, Klatskin G. Duration and survival in patients with Laennec's cirrhosis. Influence of alcohol withdrawal, and possible effects of recent changes in general management of the disease. Am J Med 1968;44(3):406–20.
96. de Franchis R. Updating consensus in portal hypertension: report of the Baveno III consensus workshop on definitions, methodology and therapeutic strategies in portal hypertension. J Hepatol 2000;33(5):846–52.
97. Garcia-Tsao G, Sanyal AJ, Grace ND, et al. AASLD practice guidelines: prevention and management of gastroesophageal varices and variceal hemorrhage in cirrhosis. Hepatology 2007;46(3):922–38.
98. Sanyal AJ, Freedman AM, Luketic VA, et al. Transjugular intrahepatic portosystemic shunts for patients with active variceal hemorrhage unresponsive to sclerotherapy. Gastroenterology 1996;111(1):138–46.
99. McCormick PA, Dick R, Panagou EB, et al. Emergency transjugular intrahepatic portosystemic stent shunting as a salvage treatment for uncontrolled variceal hemorrhage. Br J Surg 1994;81(9):1324–7.
100. Gines P, Quintero E, Arroyo V, et al. Compensated cirrhosis: natural history and prognostic factors. Hepatology 1987;7(1):122–8.

101. Runyon BA. Ascites and spontaneous bacterial peritonitis. In: Feldman M, Friedman LS, Sleisenger MH, editors. Sleisenger and Fordtran's gastrointestinal and liver disease. 7th edition. Philadelphia: Saunders; 2002. p. 1517–42.
102. Runyon BA. AASLD practice guideline: management of adult patients with ascites due to cirrhosis. Hepatology 2004;39(3):841–56.
103. Starr SP, Raines D. Cirrhosis: diagnosis, management, and prevention. Am Fam Physician 2011;84(12):1353–9.
104. Schafer DF, Jones EA. Hepatic encephalopathy. In: Zakim D, Boyer TD, editors. Hepatology. A textbook of liver disease. Philadelphia: W. B. Saunders; 1990. p. 447–60.
105. de Melo RT, Charneski L, Hilas O. Rifaximin for the treatment of hepatic encephalopathy. Am J Health Syst Pharm 2008;65(9):818–22.
106. Fitz G. Hepatic encephalopathy, hepatopulmonary syndrome, coagulopathy and other complications of chronic liver disease. In: Feldman M, Friedman LS, Sleisenger MH, editors. Sleisenger and Fordtran's gastrointestinal and liver disease. 7th edition. Philadelphia: Saunders; 2002.
107. Schiano TD. Complications of chronic liver disease. In: Friedman S, Grendell J, McQuaid K, editors. Current diagnosis and treatment in gastroenterology. 2nd edition. Lange Current Series. USA: McGraw-Hill Companies; 2002. p. 639–63.
108. Blei AT, Córdoba J. Hepatic encephalopathy. Am J Gastroenterol 2001;96(7):1968–76.
109. Abou-Assi S, Vlahcevic ZR. Hepatic encephalopathy. Metabolic consequence of cirrhosis often is reversible. Postgrad Med 2001;109(2):52–4.
110. Arroyo V, Ginès P, Gerbes AL, et al. Definition and diagnostic criteria of refractory ascites and hepatorenal syndrome in cirrhosis. International Ascites Club. Hepatology 1996;23(1):164–76.
111. Magan AA, Khalil AA, Ahmed MH. Terlipressin and hepatorenal syndrome: what is important for nephrologists and hepatologists. World J Gastroenterol 2010;16(41):5139–47.
112. Garcia-Tsao G, Lim JK, Members of Veterans Affairs Hepatitis C Resource Center Program. Management and treatment of patients with cirrhosis and portal hypertension: recommendations from the Department of Veterans Affairs hepatitis C Resource Center program and the national hepatitis C program. Am J Gastroenterol 2009;104(7):1802–29.
113. Ginès P, Guevara M, Arroyo V, et al. Hepatorenal syndrome. Lancet 2003;362(9398):1819–27.
114. Bruix J, Sherman M. AASLD practice guideline: management of hepatocellular carcinoma. Hepatology 2005;42(5):1208–36.
115. Hassan MM, Hwang LY, Hatten CJ, et al. Risk factors for hepatocellular carcinoma: synergism of alcohol with viral hepatitis and diabetes mellitus. Hepatology 2002;36(5):1206–13.
116. Schoniger-Hekele M, Muller C, Kutilek M, et al. Hepatocellular carcinoma in Austria: aetiological and clinical characteristics at presentation. Eur J Gastroenterol Hepatol 2000;12(8):941–8.
117. Zhang BH, Yang BH, Tang ZY. Randomized controlled trial of screening for hepatocellular carcinoma. J Cancer Res Clin Oncol 2004;130(7):417–22.
118. Trevisani F, De NS, Rapaccini G, et al. Semiannual and annual surveillance of cirrhotic patients for hepatocellular carcinoma: effects on cancer stage and patient survival (Italian experience). Am J Gastroenterol 2002;97(3):734–44.
119. López-Larramona G, Lucendo AJ, González-Castillo S, et al. Hepatic osteodystrophy: an important matter for consideration in chronic liver disease. World J Hepatol 2011;3(12):300–7.

120. Gonzalez-Reimers E, Alvisa-Negrin J, Santolaria-Fernandez F, et al. Vitamin D and nutritional status are related to bone fractures in alcoholics. Alcohol Alcohol 2011;46(2):148–55.
121. Bhagat V, Mindikoglu AL, Nudo CG, et al. Outcomes of liver transplantation in patients with cirrhosis due to nonalcoholic steatohepatitis versus patients with cirrhosis due to alcoholic liver disease. Liver Transpl 2009;15(12):1814–20.
122. Berlakovich GA. Wasting your organ with your lifestyle and receiving a new one? Ann Transplant 2005;10(1):38–43.
123. Lucey MR. Liver transplantation in patients with alcoholic liver disease. Liver Transpl 2011;17(7):751–9.
124. Vaillant GE. A 60-year follow-up of alcoholic men. Addiction 2003;98(8):1043–51.
125. Burra P, Senzolo M, Adam R, et al. Liver transplantation for alcoholic liver disease in Europe: a study from the ELTR (European Liver Transplant Registry). Am J Transplant 2010;10(1):138–48.
126. Watt KD, Pedersen RA, Kremers WK, et al. Evolution of causes and risk factors for mortality post-liver transplant: results of the NIDDK long-term follow-up study. Am J Transplant 2010;10(6):1420–7.

Infections in Alcoholic Liver Disease

Angela C. Kim, MD[a],*, Marcia E. Epstein, MD[a],
Pranisha Gautam-Goyal, MD[a], Thien-Ly Doan, PharmD[b]

KEYWORDS

- Alcoholism • Lung abscess • Spontaneous bacterial peritonitis • Tuberculosis
- *Klebsiella pneumoniae* • *Bartonella quintana* • *Vibrio vulnificus*
- *Capnocytophaga canimorus*

KEY POINTS

- Alcoholic individuals are at increased risk of infection by its direct effects in altering immune parameters. Alcohol may also result in depressed mental status with aspiration leading to lung abscess and empyema.
- Both community acquired infections and specific syndromes occur with increased frequency among alcoholics.
- Social and behavioral factors often linked to alcoholism such as hygiene and living situations may predispose to infection with hepatitis B and/or C viruses, HIV, *Mycobacterium tuberculosis*, and *Bartonella quintana*.
- Infection with specific pathogens such as *Vibrio vulnificus*, *Capnocytophaga canimorus* and Rickettsiae, occur with increased morbidity and mortality among alcoholics.
- Depending on degree of liver dysfunction due to alcohol, certain antimicrobial agents require dosage adjustments.

INTRODUCTION

Patients with alcoholic liver disease are predisposed to infections for a multitude of reasons. The main reasons include the altered immune parameters in the chronic alcoholic patient; altered mental status and increased risk of aspiration of oropharyngeal contents; the development of cirrhosis and its infectious complications; and the altered social and behavioral factors in the alcoholic patient, which can be associated with unfavorable living situations, poor oral and general hygiene, poor nutrition, and risky sexual practices. These social and behavioral factors predispose to coinfections with hepatitis B and C, HIV, sexually transmitted infections, tuberculosis, and trench

Disclosures: None.
[a] Department of Medicine, North Shore LIJ Health System, Division of Infectious Disease, 400 Community Drive, Manhasset, NY 11030, USA; [b] Pharmacy Department, Long Island Jewish Medical Center, 270-05 76th Avenue, New Hyde Park, NY 11040, USA
* Corresponding author.
E-mail address: akim@nshs.edu

fever. Finally, even mild to moderate alcohol consumption can affect iron homeostasis and has been associated with iron overload, which itself predisposes to infections. **Box 1** outlines some of the clinical syndromes and associated pathogens known to occur with increased frequency in alcoholic individuals.

CLINICAL SYNDROMES BY ORGAN SYSTEM
Respiratory Tract

Local host defenses of the upper respiratory tract help to avoid infection of the lungs. Some mechanisms include ciliated epithelial cells that can contain and clear organisms,

---

Box 1
Infections by syndrome (*pathogens*)

Pulmonary

Streptococcus anginosis pulmonary infections

Community acquired pneumonia: *Staphylococcus aureus, Acinetobacter* sp, *Klebsiella pneumonia*

Nosocomial pneumonia

Bacterial lung abscess

Chronic pneumonia

Viridans streptococcal community-acquired pneumonia and empyema

Anaerobic lung infections: *Bacteroides* sp, *Prevotella* sp, *Porphyromonas* sp, *Fusobacterium* sp

Actinobacillus sp and *Aggregatibacter* sp Infections: pulmonary infections, endocarditis

Mycobacteria tuberculosis: including military tuberculosis

Cardiovascular

Endocarditis: *Streptococcal agalactiae, Actinobacillus* sp, and *Aggregatibacter* sp, *Capnocytophaga canimorus, Bartonella quintana*

Gastrointestinal

Spontaneous bacterial peritonitis

Infected pancreatic pseudocyst

Nervous System

Meningitis: *Staphylococcus aureus, Haemophilus influenza, Streptococcus agalactiae, Listeria monocytogenes*

Spinal epidural abscess

Balamuthiasis (amebic)

Systemic

Postsplenectomy sepsis: "functional hyposplenism," *Haemophilus influenza*, pneumococcus, meningococcus, *Capnocytophaga canimorus*, severe salmonellosis

Streptococcal toxic shock syndrome

Vibrio vulnificus

Rickettsioses

Skin

Vibrio vulnificus

coughing or ingestion of organisms, and secretory immunoglobulin (Ig)A antibodies.[1] Any barrier to this process may predispose to infection of the lung. Alcohol, by altering level of consciousness, can diminish epiglottic closure and cough reflexes, increasing risk of aspiration of oral flora, thereby predisposing to pneumonia and its complications of lung abscess and empyema. Impaired neutrophilic mobilization and cytokine response aggravate this process.[1] Alcoholic individuals also tend to be colonized in the oropharynx with more virulent organisms including *Klebsiella pneumoniae, Pseudomonas aeruginosa,* and *Enterobacter* species.[1]

Community-acquired pneumonia

Acute community-acquired pneumonia (CAP) classically presents with fever, chills, pleuritic chest pain, and cough with mucopurulent sputum. A chest radiograph may show a lobar, multilobar, nodular, or interstitial pattern depending on the etiologic agent. *Streptococcus pneumoniae, Haemophilus influenza, Staphylococcus aureus,* including community-acquired *S aureus, Morexella catarrhalis,* and *Legionella* species are common causes of CAP.[1] Presentations are similar among alcoholic individuals and nondrinkers; however, an increased severity of infection as well as complications are more likely in the former.

Klebsiella pneumoniae has a particularly strong association with alcohol consumption and is responsible for 6.0% to 8.6% of all CAP.[2] Thirty-five percent to sixty-five percent of those dying of infection with this microorganism are alcoholic individuals.[3] Other comorbidities for *K pneumoniae* pneumonia include diabetes or severe chronic obstructive pulmonary disease (COPD). Although the prevalence is low, infections are more severe with a higher incidence of septic shock. Mortality rates are as high as 50% and approach 100% in those with associated alcoholism and bacteremia in spite of early and appropriate antibiotic therapy.[4]

The principal virulence factor that has been described for *K pneumoniae* is its polysaccharide capsule that is thought to elude phagocytosis. Other factors are variety of fimbrial types, including type 1 pili that are involved in adherence to host cells.

The sputum of *K pneumoniae* pneumonia appears thick, mucoid, and blood-tinged, referred to as "currant jelly" sputum, owing to marked inflammation and necrosis. Gram stain reveals short, plump gram-negative bacilli that are usually surrounded by a capsule that appears as a clear space.

All strains of *K pneumoniae* are intrinsically resistant to ampicillin. Therapeutic options for infections caused by non–multidrug-resistant strains include first-generation cephalosporins, penicillin/β-lactamase inhibitor combinations, trimethoprim-sulfamethoxazole, fluoroquinolones, and aminoglycosides. For multidrug-resistant strains, especially those expressing extended-spectrum β-lactamases, treatment options are often limited to carbapenems.

Lung abscess/empyema

When lung tissue necroses secondary to infection, a cavity is formed. A lung abscess most often occurs as a result of depressed consciousness and aspiration of contents from stomach or oral cavity including microorganisms or subsequent infection of the area. Poor oral hygiene may also increase risk of infection owing to higher bacterial load with or without more pathogenic organisms, such as *K pneumonia*. Other risk factors include extrinsic compression of the bronchial tree, intrinsic obstruction by tumor, and immunocompromised states. Bronchiectasis, secondarily infected pulmonary emboli, and right-sided endocarditis with septic emboli are other conditions that may lead to lung abscess.

Oral anaerobes, both-gram positive and gram-negative, cause most infections, including *Peptostreptococcus* spp, *Fusobacterium neucleatum*, and *Prevotella melaninogenica*.[5] Infection is often mixed; however, single organisms can also cause lung abscess which more often occur in the hospital setting or in otherwise immunosuppressed patients.

Typically, symptom onset is more subacute to chronic compared with CAP. Fever, sweats, productive cough, chest pain, and weight loss are common symptoms. Examination may reveal halitosis. Radiograph reveals cavitary infiltrate(s) with an air-fluid level and possible associated empyema. Expectorated sputum may not be helpful in microbiologic diagnosis, whereas bronchoalveolar lavage or protected brush specimens provide more accurate results. If lung abscess occurs in the absence of aspiration, seizure, or other period of diminished consciousness, other organisms to consider include *S aureus*, *Klebsiella* spp, *Pseudomonas* spp, and, of course *Mycobacterium tuberculosis*. In the immunocompromised population, *Aspergillus*, *Nocardia*, and *Rhodococcus* are possible culprits.[6]

If oral therapy is chosen, amoxicillin-clavulanate, clindamycin, or moxifloxacin are suggested. Clindamycin is preferred over metronidazole for anaerobic coverage. β-lactams with β-lactamase inhibitor, carbapenems, and fluoroquinolones with anaerobic activity are alternatives. Generally, several weeks of treatment are required with serial films. Rarely is surgical intervention indicated unless the abscess is large, infected with highly resistant pathogens or an underlying malignancy is the cause.[6] Empyema requires surgical drainage in conjunction with a prolonged antibiotic course of therapy.

Tuberculosis

An association between alcohol use and tuberculosis (TB) has been well documented. One study from the 1950s found that the risk of active pulmonary tuberculosis was significantly more prevalent in alcoholic individuals then the general population.[7] In the 1980s, Friedman and colleagues[8] reported a prevalence of tuberculosis of 46 times higher in people with alcohol use disorders (who did not use other drugs) in New York.

Possible explanations for increased tuberculosis in this population are likely attributable to a combination of social factors and immune disorders related to alcohol use. Specifically, social mixing patterns of alcoholic individuals may increase the risk of exposure others with infectious TB in settings such as shelters for the homeless, prisons, social institutions, and bars.[9,10] Animal studies demonstrate that alcohol has a direct toxic effect on the immune system. Studies suggest that some of the changes in cell-mediated immunity seen in alcoholic individuals are more pronounced because of malnutrition.[11]

Clinical response to treatment does not seem to differ among alcoholic individuals but the compliance rate among alcohol users can be a major issue. In one study, as a result of inability to complete a treatment course, alcoholic individuals had a twofold to threefold higher relapse rate than nonalcoholic individuals.[12] The failure to complete a course of therapy and intermittent compliance can lead to the development of multiple drug-resistant strains of tuberculosis. Therefore, it is recommended that these patients be monitored very closely for compliance and tolerance of the medications, such as through directly observed therapy on a daily or intermittent basis through the Department of Health. Finally, all alcoholic individuals should be monitored for the risk of reactivation and should receive testing to demonstrate prior exposure to TB and should receive isoniazid prophylaxis with vitamin B6, if they test positive. These patients need to be carefully monitored for both compliance and tolerance, especially monitoring of liver enzymes to avoid drug-induced hepatitis.[13]

Cardiovascular System

Endocarditis

In general, alcoholic individuals are not necessarily more prone to endocarditis; however, because of a combination of immunodeficiencies from the alcoholism or because of social and lifestyle situations, alcoholic individuals are at increased risk of certain microbiologic etiologies of endocarditis. In particular, 3 microorganisms are more highly associated with endocarditis in alcoholic individuals: *Pneumococcus*, *Bartonella quintana*, and *Capnocytophaga* spp.

Pneumococcal endocarditis is a rare cause of endocarditis.[14,15] Alcoholism is considered one of the strongest risk factors for this illness. Patients usually develop pneumococcal endocarditis following pneumococcal infection elsewhere. The typical portal of entry is the lung, but the disease can occur after sinusitis, mastoiditis, otitis media, and tooth extraction.[14] Infection sometimes occurs in association with meningitis and pneumonia (Austrian's triad).[16] Pneumococcal endocarditis is an aggressive disease with rapid destruction of endothelial tissue. It can affect native or prosthetic valves and has a predilection for the aortic valve with a tendency toward the formation of large vegetations that can cause septic emboli.[14,17] An effective antibiotic regimen should be initiated as soon as possible. In view of increasing prevalence of penicillin-resistant pneumococcus, initial regimens should consist of a third-generation cephalosporin, with or without vancomycin (if strains fully resistant to penicillin are circulating) or the new-generation quinolones. Penicillin G sodium (12–24 million units/day) or a third-generation cephalosporin are effective therapy for penicillin-sensitive *S pneumoniae* (minimum inhibitory concentration <0.1 mg/mL).[18] Surgical management has a major role in the treatment of pneumococcal endocarditis. Finally, pneumococcal vaccination should be promoted in patients with a history of alcoholism.

Capnocytophaga canimorsus and *Capnocytophaga cynodegmi* are normal inhabitants of the oral cavity of dogs and cats. Most serious infections occur owing to *C. canimorsus* and are introduced via the bite of an animal or from inapparent introduction of the bacteria into abraded tissue via intimate contact with pets. This bacterium is known to cause fulminant sepsis in patients from dog bites, mostly in asplenic patients and in alcoholic individuals but is also an uncommon cause of endocarditis.[19] *Capnocytophaga* can cause an acute or subacute "culture-negative" endocarditis or myocarditis. Patients may have no history of cardiac pathology and typical symptoms, such as fever and heart murmur, may be absent. Blood cultures may be negative initially taking 7 days of incubation in CO_2 before visible growth is apparent. Susceptibility testing is difficult and standardized methods are not available. A variety of antibiotic regimens have successfully treated *C canimorsus* endocarditis. The organism is susceptible to many antimicrobial agents but has been known to produce a β-lactamase in some strains.

Bartonella quintana is another pathogen that may cause endocarditis in alcoholic individuals. *Bartonella* species are generally infectious agents of animals, and humans are incidental hosts in most situations. Transmission occurs through arthropod vectors.[20] *Bartonella* spp are small, fastidious, intracellular gram-negative organisms. The genus includes more than 15 distinct species of which 5 are felt to be capable of causing human disease.[21] The diagnosis of most *Bartonella* infections is made serologically. Unlike other members of the Rickettsial family, *Bartonella* spp can be cultured on cell-free media. Various forms of blood or chocolate agar will support their growth, and yield is improved with fresh media. Incubation often requires more than 7 days before growth occurs, usually at temperatures of 35° to 37°C under 5% to 10% CO_2 and greater than 40% humidity.

B quintana was identified as the cause of epidemic trench fever in Europe after World War I.[22] The descriptions of the clinical manifestations of this disease vary from one of an insidious onset to an abrupt-onset illness characterized by fever, malaise, headache, bone pain, and a transient macular rash. Patterns of fever range from a single fever, continuous fever for 5 to 7 days, and to recurrent febrile episodes recurring every 4 to 5 days.[22] The incubation period ranges from 5 to 20 days and is dependent on the inoculum size.[23]

In the mid 1990s, there were several articles describing clusters of *B quintana* bacteremia in the urban poor. Most patients were homeless, alcoholic men. The reason for this change in epidemiology remains unclear. A potential explanation may include availability of better techniques for microbiological detection of the organism. Other factors possibly involve changes in virulence within the bacterium and potential other vectors that influence the epidemiology. For *B quintana,* perhaps there are arthropod vectors other than lice and reservoirs, such as small rodents, that can be associated with the poor social conditions among this affected population.[24]

Diagnosis of bacterial endocarditis caused by *B quintana* remains challenging and presentation may be subacute with a significant proportion of the patients being afebrile at the time of presentation (17% in one study).[25] More than half of the patients have previous valvular disease and three-quarters of the patients require valvular surgery. Diagnosis in culture-negative cases is made with serology, DNA amplification from valvular tissues, and immunohistochemistry, or all 3. Treatment for *Bartonella* endocarditis is unclear, and antibiotic susceptibility does not necessarily predict in vivo response to therapy. A current accepted regimen include 6 weeks of doxycycline with 2 weeks of parental gentamicin at the beginning of the course.[25]

Gastrointestinal System

The direct and indirect effects of alcohol on infectious complications within the gastrointestinal system are wide ranging. Acute effects include pancreatitis and infected pancreatic pseudocyst, whereas the long-term consequence of alcohol on the liver and resulting cirrhosis can predispose to spontaneous bacterial peritonitis (SBP). Viral hepatitides may be particularly detrimental to the liver in the setting of alcoholism. Fortunately, not all effects of alcohol are detrimental. In fact, alcohol may be bactericidal to certain enteric infections.

Infected pancreatic pseudocyst

Acute and chronic pancreatitis is known to be associated with alcohol abuse, but interestingly only a small proportion of persons (10%–20%) who abuse alcohol develop symptomatic pancreatitis. Another 10% are attributed to hyperlipidemia, viral infection, drugs, hypercalcemia, ischemia, and 10% are idiopathic.[26]

Studies have suggested that viral infections are important cofactors for the development of alcoholic pancreatitis. A number of viruses have shown to infect the pancreas and induce acute and chronic pancreatitis such as Epstein-Barr virus, cytomegalovirus (CMV), mumps, coxsackie, rubella, HIV, and hepatitis A and B viruses. CMV has been shown to be important in the development of pancreatitis, especially in immunodeficient persons. Jerrells and colleagues[27] performed a study on mice infected with coxsackievirus B3-CO, showing that relatively short-term and chronic (ie, 6–8 weeks) ethanol consumption by mice resulted in a more severe pancreatitis mediated by a pancreas-specific virus (ie, CVB3-CO) in comparison with the pancreatitis in the appropriate control groups. This group found that ethanol consumption resulted in a continued inflammatory response that persisted after the infectious virus was no longer demonstrable in the pancreas. The chronic pancreatitis was clearly associated with the development of fibrosis in the pancreas, which was one of the key pathologic features of chronic pancreatitis.[27] The infection of pancreatic and peripancreatic tissue in severe acute pancreatitis occurs most frequently in patients with extensive pancreatic necrosis, beginning approximately 2 weeks after the onset of the disease, with mortality reaching 25% in cases of infected necrosis.[28] Another complication of acute pancreatitis is development of pseudocysts, which is associated with increased morbidity and mortality.

Infected pancreatic pseudocysts are more frequently polymicrobial (57%), whereas infected pancreatic necrosis is usually monomicrobial (43%).[29] The pathogens infecting the pancreas suggest an enteric origin in both conditions. Several mechanisms have been proposed to explain how these enteric bacteria reach the pancreas: (1) translocation of bacteria from the gut, (2) infection from the biliary tree or duodenum, and (3) hematogenous or lymphatic spread.[29]

The commonly isolated microorganisms in pancreatic infections include *Escherichia coli*, *Enterococcus* spp, *K pneumoniae*, and *Enterobacter* spp; less frequently *Staphylococcus* spp, *P aeruginosa*, *Streptococcus* spp, and *Bacteroides*.[29] Other organisms include *Citrobacter freundii*, *Escherichia fergusonii*, *Brucella maletiensis*, *M tuberculosis*, and *Candida albicans*.[30] There are case reports of pseudocyst infection and superinfection of necrotizing pancreatitis by *Achromobacter xylosoxidans*.[31]

The diagnosis of an infected pancreatic pseudocyst is based on clinical presentation, imaging modalities including computed tomography (CT) scan and, if possible, demonstration of infection by performance of a fine-needle aspiration. Because clinical presentation may be nonspecific, any patient with fever with signs or symptoms suggestive of sepsis should be assumed to have pancreatic infection in the context of pancreatic necrosis or pancreatic pseudocyst.

Appropriate antibiotic therapy should be initiated empirically. Intravenous administration of imipenem–cilastatin is currently recommended, and therapy should begin as soon as the diagnosis of acute necrotizing pancreatitis is made and should continue for at least 2 to 4 weeks.[32] Others include a combination of ceftazidime and clindamycin; a combination of ciprofloxacin and metronidazole.

In addition to antibiotics, definitive treatment often requires complete drainage of the pseudocyst and debridement of the necrotic tissue. Currently, three different approaches for primary drainage of a pancreatic pseudocyst and infected pancreatic necrosis include (1) CT-guided or ultrasound-guided percutaneous drainage, (2) transgastric or transduodenal endoscopic drainage, or (3) minimally invasive laparoscopy.[28]

Spontaneous bacterial peritonitis

SBP is an infection of ascitic fluid (AF) and a well-known complication in patients with cirrhosis, and its development is associated with a poor long-term prognosis. Although SBP has been described in different clinical settings, such as nephrotic syndrome or heart failure, most SBP episodes develop in patients with advanced cirrhosis secondary to altered hepatic function. Peritonitis is considered the most frequent infectious complication among patients with cirrhosis and ascites, making up 31% of all bacterial infections.[33]

Evaluation of ascitic fluid in SBP may reveal a positive bacterial culture and a polymorphonuclear cell count of 250 cells/mm^3 or more, in the absence of a surgically treatable intra-abdominal source of infection. Usually, infections are caused by one organism, and the growth of more than one organism should raise the suspicion of secondary peritonitis. More than 60% of cases of SBP are caused by gram-negative enteric bacteria. *E coli* and *K pneumoniae* are the organisms most frequently isolated. Gram-positive cocci account for approximately 25% of episodes. Anaerobes are infrequently isolated presumptively because of the high oxygen content of the intestinal wall and surrounding tissue and with the difficulty of the anaerobes to translocate across the intestinal mucosa.

The pathogenesis of SBP is complex. Essentially, individuals with cirrhosis often have intestinal bacterial overgrowth thought to be related to altered local IgA immune response and delayed intestinal transit.[33] The intestinal bacteria then can translocate across the mucosa, and, in escaping the intestines, spread to other tissues, including the bloodstream. Normally, the bacteria would be killed by the intestinal lymph nodes but there is altered immunity in patients with cirrhosis. Several humoral and cellular abnormalities have been described, including decreased complement, impaired chemotaxis, altered phagocytic function of neutrophils and altered macrophage function, and altered Kupffer cells (the stationary macrophages of the liver). Furthermore, the presence of intrahepatic and extrahepatic portosystemic shunts, as a result of portal hypertension, prevents circulating bacteria from interacting with the Kupffer cells. Finally, not all bacteria that invade the ascitic fluid cause SBP. Patients with cirrhosis may be capable of humoral self-defense, if the complement system is effective. It has been demonstrated, however, that when AF complement level is less than 13 mg/dL and/or AF protein level is less than 1 g/dL, there is an increased risk of infection.

Other factors that predispose patients with cirrhosis to SBP include Child-Pugh class C status (more than 70% are, the remainder being class B) and serum bilirubin higher than 2.5 mg/dL. An ascitic fluid total protein level lower than 1 g/dL is a risk factor for development of ascitic fluid infection, as it likely correlates with worsening complement and opsonic activity. Bacteriuria is common among patients with cirrhosis, particularly females and can also predispose to infection. These patients should be screened for urinary tract infections. Finally, patients with SBP are at a high risk for recurrence. Seventy-four percent are said to recur within 2 years.[33]

The clinical symptoms of SBP include fever (69%) and abdominal pain (59%). Patients do not generally develop a rigid abdomen, which is thought to be a result of the large volume of ascites that prevents contact of the viscera and parietal peritoneal surfaces to sufficiently elicit a rigid reflex. Other prominent signs and symptoms include hepatic encephalopathy, abdominal tenderness, diarrhea, ileus, shock, and hypothermia. Approximately 10% have no clinical symptoms or signs other than unexplained deterioration in status.

A diagnosis of SBP is suspected when the neutrophil count is higher than $250/mm^3$. Usually, about 10 mL per each 100-mL bottle is needed, and the use of blood culture bottles significantly increases the yield. The serum-ascites albumin gradient of greater than 1.1 g/dL is helpful in determining whether the patient has portal hypertension.[34] Other recommended tests in addition to cell count and fluid ascites include Gram stain, adenosine deaminase level, acid-fast bacilli smear and culture, ascites protein, and cytology. Other data with potential diagnostic utility includes pH, lactate dehydrogenase (LDH), glucose, and amylase.[35] Measurement of tumor necrosis factor α and interleukin 6 are possible useful markers for diagnosis and in monitoring response to treatment, although this is not standard practice.[36] In differentiating secondary peritonitis from SBP, the ascitic fluid analysis can be helpful. SBP tends to be monomicrobial more than 90% of the time.[37]

The treatment for SBP is usually empiric, based on the most likely pathogens. Gram stain of the fluid can sometimes help guide therapy, but usually antibiotics are modified only when culture and sensitivity results become available. If possible, aminoglycosides should be avoided to minimize the risk of nephrotoxicity. Usually, a third-generation cephalosporin, β-lactam/β-lactamase inhibitor combinations, carbapenems, or the newer quinolones are effective. Some of these choices may depend on the emergence of resistance pathogens in the patient's hospital, known colonization with resistant organisms, previous treatment or prophylaxis history, history of allergy to certain classes of antimicrobials, and cost. In cases in which there is a strong clinical suspicion of bacterial peritonitis but cultures are negative, antimicrobials should be continued and the ascitic fluid monitored for response (leukocyte count should decline in the fluid after 24–48 hours of antimicrobial therapy). The duration of therapy should be a minimum of 5 days.

Certain patients with cirrhosis have been identified at high risk for SBP. Risk factors include previous episode of SBP, AF protein levels lower than 1 g/dL, and those with gastrointestinal bleeding. Patients with an episode of SBP have a 1-year recurrence rate of 40% to 70%. Selective intestinal decontamination has been shown to lower the frequency of infections in these patients; however, there is concern about selecting out for more resistant infections and the development of complications of antibiotic use (Clostridium difficile, side effects, and so forth). Regimens include norfloxacin[38] and trimethoprim-sulfamethoxazole.[39] Prolonged antibiotic prophylaxis is generally limited to patients who have had one or more episodes of SBP. Prophylaxis should be used during acute events like gastrointestinal bleeds to minimize bacterial translocation and possible infection.

Coinfection viral hepatitis

Although it beyond the scope of this article to review the treatment options for hepatitis B and C, it is important to understand how alcohol abuse affects the rate of progression in patients with viral hepatitis. Mota and colleagues[40] investigated 298 patients chronically infected with hepatitis B in Portugal. Patients underwent HBV genotyping and liver biopsy and were graded by habits of alcohol intake (more or less than 20 g/day). A positive association was found between liver damage (by biopsy) and alcohol intake, increasing with age ($P<.001$). The differences were more pronounced in alcoholic women older than 45 and were unrelated to genotype. Studies have also demonstrated that heavy alcohol consumption in patients with hepatitis C has been associated with a more rapid progression to cirrhosis and to hepatocellular carcinoma (HCC). In addition, the evidence suggests that heavy alcohol use during treatment of hepatitis C with pegylated interferon adversely affects treatment effectiveness.[41] Even in patients who have stopped drinking, the response to interferon-alpha is less than that of nonalcoholic individuals.[42]

Oliveira and colleagues[43] demonstrated that in alcoholic individuals, without clinically evident cirrhosis, the response to hepatitis B vaccine was similar to nonalcoholic individuals. In view of the more rapid progression to cirrhosis and HCC in patients who are alcoholic and develop hepatitis B, vaccination to prevent hepatitis B is advocated for all alcoholic patients.

Enteric infections

Alcoholic beverages, especially wine, have been shown to have bactericidal effects on enteropathogenic bacteria, including Helicobacter pylori. Historical records show that during the Prussian war, wine was consumed to help prevent dysentery.[44] In 1988, Sheth and colleagues[45] conducted an in vitro study to determine the potential for survival of enteric pathogens in common drinking beverages (carbonated drinks, 2 alcoholic beverages: wine and beer, skim milk, and water). These beverages were inoculated with Salmonella, Shigella, and enterotoxigenic E coli and quantitative counts were performed over 2 days. The investigators showed the poorest survival of organisms in red wine, the effects of beer were inferior to those of wine. The greatest growth of organisms occurred in milk and water.

In recent years, an inverse correlation between alcohol consumption and the prevalence of H pylori infections has been established.[46] Red wine has been found to exert a more marked bactericidal effect on H pylori than other alcoholic beverages. Soleas and others[47] quantified the levels of various phenolic compounds (cis- and trans-resveratrol, gallic acid, caffeic acid, p-coumaric acid, vanillic acid, ferulic acid, and gentisic acid) in a number of red and white wines made in Ontario. Red wines contain much higher levels of many of these compounds. Phenolic extractions from wines have been shown to have marked antimicrobial activity and perhaps enhance the antimicrobial properties of the wine.[48]

Nervous System

There is a general perception that there is an increased risk of meningitis in alcoholic individuals than in the general population, but this has never been proven in a controlled study. Studies of patients with meningitis, however, show an overrepresentation of alcoholic individuals. In Carpenter and Petersdorf's series on meningitis, there were 118 adult patients, of whom 22% were alcoholic individuals; and of pneumococcal cases, 29% were alcoholic individuals.[49] In the classic review by Swartz and Dodge,[50] the mortality from meningitis was higher among alcoholic individuals than nondrinkers. In another series, alcoholic individuals represented a high proportion of E coli meningitis that occurred in patients without obvious cause (ie, trauma or neurosurgery). This was felt to be possibly related to the higher risk of "spontaneous" bacteremias in alcoholic individuals with liver disease.[51]

Listeria monocytogenes is also often linked to alcoholism. The organism is a facultative intracellular organism, and infection is controlled by macrophages and T-cell–mediated immunity. In a review of central nervous system listeriosis, alcoholism/liver disease was the third most common predisposing factor for developing Listeria meningitis, representing 13% of the cases outside of the neonatal period and pregnancy (malignancy 24%; transplantation 21%; alcoholism/liver disease 13%; immunosuppression/steroids for various reasons 11%; diabetes mellitus 8%; HIV/AIDS 7%; no risk factor 36%).[52] In contrast to other organisms that most commonly cause bacterial meningitis, L monocytogenes has a tropism for the brain stem causing encephalitis (rhomboencephalitis) and brain abscess. A surveillance study by the Centers for Disease Control and Prevention in the 1990s showed that L monocytogenes was the fifth most common cause of meningitis but had the highest mortality at 22%. A prospective study of Listeria meningitis reported headache in 88%, nausea in 83%, and fever in 90%, but only 75% of patients had a stiff neck. A focal neurologic defect was found in 37% of the patients. Only 28% of patients had a positive Gram stain but 46% had positive blood cultures.[53] In comparison with nondrinkers of culture-proven bacterial meningitis, alcoholic individuals more likely developed complications (82% vs 62%, P = .04) resulting in higher morbidity and mortality rates. Complications included cardiorespiratory failures owing to underlying pneumonia.[54]

A rare but fatal cause of encephalitis is infection caused by the amoeba, Balamuthia mandrillaris. This organism was first described in 1986, and there have only been 70 confirmed cases described in the United States. There is suspicion that this etiology is underrepresented secondary to misdiagnosis. B mandrillaris infects humans when organisms contaminating soil enter the body through skin cuts and wounds. Once inside the body, the amoebas can travel to the brain and cause Granulomatous amoebic encephalitis that is fatal in more than 95% of the cases. Several case reports of B mandrillaris infection have been reported in chronic alcoholism, suggesting a possible predisposition.[55]

Systemic Infections

Both acute alcohol ingestion and chronic alcohol abuse effect host immunity. Acutely, neutrophil adhesion, margination, and emigration are affected.[56] Chronically, cell-mediated immunity is affected at different levels. Lymphocyte proliferative response, monocyte production of proinflammatory cytokines, antibody-directed cellular cytotoxicity, and B-cell antibody-specific proliferation and production are all diminished.[56] Together, these events increase the chance of acquiring a variety of infections, and this group of patients is more at risk of developing sepsis and progressing to septic shock in comparison with nonalcoholic individuals.

Bacterial infections more commonly associated with the development of sepsis and septic shock in patients who abuse alcohol use in the setting of alcoholic liver disease with or without cirrhosis include the following pathogens: *Vibrio vulnificus*, *Capnocytophaga canimorsus*, *Bartonella quintana*, and *Rickettsia* spp.

Vibrio vulnificus

V vulnificus is a gram-negative bacterium that causes severe wound and skin/soft tissue infections, as well as septicemia. It is present in normal marine flora and can be isolated from virtually all oysters harvested in the Chesapeake Bay and the US Gulf Coast when water temperatures exceed 20°C.[57] *V vulnificus* is estimated to account for 90% of all seafood-related deaths in the United States. Wound infection with or without septicemia is preceded by exposure of wound to salt or brackish water contaminated with *V vulnificus* or consumption of contaminated raw oysters in most of the cases.[58]

A major virulence factor is its polysaccharide capsule that stimulates inflammatory cytokines and inhibits phagocytosis and opsonization. In chronic alcoholic individuals undergoing treatment for substance abuse, reduced levels of glutathione correlated with decreased cytokine production by peripheral blood mononuclear cells after exposure in vitro to *V vulnificus*.[59] Such a weak cytokine response likely contributes to the poor bloodstream clearance and resulting high frequency of bacteremia in *V vulnificus* infections. The organism's ability to cause infection in liver disease with iron overload is also because of its ability to sequester iron from hemoglobin and fully saturated transferrin and grow exponentially. The relationship between iron and virulence in *V vulnificus* may account for the enhanced susceptibility to serious infections with this pathogen in patients with hemochromatosis; however, most patients with serious *V vulnificus* infections have normal iron and iron saturation levels.[60]

V vulnificus is the most virulent of the noncholera vibrios species primarily associated with a severe, distinctive soft tissue infection and/or septicemia. In patients with cirrhosis, *V vulnificus* has the unique ability to invade the bloodstream without causing gastrointestinal symptoms.[57] Primary *V vulnificus* septicemia is a serious illness with a high mortality rate. Among all reported foodborne infections in the United States, *V vulnificus* is associated with the highest case fatality rate of 39%.[61]

Patients present with an abrupt onset of chills and fever, followed by hypotension and the development of metastatic cutaneous lesions within 36 hours after onset of symptoms. Skin involvement starts with erythematous lesions that rapidly evolve to hemorrhagic bullae or vesicles, **Fig. 1**, and then to necrotic ulcerations. *V vulnificus* bacteremia is fatal in more than 50% of patients in whom this syndrome has been identified, including 100% of patients with hypotension.[62]

In skin and soft tissue, infection begins after contamination of a superficial wound by warm seawater. The cellulitis can be mild or rapidly develop into an intense cellulitis, necrotizing vasculitis, and ulcerative process in both healthy persons and

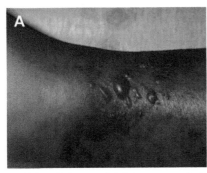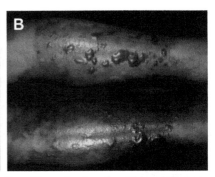

Fig. 1. (A) Cellulitis and (B) hemorrhagic bullae. (*From* Centers for Disease Control and Prevention [CDC]. Vibrio illnesses after Hurricane Katrina—multiple states, August–September, 2005. MMWR Morb Mortal Wkly Rep 2005;54:928–31; with permission.)

compromised hosts.[57] In high-risk individuals, the infection may produce severe myositis and fasciitis.

V vulnificus grows readily on MacConkey agar and the more selective thiosulfate-citrate-bile-sucrose medium. Final identification is made by standard biochemical tests. A real-time quantitative polymerase chain reaction (PCR) assay has been developed to detect the *ToxR* of *V vulnificus*, a gene encoding a transmembrane DNA binding regulatory protein in *Vibrio* species.

Mortality was lowest for bacteremic patients initiated on antibiotics within 24 hours of onset of illness but was still unacceptably as high as 33%.[62] Mild wound infections in patients who do not have significant underlying diseases generally respond well to local care and oral antibiotics, such as tetracyclines or fluoroquinolones. In high-risk patients, more serious wound infections may require aggressive debridement in addition to parenteral antibiotics with either a third-generation cephalosporin plus minocycline, or ciprofloxacin with or without minocycline, which had lower mortality rates than those who received a third-generation cephalosporin alone. Combination therapy applies to patients with septicemia as well (either minocycline or doxycycline [100 mg orally twice daily] plus either cefotaxime [2 g intravenously every 8 hours] or ceftriaxone [1 g intravenously daily]) with appropriate dosing adjustment for underlying renal or hepatic disease.[63] A reasonable alternative is levofloxacin (500 mg orally or intravenously once daily).

Patients with underlying liver disease and other chronic illnesses should avoid ingestion of raw oysters. At present, thorough cooking of seafood remains the only effective means of prevention.[64]

Capnocytophaga canimorus

Capnocytophaga species are fusiform, fastidious, gram-negative bacilli found in the oral cavity of humans and dogs. In humans, species include *Capnocytophaga ochracea* (cause of most infections), *Capnocytophaga gingivalis*, *Capnocytophaga sputigena*, *Capnocytophaga haemolytica*, and *Capnocytophaga granulose*. And in dogs, *C canimorus* (Latin for dog bite) and *Capnocytophaga cynodegmi* (Greek for dog bite) are the predominant species encountered.[65] *Capnocytophaga* translates to "eater of carbon dioxide" as the pathogens are facultatively anaerobic.[66] *C canimorus* was originally called DF-2 for dysgenic fermenter (slow growth and fermentation of carbohydrates). To identify organisms in clinical specimens, blood cultures should be CO2 enriched 5% or 10% and possibly with heart infusion agar with rabbit or sheep blood and incubated 5 to 7 days.[65]

In general, patients without evidence of immune system defects present with cellulitis or wound infection, periodontitis, bacteremia, endocarditis, keratitis, subphrenic abscess, empyema, septic arthritis, cervical and inguinal lymphadenitis, sinusitis, thyroiditis, osteomyelitis, peritonitis, abdominal abscess, or peripartum infection.[65] However, alcoholism has been identified as a risk factor for septicemia caused by *C canimorus*.[67,68] A review by Kullberg and colleagues[67] noted that 33% of patients were asplenic and 22% had an associated alcohol history. Other syndromes associated with the reviewed septicemic patients include brain abscess, endocarditis, meningitis, acute respiratory distress syndrome, pneumonia, and wound necrosis.[67] Both splenectomy and corticosteroid use contributed to the development of septicemia from *C canimorus*.[67] In the review by Pers and colleagues,[68] 7 of 39 subjects with septicemia from *C canimorus* were alcoholic individuals. One patient was caring for a dog and 5 owned dogs; however, 7 had no exposure at all.[68] In this series, disseminated intravascular coagulation (DIC) occurred in 14 of the patients; 5 patients developed meningitis and 1 endocarditis. Unfortunately, 12 (31%) patients actually died of infection.[68] Physical examination may reveal an eschar or gangrene at the site of bite. Chest imaging may show pulmonary infiltrates.

In mild infections, amoxicillin-clavulanate is the drug of choice owing to increasing β-lactamase production. Penicillins, imipenem, erythromycin, vancomycin, clindamycin, cephalosporins, chloramphenicol, tetracyclines, and fluoroquinolones can all be used for treatment. There is resistance to aztreonam, and both aminoglycosides and trimethoprim-sulfamethoxizole are less reliable.[65,67] There is some suggestion that in severe, fulminant infections with DIC, there may be efficacy in adjunctive plasmapheresis, leukopheresis, or complete blood exchange.[67] Prophylactic penicillin after dog bite is suggested.

Bartonella quintana
Reviewed in section on endocarditis.

Rickettsioses
Rickettsiae are small gram-negative bacteria associated with arthropods (**Fig. 2**). Alcoholism is a risk factor for more serious outcomes of some of the rickettsial infections especially Rocky Mountain Spotted Fever (RMSF) caused by *Rickettsia rickettsii*, epidemic typhus caused by *Rickettsia prowazekii*, and Boutonneuse fever caused by

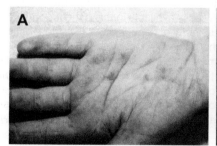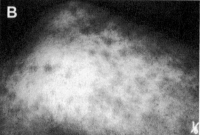

Fig. 2. (*A*) The wrist and palm manifest the rash of Rocky Mountain Spotted Fever with central petechiae in some of the maculopapules. (*B*) Early petechial rash on arm. (*From* Walker DH. *Rickettsia rickettsii* and other spotted fever group Rickettsiae (Rocky Mountain Spotted Fever and other spotted fevers). In: Mandell GL, Bennett JE, Dolin R, editors. *Principles and practice of infectious diseases.* 7th edition. Philadelphia: Elsevier; p. 2789; with permission.)

Rickettsia conorii.[69] Alcoholism has also been linked to an increased chronicity of Q fever, the causative agent *Coxiella burnetti*. Other risk factors for a fatal outcome in rickettsiosis include older age. In a case series, the Malish strain of *R conorii* in the population investigated was found to have alcoholism as a risk factor for fatal outcome in Mediterranean Spotted Fever.[70]

Fever, rash, and headache are classic diagnostic clues for rickettsial diseases (**Fig. 2**). Major findings in rickettsioses include fever in a patient with vector exposure presenting with rash, inoculation eschar, or localized lymphadenopathy. In RMSF, the headache is often accompanied by intense myalgias and malaise. The rash of RMSF classically is described as beginning on the ankles and wrists and spreading centrally involving palms and soles. In comparison, the rash in epidemic typhus progresses from macules that disappear on pressure to maculopapules with petechiae. The face, palms, and soles are usually spared. In severe rickettsiosis, multiorgan failure occurs with a rapid and fulminant course presenting with stupor, ataxia, splenomegaly, hepatomegaly, jaundice, pneumonitis, seizures, arrhythmias, myocarditis, and/or azotemia.[71] Neutropenia, thrombocytopenia, moderate increases in liver enzymes, hyponatremia, and hypocalcaemia are common. Culture is extremely difficult, and diagnosis is mainly by serology and PCR.[72] The reference technique for serology is the indirect fluorescent antibody test. The diagnosis of louse-borne typhus is generally based on the detection of antibodies with a fourfold rise in titer in convalescence. Rickettsiae may also be isolated most effectively from blood, Buffy coat, plasma, or tissue in shell-vial cell culture. In rickettsiosis, biopsies of skin lesions are helpful, especially with the use of immunohistochemistry.[73] Most patients with rickettsiosis are treated for 7 to 10 days with doxycycline. The only other antimicrobial agent that is recommended for treatment is chloramphenicol.

ANTIBIOTIC DOSING IN LIVER DYSFUNCTION AND DRUG TOXICITY
Altered Pharmacokinetics in Liver Dysfunction that Influence Drug Dosing

Drug dosing in patients with liver impairment can be complex because of the various physiologic changes that occur, especially in the setting of advanced hepatic disease.[74] Summarized in **Table 1**, are some potential effects that chronic liver impairment may cause.[75]

Antibiotic Adjustments for Liver Dysfunction

The challenge of appropriate antimicrobial dosing is further complicated by impaired hepatic function because of the pharmacokinetic alterations noted in **Table 1**, but also because of the lack of clinical data that are readily available in this patient population. Unlike renal impairment, the degree and/or severity of hepatic disease is more difficult to quantify and monitor. Extreme caution should be exercised in the administration of agents that are largely cleared by hepatic metabolism. In cases in which the benefits outweigh the risks, agents with a narrow therapeutic window and those potentially hepatotoxic, should be initiated at a low dose, without compromising the efficacy of the antimicrobial or promoting the development of resistance. **Table 2** suggests adjustments for commonly prescribed antimicrobials in the setting of hepatic impairment.

Antibiotics and Liver Toxicity

Because the liver is a vital organ with the primary responsibility of metabolizing and removing drugs, it is susceptible to damage and toxicity. The hepatic injury induced by some hepatotoxic antimicrobials could be the result from short-term

Table 1
Pharmacokinetic (PK) alterations in liver dysfunction

PK Process	Changes in Liver Dysfunction	Potential Effect
Absorption	• Reduction in presystemic hepatic metabolism • First-pass effect decreased for drugs with intermediate and high hepatic extraction ratio	• Increased bioavailability of orally administered drugs with high hepatic extraction ratio
Distribution	• Reduction of plasma protein binding from decreased albumin synthesis • Increase in volume of distribution of hydrophilic drugs secondary to ascites	• Increased unbound (active) drug found in body
Metabolism	• Decrease in liver mass and/or activity owing to alteration in function • Oxidative metabolic reactions (cytochrome P450 pathyway) affected more than glucuronidation	• Inability of unbound drug to be cleared • Impaired drug metabolism
Elimination	• Impaired metabolism of creatine to creatinine in severe liver disease, estimation of creatinine clearance can be inaccurate • Advanced liver disease is commonly complicated by impaired renal function	• Inaccurate estimation of creatinine clearance • Impaired renal elimination of drugs in patients with concurrent liver and renal disease

or long-term exposure. Drug-induced liver injury can range from asymptomatic transient liver enzyme elevations to fulminant liver failure.[76] Most commonly, patients develop hepatitis, which can also be termed hepatocellular or cytotoxic injury. Commonly used antimicrobials that have been associated with hepatic injury are noted in **Table 3**.[77] Frequency of drug-induced liver injury is often difficult to quantify because of the presence confounding variables (eg, the use of multiple agents in the treatment of TB).

Other agents to avoid in patients with a history of alcohol consumption are those drugs that can induce a disulfiramlike reaction as a result of the accumulation of acetaldehyde. Patients with disulfiramlike reaction most likely present with nausea, vomiting, and abdominal pain. In addition, some patients complain of flushing, generalized body warmth, diaphoresis, lightheadedness, hypotension, and tachycardia. Antimicrobials that have been associated with disulfiramlike reaction in the presence of alcohol include second-generation cephalosporins that contain the N-methylthiotetrazole (nMTT) side chain, which is released as these agents undergo metabolism, and metronidazole. The free nMTT inhibits the enzyme aldehyde dehydrogenase that induces the disulfiramlike reaction in the presence of alcohol.[78] Cefotetan is the more frequently encountered cephalosporin in the United States that contains the nMTT side chain that has been associated with disulfiramlike reactions.[79] Metronidazole is another regularly used antimicrobial agent that has been reported to cause disulfiramlike reactions, when taken together with alcohol.[80] Interestingly, a small double-blind study that included 12 moderate consumers of ethanol who received either metronidazole 200

Table 2
Antimicrobials and hepatic dosing considerations[a]

Antimicrobials		Hepatic Adjustment
Azithromycin	Child-Pugh class A, B, C	No specific guidelines available. Use with caution owing to potential for rare hepatotoxicity
Caspofungin	Child-Pugh score 5–6	No adjustments required
	Child-Pugh score 7–9	70-mg IV loading dose, then 35 mg IV daily
	Child-Pugh >9	No clinical experience
Ceftriaxone	Concurrent liver and renal impairment	Ceftriaxone dosing should not exceed 2 g per day
Clindamycin	Severe liver disease	Consider dosage reduction
Daptomycin	Child-Pugh class A and B	No adjustments required
	Child-Pugh class C	Not evaluated
Isoniazid	Child-Pugh class A, B, C	No adjustments required; however, use with caution because of accumulation in those with preexisting liver damage
Linezolid	Child-Pugh class A and B	No adjustments required
	Child-Pugh class C	Not evaluated
Metronidazole	Mild liver disease	No adjustments required
	Severe liver disease	Consider dosage reduction
Moxifloxacin	Child-Pugh class A, B, C	No adjustments needed, however increased risk of QT prolongation may occur
Nafcillin	Concurrent liver and renal impairment	Modification may be necessary
Posaconazole	Child-Pugh class A, B, C	No adjustment required, but if clinical signs and symptoms of liver disease secondary to posaconazole, then stop
Rifampin	Child-Pugh class A, B, C	Dose reduction may be necessary to reduce hepatotoxicity
Rifaximin	Child-Pugh class A, B, C	No adjustments required, but use caution in severe impairment as systemic absorption does occur
Telithromycin	Concurrent liver and renal impairment	Consider dosage reduction
Tigecycline	Child-Pugh class A and B	No adjustments required
	Child-Pugh class C	100 mg IV loading dose, then 25 mg IV every 12 h
Voriconazole	Child-Pugh class A and B	Standard loading dose, but reduce maintenance dose by 50%
	Child-Pugh class C	Should only be used if benefit outweighs risk; monitor closely for toxicity

Abbreviation: IV, intravenous.
[a] Information from table derived from individual agents' package insert information.

mg 3 times daily or placebo, found that those receiving metronidazole did not exhibit any objective reactions (increased blood pressure, elevated body temperature, elevations in acetaldehyde concentrations). None of the subjects reported any headache, nausea, dyspnea, or vertigo.[81] Other antimicrobial agents that have been reported to possibly induce a disulfiramlike reaction include chloramphenicol, griseofulvin, nitrofurantoin, and sulfonamides.[78]

Table 3
Common antimicrobials and the type of hepatic injury reported in the literature

Antimicrobial Agent(s)	Pattern of Hepatic Damage
Beta-lactams	
Amoxicillin	Hepatocellular
Amoxicillin/clavulanate, cephalosporins	Cholestasis (can be irreversible with amoxicillin/clavulanate)
Ampicillin	Hepatocellular, cholestasis
Ceftriaxone	Biliary sludge
Oxacillin, penicillin	Hepatocellular
Fluoroquinolones	
Ciprofloxacin, norfloxacin	Hepatocellular, cholestasis, fulminant hepatic failure
Moxifloxacin	Hepatic necrosis, hepatocellular, cholestasis, liver failure
Trovafloxacin	Fulminant hepatic failure
Macrolides	
Azithromycin	Cholestasis
Clarithromycin Telithromycin	Hepatocellular, acute liver failure
Erythromycin	Cholestasis, liver failure
Tetracyclines	
Doxycycline, minocycline	Cholestasis, autoimmune hepatitis, hepatocellular, fulminant liver failure
Tigecycline	Cholestasis
Antifungals	
Caspofungin	Hepatic necrosis, liver failure
Fluconazole	Hepatocellular, cholestasis, fulminant liver failure
Itraconazole	Cholestasis, liver failure
Micafungin, voriconazole	Hepatocellular, cholestasis, liver failure
Antituberculous agents and miscellaneous agents	
Chloramphenicol, ethambutol, rifampin	Hepatocellular
Clindamycin, SMX/TMP	Cholestasis
Isoniazid	Hepatocellular, severe hepatitis
Nitrofurantoin	Hepatocellular, cholestasis, chronic hepatitis
Pyrazinamide	Hepatic necrosis, dose-dependent hepatocellular

Abbreviation: SMX/TMP, sulfamethoxazole/trimethoprim.

REFERENCES

1. Donowitz GR. Acute pneumonia. In: Mandell GL, Bennett JE, Dolin R, editors. Principles and practice of infectious diseases. 7th edition. Philadelphia: Elsevier; 2010. p. 891–916.
2. Manfredi F, Daly WJ, Behnke RH. Clinical observations of acute friedlander pneumonia. Ann Intern Med 1963;58:642–53.
3. Pierce AK, Sanford JP. Aerobic gram-negative bacillary pneumonias. Am Rev Respir Dis 1974;110:647–58.

4. Jong GM, Hsiue TR, Chen CR, et al. Rapidly fatal outcome of bacteremic *klebsiella pneumonia* pneumonia in alcoholics. Chest 1995;107(1):214–7.

5. Marina M, Strong CA, Cliven R, et al. Bacteriology of anaerobic pleuropulmonary infections: preliminary report. Clin Infect Dis 1993;16(Suppl 4):S256–62.

6. Lorber B. Bacterial lung abscess. In: Mandell GL, Bennett JE, Dolin R, editors. Principles and practice of infectious diseases. 7th edition. Philadelphia: Elsevier; 2010. p. 925–9.

7. Jones HW, Roberts J, Brantner J. Incidence of tuberculosis among homeless men. JAMA 1954;155:222–3.

8. Friedman LN, Sullivan GM, Bovilaqua RP, et al. Tuberculosis screening in alcoholics and drug addicts. Am Rev Respir Dis 1987;136:1188–92.

9. Diel RS, Schneider K, Meywald-Walter K, et al. Epidemiology of tuberculosis in Hamburg, Germany: long-term population-based analysis applying classical and molecular epidemiological techniques. J Clin Microbiol 2002;40:532–9.

10. Bobrik A, Danishevski K, Ershina K, et al. Prison health in Russia: the larger picture. J Public Health Policy 2005;26:30–59.

11. Mendenhall CL, Moritz TE, Roselle GA, et al. A study of nutritional support with oxandrolone in malnourished patient with alcoholic hepatitis: results of a Department of Veterans Affairs cooperative study. Hepatology 1993;17:564–76.

12. Segarra F, Sherman DS. Relapses in pulmonary tuberculosis. Dis Chest 1967;51: 59–63.

13. Advisory Committee for Elimination of TB. Use of preventative therapy for tuberculosis infection in the United States. MMWR Recomm Rep 1990;39:9–12.

14. Aronin SI, Mukherjee SK, West JC. Review of pneumococcal endocarditis in adults in the penicillin era. Clin Infect Dis 1998;26:165–71.

15. Powderly WG, Stanley SL, Medoff G. Pneumococcal endocarditis: report of a series and review of the literature. Rev Infect Dis 1986;8:786–91.

16. Buchbinder AN, Roberts WC. Alcoholism—an important but unemphasized factor predisposing to infective endocarditis. Arch Intern Med 1973;132:689–92.

17. Wolff M, Regnier B, Witchitz S, et al. Pneumococcal endocarditis. Eur Heart J 1984;5(Supp C):77–80.

18. Martinez E, Miro JM, Almirante B, et al. Effect of penicillin resistance of *Streptococcus pneumoniae* on the presentation, prognosis, and treatment of pneumococcal endocarditis in adults. Clin Infect Dis 2001;35:130–9.

19. Sandoe JA. *Capnocytophaga canimorus* endocarditis. J Med Microbiol 2004;53: 245–8.

20. Slater LN, Welch DF. Bartonella, including cat-scratch. In: Mandell GL, Bennett JE, Dolin R, editors. Principles and practice of infectious diseases. 7th edition. Philadelphia: Elsevier; 2010. p. 2995–3009.

21. Maguina C, Garcia PJ, Gotuzzo E, et al. Bartonellosis (Carrión's disease) in the modern era. Clin Infect Dis 2001;33(6):772–9.

22. Spach DH, Kanter AS, Dougherty MJ, et al. *Bartonella* (rochalimaea) *quintana* bacteremia in inner-city patients with chronic alcoholism. N Engl J Med 1995;332:424–8.

23. Vinson JW, Varela G, Molina-Pasquel C. Trench fever. III. Induction of clinical disease in volunteers inoculated with *Rickettsia quintana* propagated on blood agar. Am J Trop Med Hyg 1969;18:713–22.

24. Relman DA. Has trench fever returned? N Engl J Med 1995;332(7):463–4.

25. Raoult D, Fournier PE, Vandenesch F, et al. Outcome and treatment of *Bartonella* endocarditis. Arch Intern Med 2003;163:226–30.

26. Sakorafas GH, Tsiotou AG. Etiology and pathogenesis of acute pancreatitis: current concepts. J Clin Gastroenterol 2000;30(4):343–56.

27. Jerrells TR, Vidlak D, Strachota JM. Alcoholic pancreatitis: mechanisms of viral infections as cofactors in the development of acute and chronic pancreatitis and fibrosis. J Leukoc Biol 2007;81(2):430–9.
28. Frossard JL, Steer ML, Pastor CM. Acute pancreatitis. Lancet 2008;371(9607):143–52.
29. Lozano-Leon A, Iglesias-Canle J, Iglesias-Garcia J, et al. *Citrobacter freundii* infection after acute necrotizing pancreatitis in a patient with a pancreatic pseudocyst. J Med Case Rep 2011;7(5):51.
30. Foust RT. Infection of a pancreatic pseudocyst due to *Candida albicans*. South Med J 1996;89(11):1104–7.
31. Eshwara VK, Mukhopadhyay C, Mohan S, et al. Two unique presentations of *Achromobacter xylosoxidans* infections in clinical settings. J Infect Dev Ctries 2011; 5(2):138–41.
32. Baron TH, Morgan DE. Acute necrotizing pancreatitis. N Engl J Med 1999;340: 1412–7.
33. Such J, Runyon BA. Spontaneous bacterial peritonitis. Clin Infect Dis 1998;27:669–76.
34. Runyon BA, Montano AA, Akriviadis EA, et al. The serum-ascites albumin gradient is superior to the exudate-transudate concept in the differential diagnosis of ascites. Ann Intern Med 1992;117:215–20.
35. Brook I. The importance of lactic acid levels in body fluids in the detection of bacterial infections. Rev Infect Dis 1981;1(3):470–8.
36. Zeni F, Tardy B, Vindimian M, et al. High levels of tumor necrosis factor-α and interleukin 6 in the ascitic fluid of cirrhotic patients with spontaneous bacterial peritonitis. Clin Infect Dis 1993;17:218–23.
37. Alaniz C, Regal RE. Spontaneous bacterial peritonitis: a review of treatment options. P T 2009;34(4):204–10.
38. Gines P, Rimol A, Planas, et al. Norfloxacin prevents spontaneous bacterial peritonitis recurrence in cirrhosis: results of a double-blind, placebo controlled trial. Hepatology 1990;12:716–24.
39. Lontos S, Gow PJ, Vaughan RB, et al. Norfloxacin and trimethoprim-sulfamethoxazole have similar efficacy in the prevention of spontaneous bacterial peritonitis. Hepatology 2008;23:252–5.
40. Mota A, Guedes F, Areias J, et al. Alcohol consumption among patients with hepatitis b infection in northern Portugal considering gender and hepatitis B virus genotype difference. Alcohol 2010;44(2):149–56.
41. Schiff ER, Ozden N. Hepatitis C and alcohol. Alcohol Res Health 2003;27(3):232–9.
42. Okazaki T, Yoshihara H, Suzuki K, et al. Efficacy of interferon therapy in patients with chronic hepatitis C. Comparison between non-drinkers and drinkers. Scand J Gastroenterol 1994;29:1039–43.
43. Oliveira LC, Silva TE, Alves MH. Response to hepatitis B vaccine in alcoholics without clinically evident liver cirrhosis. Arq Gastroenterol 2007;44(3):195–200 [in Portuguese].
44. Bujanda L. The effects of alcohol consumption upon the gastrointestinal tract. Am J Gastroenterol 2000;95(12):3374–82.
45. Sheth NK, Wisniewski TR, Franson TR. Survival of enteric pathogens in common beverages: an in vitro study. Am J Gastroenterol 1988;83(6):658–60.
46. Brenner H, Rothenbacher D, Bode G, et al. Inverse graded relation between alcohol consumption and active infection with *Helicobacter pylori*. Am J Epidemiol 1999;149:571–6.
47. Soleas GJ, Dam J, Carey M, et al. Toward the fingerprinting of wine: cultivar-related patterns of polyphenolic constituents in Ontario wines. J Agric Food Chem 1997;45(10):3871–80.

48. Vaquero MJ, Alberto MR, Manca de Nadra MC. Antibacterial effects of phenolic compounds from different wines. Food Contr 2007;18:93–101.
49. Carpenter RR, Petersdorf RG. The clinical spectrum of bacterial meningitis. Am J Med 1962;33:262–75.
50. Swartz MN, Dodge PR. Bacterial meningitis: a review of selected aspects. N Engl J Med 1965;272:725–31.
51. Cherubin CE, Marr JS, Sierra MF, et al. *Listeria* and gram-negative bacillary meningitis in New York City, 1972-1979. Am J Med 1981;71:199–209.
52. Mylonakis E, Hohmann EL, Calderwood SB. Central nervous system infection with *Listeria monocytogenes*: 33 years' experience at a general hospital and review of 776 episodes from the literature. Medicine 1998;77:313–36.
53. Brouwer MC, van de Beek D, Heckenberg SG, et al. Community-acquired *Listeria monocytogenes* meningitis in adults. Clin Infect Dis 2006;43:1233–8.
54. Weisfeld M, de Gans J, van der Ende A, et al. Community-acquired bacterial meningitis in alcoholic patients. PLoS One 2010;5(2):e9102.
55. Denney CF, Iragui VJ, Uher-Zak LD, et al. Amebic meningoencephalitis caused by *Balamuthia mandrillaris*: case report and review. Clin Infect Dis 1997;25:1354–8.
56. MacGregor RR, Louria DB. Alcohol and infection. Curr Clin Top Infect Dis 1997; 17:291–315.
57. Neill M, Carpenter CJ. Other pathogenic vibrios. In: Mandell GL, Bennett JE, Dolin R, editors. Principles and practice of infectious diseases. 7th edition. Philadelphia: Elsevier; 2010. p. 2787–9.
58. Jones MK, Oliver JD. *Vibrio vulnificus*: disease and pathogenesis. Infect Immun 2009;77(5):1723–33.
59. Powell JL, Wright AC, Wasserman SS, et al. Release of tumor necrosis factor alpha in response to *Vibrio vulnificus* capsular polysaccharide in vivo and in vitro models. Infect Immun 1997;65:3713–8.
60. Shin SH, Shin DH, Ryu PY, et al. Proinflammatory cytokine profile in *Vibrio vulnificus* septicemic patients' sera. FEMS Immunol Med Microbiol 2002;33:133–8.
61. Mead PS, Slutsker L, Dietz V, et al. Food-related illness and death in the United States. Emerg Infect Dis 1999;5(5):607–25.
62. Klontz KC, Lieb S, Schreiber M, et al. Syndromes of *Vibrio vulnificus* infections: clinical and epidemiologic features in Florida cases, 1981-1987. Ann Intern Med 1988;109:318–23.
63. Chen SC, Lee YT, Tsai SJ, et al. Antibiotic therapy for necrotizing fasciitis caused by *Vibrio vulnificus*: retrospective analysis of an 8 year period. J Antimicrob Chemother 2012;67(2):488–93.
64. Mouzin E, Mascola L, Tormey M, et al. Prevention of *Vibrio vulnificus* infections: assessment of regulatory educational strategies. JAMA 1997;278:576–8.
65. Janda JM, Graves M. Capnocytophaga. In: Mandell GL, Bennett JE, Dolin R, editors. Principles and practice of infectious diseases. 7th edition. Philadelphia: Elsevier; 2010. p. 2991–4.
66. Butler T, Weaver RE, Ramani TK, et al. Unidentified gram-negative rod infection: a new disease of man. Ann Intern Med 1977;86:1–5.
67. Kullberg BJ, Westendorp RJ, Van't Wout JW, et al. Purpura fulminans and symmetrical peripheral gangrene caused by *Capnocytophaga canimorus* (formerly df-2) septicemia—A complication of dog bite. Medicine 1991;70(5):287–92.
68. Pers C, Gahrn-Hansen B, Frederiksen W. *Capnocytophaga canimorus* septicemia in Denmark, 1982-1995: review of 39 Cases. Clin Infect Dis 1996;23:71–5.
69. Walker DH. The role of host factors in the severity of spotted fever and typhus rickettsioses. Ann N Y Acad Sci 1990;590:10–9.

70. Sousa R, França A, Dória Nòbrega S, et al. Host- and microbe-related risk factors for and pathophysiology of fatal *Rickettsia conorii* infection in Portuguese patients. J Infect Dis 2008;198(4):576–85.
71. Walker DH. *Rickettsia rickettsii* and other spotted fever group rickettsiae (Rocky Mountain spotted fever and other spotted fevers). In: Mandell GL, Bennett JE, Dolin R, editors. Principles and practice of infectious diseases. 7th edition. Philadelphia: Elsevier; 2010. p. 2499–507.
72. Raoult D, Fournier PE, Fenollar F, et al. *Rickettsia africae*, a tick-borne pathogen in travelers to sub-Saharan Africa. N Engl J Med 2001;344:1504–10.
73. Walker DH, Feng HM, Ladner S, et al. Immunohistochemical diagnosis of typhus rickettsioses using an anti-lipopolysaccharide monoclonal antibody. Mod Pathol 1997;10:1038–42.
74. Verbeeck RK. Pharmacokinetics and dosage adjustment in patients with hepatic dysfunction. Eur. J Clin Pharmacol 2008;64:1147–61.
75. Rodighiero V. Effects of liver disease on pharmacokinetics. An update. Clin Pharm 1999;37(5):399–431.
76. Robles M, Toscano E, Cotta J, et al. Antibiotic-induced liver toxicity: mechanisms, clinical features and causality assessment. Curr Drug Saf 2010;5:212–22.
77. MacLaren R. Hepatic and cholestatic diseases. In: Tisdale JE, Miller DA, editors. Drug-induced diseases: prevention, detection, and management. 2nd edition. Bethesda (MD): American Society of Health-System Pharmacists, Inc; 2010. p. 771–98.
78. Kuffner E. Disulfiram and disulfiram-like reactions. In: Nelson LS, Lewin NA, Howland MA, et al, editors. Goldfrank's toxicologic emergencies. 9th edition. New York: The McGraw-Hill Companies; 2011. p. 1143–6.
79. Kline SS, Mauro VF, Forney RB, et al. Cefotetan-induced disulfiram-type reactions and hypoprothrombinemia. Antimicrobial Agents Chemother 1987;31(9):1328–31.
80. Williams CS, Woodcock KR. Do ethanol and metronidazole interact to produce a disulfiram-like reaction? Ann Pharmacother 2000;34:255–7.
81. Visapää JP, Tillonen JS, Kaihovaara PS. Lack of disulfiram-like reaction with metronidazole and ethanol. Ann Pharmacother 2002;36:971–4.

Nutrition in Alcoholic Liver Disease

Ashwani K. Singal, MD, Michael R. Charlton, MD*

KEYWORDS

- Metabolism • Nutrition • Alcohol • Cirrhosis

KEY POINTS

- The liver plays an important role in the metabolism, synthesis, storage, and absorption of nutrients. Hence, patients with cirrhosis are prone to nutritional deficiencies and malnutrition, with a higher prevalence among patients with decompensated disease compared with compensated cirrhosis.
- Mechanisms of nutritional deficiencies in patients with liver disease are multifactorial.
- Assessment of nutritional status should be a routine recurring part of the care of patients with alcoholic liver disease.
- Malnutrition among patients with cirrhosis in general and alcoholic liver disease in particular correlates with poor quality of life, increased risk of infections, frequent hospitalizations, complications (ascites, encephalopathy, hepatorenal syndrome, and variceal bleeding), mortality, poor graft and patient survival after liver transplantation, and economic burden.
- Physicians, including gastroenterologists and hepatologists, should be conversant with management of malnutrition and nutritional supplementation.

PREVALENCE AND MAGNITUDE

The prevalence of protein calorie malnutrition in patients with alcoholic liver disease has been reported as from between 20% to 60% in outpatients with alcoholic cirrhosis to almost 100% in hospitalized patients with acute alcoholic hepatitis (AH).[1–5] In a detailed multivariate analysis of 74 patients evaluated for orthotopic liver transplantation (15% with alcoholic cirrhosis), evidence of malnutrition as assessed by anthropometric measurements was ubiquitous.[6] Similar results were obtained in a much smaller study of prospective transplant recipients.[7]

Although reports vary, the preponderance of evidence suggests that the prevalence of malnutrition is similar among patients with alcoholic compared with nonalcoholic cirrhosis.[6,8–10] Malnutrition correlates better than etiology with the severity of liver

Division of Gastroenterology and Hepatology, Department of Internal Medicine, Mayo Clinic, 200 First Street Southwest, Rochester, MN 55905-0001, USA
* Corresponding author.
E-mail address: charlton.michael@mayo.edu

Clin Liver Dis 16 (2012) 805–826
http://dx.doi.org/10.1016/j.cld.2012.08.009
1089-3261/12/$ – see front matter © 2012 Elsevier Inc. All rights reserved.
liver.theclinics.com

disease. In one study, 46%, 84%, and 95% of Child-Turcotte-Pugh stages A, B, and C alcoholic cirrhotics, respectively, were malnourished.[11,12] The prevalence and severity of malnutrition are also higher, with increasing amounts of alcohol use, lower socio-economic status, and lack of employment.[13,14]

Presence of malnutrition is associated with higher rate of complications (variceal bleeding, ascites, encephalopathy, infections, and hepatorenal syndrome) and mortality.[12,15,16] In a study of male veterans with acute AH, mortality was reported more than 80%, with a voluntary intake of less than 1000 calories per day, and almost no mortality with voluntary intake of greater than 3000 calories per day.[17] Nutrition is also important in compensated liver disease, with higher mortality and complication rates at 1 year in the presence of malnutrition compared with adequately nourished patients (20% vs 0% and 65% vs 13%, respectively).[16] Malnutrition has also been associated with longer stay in intensive care, longer overall hospitalization, and higher mortality after liver transplantation.[18,19]

MECHANISMS OF MALNUTRITION

Malnutrition in patients with liver disease is multifactorial (**Fig. 1**).

Decreased Oral Intake

Patients with chronic alcoholism consume a disproportionate amount of calories from alcohol and do not take adequate food calories (alcohol substitution). The caloric value of alcohol (average approximately 7.1 calories per gram of alcohol) decreases when more than 25% of total calories are derived from alcohol.[13] Anorexia is a frequent symptom in patients with cirrhosis, with an incidence as high as 90%.[4] This is exacerbated by altered taste from zinc deficiency and less palatable diet due to dietary salt or protein restrictions.[20] Abdominal distention from ascites and decreased gastric emptying in cirrhosis further cause postprandial fullness, adding fuel to the fire.[21–23] Prevalence of malnutrition increases during hospitalization due to the need for fasting for investigations and dietary restrictions, with reported dietary intake of approximately 48% to 80% and protein intake of 34% to 63% among hospitalized

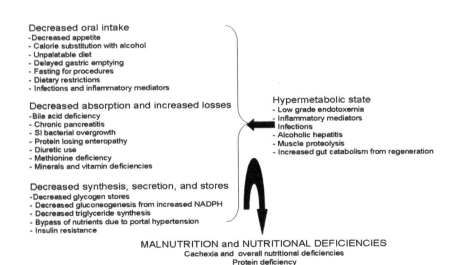

Fig. 1. Mechanisms of malnutrition in patients with alcoholic liver disease.

alcoholic cirrhotics of varying severity.[1,12] Catabolic state with elevated cytokines, such as tumor necrosis factor and leptin, may contribute to anorexia.[24,25] Role of ghrelin, a hormone involved in satiety and food intake, is controversial.[24,26]

Decreased Absorption

Alcohol impairs gastrointestinal mucosal absorption of nutrients, especially folate and vitamin B_{12}. Protein-losing enteropathy may occur in approximately 40% to 50% of patients with cirrhosis.[27,28] Alcohol-induced mucosal damage can cause loss of proteins, as evidenced by increased fecal loss of nitrogen in chronic alcoholics with and without liver disease. Whether congestion of the gastrointestinal mucosa due to portal hypertension plays a role is controversial. Correlation with portal pressures[29,30] and improvement after portacaval shunting support this mechanism.[31] Lack of correlation of protein-losing enteropathy, however, with severity of underlying liver disease speaks against this mechanism.[32] Steatorrhea may occur in approximately 45% of cirrhotics by alcohol-induced mucosal damage, small bowel bacterial overgrowth, chronic pancreatitis, and cholestasis.[33,34]

Decreased Synthesis, Secretion, and Stores

Amino acids

Alcohol inhibits protein synthesis and stimulates protein breakdown in animal models.[35] Impaired conversion of pyruvate to acetyl coenzyme A due to vitamin B_6 deficiency results in decreased synthesis of amino acids.[36] Impaired gluconeogenesis from a high NADH/NAD$^+$ (nicotinamide adenine dinucleotide) ratio as a result of metabolism of alcohol leads to proteolysis in periods of fasting. Hyperglucagonemia, a near universal finding in chronic liver disease, attenuates protein synthesis through diversion of amino acids for gluconeogenesis.[37,38] Diminished androgenic steroids and insulinlike growth factors contribute to the overall protein catabolic state of cirrhosis.[39,40] Secretion of hepatic plasma proteins, including albumin and transferrin, is also impaired by alcohol.[41] Decreased uptake of amino acids by the liver also occurs due to direct effect of alcohol and from portosystemic shunting.[42]

These alterations in amino acid metabolism account for a characteristic pattern in alcoholic cirrhosis of elevated levels of circulating aromatic amino acids (AAAs), such as phenylalanine, tyrosine, and methionine, and low levels of circulating branched-chain amino acids (BCAAs), such as leucine, isoleucine, and valine.[43] Furthermore, increased permeability of the blood-brain barrier to AAAs occurs with precipitation of portosystemic encephalopathy.[43,44]

Fatty acid metabolism

Increased NADH/NAD$^+$ ratio from alcohol metabolism and the metabolic effects of cirrhosis (including insulin resistance) result in a net increase in free fatty acid oxidation in patients with alcoholic cirrhosis with reduced respiratory quotient.[36,45] Cholestasis and portosystemic shunting cause malabsorption of fats and fat-soluble vitamins.[46]

Carbohydrate metabolism

Carbohydrate metabolism derangement in cirrhosis includes increased gluconeogenesis from proteolysis and decreased glycogenolysis.[47] Poor glycogen storage capacity of diseased liver leads to increased rates of gluconeogenesis from fats and proteins derived from peripheral breakdown of adipose and muscular tissues, respectively. Insulin resistance in cirrhosis decreases peripheral glucose use and hepatic glycogen synthesis.[24,48,49]

Hypermetabolic State

Increased resting energy expenditure (REE), determined using the Harris Benedict equation, with hypermetabolic state (REE >110%) can occur in alcoholic liver disease. In a study of 123 cirrhotics (approximately 20% alcohol related), hypermetabolic state occurred in approximately 20% and correlated with diminished body cell mass (BCM).[50] Biochemical parameters, such as bilirubin or albumin, were not predictive of hypercatabolism. Increased REE thus is not a universal finding in the setting of alcoholic cirrhosis but should be considered while determining nutritional requirements of patients with alcoholic liver disease.

Alcohol has been shown to increase urinary and fecal nitrogen losses in humans, resulting in a net negative nitrogen balance.[51] When blood levels of alcohol exceed 100 mg/dL, the majority of alcohol metabolism occurs through microsomal oxidation rather than dehydrogenation.[41] Microsomal metabolism of alcohol involves the oxidation of NADP and is thus an energy-consuming process. In addition, the acetate generated during alcohol metabolism requires ATP for conversion to acetyl coenzyme A, adding to the net energy expenditure of oxidative alcohol metabolism.[52] Increased gut permeability in alcoholics and alcoholic liver disease sets the stage for increased translocation of gut-derived bacteria and endotoxins into the circulation.[53] This low-grade endotoxemia and consequent release of cytokines results in activation of sympathetic nervous system and catabolic state with features, such as fever, tachycardia, anorexia, hyperglycemia, and muscle wasting.[54,55] Patients with continuous active drinking are at risk for AH, resulting in exacerbation of this catabolic state.[56,57] Regeneration of gastrointestinal mucosal cells from direct toxicity of alcohol also contributes to a catabolic state. The effect of ascites on REE was shown with 9.5% reduction in REE (P<.005), as estimated with indirect calorimetry, after large volume paracentesis.[58] Spontaneous bacterial peritonitis adds to the catabolic state of alcoholic cirrhosis.

Micronutrient and Vitamin Deficiencies

Micronutrients play a major role in maintaining hepatocyte function and regeneration. Therefore, timely identification of these deficiencies is important. Thiamine deficiency, the most important cause of tissue damage in alcoholics, occurs due to impaired absorption and poor dietary intake. Folate deficiency results from combination of decreased intake, malabsorption, decreased hepatic uptake, and increased renal loss.[59] Methionine deficiency occurs as a consequence of folate, betaine, and choline deficiency. This, along with impaired activity of S-adenosyl methyltransferase in cirrhosis, leads to low levels of S-adenosylmethionine (SAM), which is essential for maintaining cell membrane integrity and synthesis of glutathione (**Fig. 2**).[36] Pyridoxine deficiency occurs due to acetaldehyde (generated from alcohol metabolism), causing competitive decrease in albumin binding, leaving the unbound vitamin to be lost in urine. This deficiency results in increased the aspartate aminotransferase (AST)/ alanine aminotransferase (ALT) ratio because ALT activity requires this vitamin and increased homocysteine levels because this vitamin is a cofactor for homocysteine transsulfuration reactions.[59] A state of oxidative stress occurs due to glutathione deficiency because pyridoxine is needed for conversion of homocysteine to glutathione. Deficiency of vitamin E, an antioxidant adds to this oxidative stress. Vitamin A deficiency occurs due to decreased dietary intake, maldigestion from pancreatic or bile deficiency, decreased retinol-binding protein from diseased liver, and increased bile loss due to cytochrome P450 stimulation by alcohol.[36] Metabolism of retinol requires the same enzymes as metabolism of alcohol, adding to this deficiency. Vitamin A deficiency promotes fibrosis and collagen deposition due to loss of negative feedback of

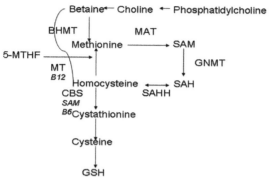

MT: Methionine synthase; MAT: Methyltransferase; MTHF: Methyltetrahydrofolate; SAM: S-adenosylmethionine; GNMT: Glycine N-methyltransferase; SAH: S-adenosylhomocysteine; SAHH: SAH hydrolase; CBS: Cystathionine Beta synthase; GSH: Glutathione; BHMT: Betaine homocysteine methyltransferase

Fig. 2. Mechanisms of methionine, SAM, and glutathione deficiency in alcoholic liver disease.

peroxisome proliferator–activated receptors and ethanol-induced signaling pathways for apoptosis.[59]

NUTRITIONAL ASSESSMENT
Clinical Assessment

Detailed history and physical examination should be obtained to assess the nutritional status of patients with liver disease (**Table 1**). Subjective global assessment (SGA) is a simple bedside tool that comprises information on weight (current weight, weight before illness, and weight range in the previous 6 months), dietary intake (appetite,

Table 1	
Clinical examination for nutritional deficiencies in patients with alcoholic liver disease	
Protein Energy Malnutrition	**Subjective Global Assessment**
Vitamin A (retinol)	Night blindness, increased fibrosis
Vitamin E	Skin changes
Vitamin D	Osteopenia and osteoporosis
Thiamine (vitamin B_1)	Wernicke encephalopathy, neuropathy, beriberi with high output heart failure
Niacin (vitamin B_3)	Pellagra: dementia diarrhea and dermatitis
Pyridoxine (vitamin B_6)	Neuropathy, sideroblastic anemia, increased AST/ALT ratio
Folic acid	Megaloblastic anemia
Cyanocobalamin (vitamin B_{12})	Megaloblastic anemia, SACD, neuropathy
Ascorbic acid (vitamin C)	Scurvy
Iron	Anemia
Calcium	Osteopenia and osteoporosis
Magnesium	Cardiomyopathy
Phosphorous	Cardiac arrhythmias, delirium tremens
Selenium	Cardiomyopathy
Zinc	Ageusia and skin changes

Abbreviation: SACD, subacute combined degeneration.

intake, and gastrointestinal symptoms), physical appearance (fat loss, muscle wasting, edema, and ascites), and existing medical conditions (encephalopathy, infections, and renal insufficiency) (**Box 1**). The SGA is scored from 0 to 3 as well nourished (0), mild malnutrition (1), moderate malnutrition (2), and severe malnutrition (3). Of the various components, muscle wasting is weighted the most.[60,61] Weight change is least reliable because it can be confounded by fluid retention frequently seen in these patients.

Bedside Anthropometry

Body mass index is unreliable in patients with fluid retention. Dry weight, if known before onset of fluid retention, or lean body mass is preferred. The latter can be

---

Box 1
Assessment of nutritional status of patients with alcoholic liver disease

1. SGA
   a. Muscle wasting
   b. Loss of subcutaneous fat
   c. Change in dry weight
   d. Change in dietary intake
   e. Functional capacity and performance
2. Anthropometric measurements
   a. Body mass index
   b. Creatinine height index
   c. Midarm circumference
   d. Triceps skinfold (TSF) thickness
   e. Arm muscle circumference
   f. Handgrip measurement
   g. Prognostic nutrition index
   h. Fat-soluble vitamin deficiencies
3. Laboratory parameters
   a. Albumin, prealbumin, and transferrin
   b. Serum cholesterol
   c. Total lymphocyte count
   d. Fat-soluble vitamins: vitamins A, D, and E levels
   e. Water-soluble vitamins: folate, vitamin B_{12}, homocysteine, and methylmalonic acid levels
   f. Mineral deficiencies: iron, calcium, magnesium, phosphorous, and zinc
   g. Delayed-type hypersensitivity
   h. Insulinlike growth factor 1 serum levels
4. Assessment of BCM or lean body mass
   a. Anthropometry and bioelectrical impedance
   b. Deuterium oxide dilution
   c. In vivo neutron activation analysis (INVAA)
   d. Dual-energy x-ray absorptiometry (DEXA)

estimated using the Hamwi equation: 106 kg for male patients and 100 kg for female patients for the first 5 feet and 6 kg for male patients and 5 kg for female patients for each incremental inch. The creatinine height index, the function of creatine synthesis by the liver, may also be confounded by fluid retention.

Arm measurements include the midarm circumference (MAC), indicating status of protein stores and measured at a point midway between acromion and medial epicondyle of humerus. At the same level, using a caliper, skinfold is pinched to provide TSF thickness representing status of fat loss. Like BMI, both these measurements may be confounded by fluid retention.[2,62–64] Using MAC and TSF, arm muscle circumference can be calculated as MAC – (TSF × 0.314) and compared with available norms derived from National Health and Nutrition Examination Survey (NHANES) data in more than 19,000 male and female subjects aged 1 to 74 years.[65]

Handgrip, measured using Jamar handgrip dynamometer (J.A. Preston Corporation, Jackson Mississippi), gives useful information on the nutritional status. A mean of 3 measurements is taken. Observed handgrip measurements can be given as proportion of predicted values calculated based on age, gender, and BMI, helping to classify identification of patients with malnutrition, defined as 2 SD below the mean of that age and gender.[16,64,66] Muscle strength correlates with malnutrition severity but not with liver disease severity, alcohol abstinence, or neuropathy.[67]

Laboratory Evaluation

Assessment of nutritional status using laboratory variables, such as albumin, prealbumin, and transferrin, lacks accuracy because these proteins are synthesized in the liver and are not shown to correlate with body mass index and lean body mass.[2,63] Furthermore, albumin products are frequently used as therapeutic agents in clinical practice masking the true albumin levels. Low insulinlike growth factor 1 levels have been shown a marker of malnutrition.[68] Serum creatinine confounded by renal function may not be accurate reflection of muscle mass in patients with renal insufficiency. Loss of muscle mass in patients with chronic illnesses, including cirrhosis, can be assessed by measuring psoas muscle thickness on CT scan. Right and left psoas muscle cross-sectional area is measured at the level of L4 vertebra on the CT scan and has been shown to be accurate in predicting post-transplant survival in cirrhotics.[69] Objective and reproducible, this may be a reliable marker of nutritional status.

Determination of BCM is accurate and is the gold standard for assessment of nutritional status. Techniques include bioelectrical impedance for determination of fat-free mass, DEXA for bone mineral density and fat-free mass, INVAA for assessment of total body nitrogen, and deuterium oxide dilution for determination of total body water.[64,70] These techniques, however, are cumbersome, expensive, and not routinely used in clinical practice. They may be of value among patients with ascites and fluid overload where routine anthropometric assessment may be confounded and be inaccurate.[71] Assessment of BCM in patients with ascites could be more simply done at bedside using the method of bioelectric impedance analysis.[72]

Recommendations for Nutritional Assessment in Routine Practice

The European Society for Clinical Nutrition and Metabolism recommends bedside nutritional assessment using SGA and anthropometric measurements.[71] SGA is a simple and inexpensive initial tool to screen patients with liver disease for malnutrition. The limitations, however, are lack of objectivity and correlation with outcomes. In one study, SGA was 82% sensitive and 72% specific compared with laboratory or anthropometric measurements.[60] In another study, SGA was only 50% as accurate as handgrip strength, with complications occurring in 65% patients classified as malnourished based on handgrip but only 36% patients classified as malnourished based on SGA.[16] Handgrip strength and arm muscle circumference can accurately predict BCM as evaluated by isotope dilution technique. A combination of less than 30-kg handgrip strength with less than 23-cm arm muscle circumference had 94% sensitivity and 97% negative predictive value for identifying patients with low BCM.[64] Assessment of sarcopenia from the measurements of psoas muscle thickening on CT scan is emerging as a novel, accurate, and objective marker of nutritional status of a patient with liver disease.[69] More studies are needed, however, in healthy volunteers to determine the norms in general population before using this method in routine practice.

NUTRITIONAL MANAGEMENT

Providing adequate nutrition is an essential component in the management of patients with liver disease for (1) improved outcome of hospitalization, surgery, and transplantation and (2) reducing complications of liver disease and hospital stay.[19,61,73–75] Goals of nutritional management are to meet basal needs and provide additional sources for hypermetabolic state. Patients not meeting their daily needs (**Table 2**) through diet should receive supplementation. Estimations of the caloric needs of patients with

Table 2
Nutritional supplementation guidelines for patients with alcoholic liver disease

Energy	25–40 kcal/kg/d[a]
Carbohydrate	50%–60% of total calories[b]
Protein	1.0–1.5 g/kg/d[c]
Fat	20%–30% of total energy intake[d]
Fluids	40–50 mL/kg/d[e]
Thiamine	100 mg/d[f]
Folic acid	1 mg/d[f]
Multivitamin	Daily
Vitamin D	50,000 U 3 times/wk
Vitamin A	10,000 U/d or 25,000 U 3 times/wk
Vitamin E	400 IU/d
Sodium	90 mEq/d fluid retention
Iron	Use only if iron deficiency
Calcium	1200–1500 mg/d
Zinc	220 mg 2 times/d

Abbreviation: TIPS, transjugular intrahepatic portosystemic shunt.
  [a] Calculated using Harris Benedict equation using actual body weight. In patients with fluid retention, lean body weight should be used as assessed using the Hamwi equation. Obese patients (BMI >30) should have 75% of basal needs and patients with ascites should add 10% to basal needs.
  [b] Monitoring for blood glucose is recommended to avoid hypoglycemia and manage hyperglycemia with insulin.
  [c] Patients in grade 3 or 4 hepatic encephalopathy or at high risk for encephalopathy (post-TIPS and past history of recurrent hepatic encephalopathy) should start with 0.6–0.8 g/kg/d protein intake and then gradually increased based on tolerance. Whole protein formula is recommended except patients in acute hepatic encephalopathy when use of BCAA is recommended.
  [d] Patients with steatorrhea should have fat intake restricted and use of medium-chain triglyceride is preferred.
  [e] Fluids are restricted to 1.0–1.5 L per day for serum sodium <125 mEq/L.
  [f] Given for at least 2 weeks after hospitalization.

alcoholic liver disease based on the Harris Benedict equation may be inaccurate, underestimating the caloric needs by 15% to 18% when compared with measurement using indirect calorimetry.[6,76] Calories are distributed as 50% to 60% carbohydrates, 25% to 30% proteins, and 15% to 20% fats.

Due to the poor reserves and inability of the liver to handle prolonged starvation as a result of reduced gluconeogenesis by the sick liver, patients with cirrhosis are instructed to eat frequent meals. It should be remembered that glucose stores are depleted in these patients after an overnight fast and, therefore, patients fasting for more than 12 hours should receive intravenous (IV) glucose at a rate of endogenous hepatic glucose production (2–3 mg/kg/d). Nighttime snacks should be encouraged to prevent muscle proteolysis during the nocturnal period of fasting.[77,78] In a randomized controlled trial (RCT), this approach resulted in increase of total body protein stores with sustained gain of 2 kg over a 12-month period compared with an equicaloric diet without a late evening meal.[78]

It was previously believed that protein should be restricted for patients with cirrhosis to avoid precipitation of hepatic encephalopathy. Later studies, however, showed that patients restricted of proteins in the diet suffer muscle catabolism, leading to rise in ammonia and worsening of encephalopathy. An RCT has demonstrated that intake of 1.2 g/kg/d protein intake prevents muscle catabolism and does not precipitate hepatic encephalopathy.[79] Although protein restriction may have a role in the management of acute hepatic encephalopathy, there is no need for this practice in the medium-term or long-term management of patients with liver disease because there is overwhelming evidence that the incidence of complications of liver disease increases with malnutrition.[80]

Patients with chronic PSE may be considered for special formulas with high BCAAs (discussed later).

Patients with steatorrhea may be considered for provision of medium-chain triglycerides as a source of fat calories. Cholesterol intake should be limited as evidenced by harmful effects from high cholesterol diet in animal studies,[81] higher risk of cirrhosis, and liver cancer with high cholesterol diet from the NHANES data[82] and improved fibrosis with the use of statins in patients with hypercholesterolemia.[83] A high-cholesterol diet increases free cholesterol within the hepatic stellate cells, increasing the Toll-like receptor 4 signaling and sensitivity to transforming growth factor β, resulting in more fibrosis.[81] Unsaturated fats, such as cholesterol, are proinflammatory and suppress the immune function.[84]

Monitoring for vitamin deficiencies should be done at baseline and replacement given for deficient ones. These could be checked annually once stable levels are achieved. Thiamine and folate supplementation are administered for at least first 2 weeks to avoid consumption of these vitamins for the glucose metabolism and precipitation of neurologic sequelae of Wernicke encephalopathy and peripheral neuropathy. Caution should be taken when replacing vitamin A because continuing alcohol intake leads to stimulation of cytochrome P450 and conversion of retinoids to toxic metabolites.[85] Patients after liver transplantation remain in negative nitrogen balance for up to approximately 28 days and this period is critical to maintaining nutritional status. Transplanted patients should have monitoring for magnesium deficiency from use of calcineurin inhibitors and receive judicious correction of sodium to avoid pontine myelinosis.[86]

Enteral Supplementation

Patients not meeting needs by oral diet should receive supplementation. The enteral route is preferred whenever possible due to its low cost, decreased risk of infections, maintenance of gut mucosal integrity, and prevention of bacterial translocation. Patients with esophageal varices can safely undergo placement of enteral tubes without any risk of variceal hemorrhage.[87] Percutaneous endoscopic gastrostomy is avoided in the presence of ascites and coagulopathy.[88]

Alcoholic hepatitis

Five RCTs have shown improvement in nutritional status with enteral supplementation without worsening hepatic encephalopathy (**Table 3**).[89–93] There was no survival benefit, however, in any study, with approximately 17% to 35% mortality in the nutritional supplementation group and 16% to 39% in the control group (see **Table 3**). In a study comparing corticosteroids (current standard of care for severe AH) and enteral supplementation, death due to infections was less frequent among patients receiving enteral nutrition.[92] In the same study, survival was better at 1 year with enteral nutritional supplementation compared with corticosteroids treated patients.[92] Similar results were shown in another study of male veterans with AH, with improved survival at 6 months with nutritional supplementation. In this study, oxandrolone treatment as an adjuvant to nutritional supplementation was used and the survival benefit at 6 months was shown for patients with moderate malnutrition but not for patients with severe malnutrition.[91] These data suggest that nutritional supplementation should be provided early and for sufficient period of time. Patients with AH are acutely sick and, therefore, need adjuvant treatment with specific drugs, such as steroids or pentoxifylline. A combination of enteral nutritional support and corticosteroids showed benefit in an open pilot study of 13 patients with severe AH. Decrease in serum bilirubin by greater than 50% at day 15 allowed tapering of steroids, and marked improvement in 3 weeks allowed discontinuation of nutritional support. Only 2 (15%) patients died during the hospital stay and another patient died at 2 months; there were no deaths due to infectious complications.[94] It would be worthwhile to study the role of combined enteral nutrition in a randomized fashion in patients with severe AH.

Alcoholic cirrhosis

Five RCTs have compared enteral nutrition supplementation to standard diet alone in alcoholic cirrhotics and shown improvement in nutritional parameters and liver function.[95–98] Data on survival, however, are conflicting with improved survival during the hospital stay (47% vs 13%; $P = .02$) in 1 study[96] and lack of survival benefit in the other 4 studies, with 1-month mortality of 12% to 13% with enteral supplementation and 24% to 26% in the control group (see **Table 3**). In 1 study analyzing 1-year outcomes, mortality rates in both groups were similar. This study was limited, however, by lack of stratification for severity of malnutrition and included patients with mild to moderate disease as evidenced by the approximately 1800-calorie intake in the control group.[99] Differences among various studies could also be related to sample size and variation in inclusion/exclusion criteria.

Parenteral Nutrition

The parenteral nutrition route is used whenever enteral or oral route is not safe or possible (**Box 2**) or when patients need to stay fasting for 72 hours or more.[100]

Alcoholic hepatitis

Based on encouraging results of a pilot study showing improved clinical outcome, nitrogen balance, and nutritional status without precipitation of encephalopathy with parenteral amino acid supplementation in patients with AH,[101] Nasrallah and Galambos[102] in an RCT showed improved survival with supplementation of 70 g to 85 g amino acids in addition to standard diet (3000 kcal/d and protein 100 g/d) in 18 patients with AH compared with standard diet alone in 17 patients with AH (0% vs 24%; P = .02). However, 6 further studies did not show this survival benefit (see **Table 3**).[103–107] Control groups in these 6 studies received a standard diet providing 30 kcal/kg of ideal body weight (IBW)/d to 3000 kcal/d and 1.0 kg/kg IBW/d to 100 g/d of proteins; the experimental group received IV supplementation with 42.5 g/d to 85 g/d amino acids. This difference could be due to inclusion of mild to moderate severity of AH in the study by Nasrallah and Galambos.[102] Furthermore, variations in sample size (15–54), proportion of male patients (32%–82%), and proportion of patients with cirrhosis (32%–100%) could have resulted in these differences. Improvement in the nutritional status and nitrogen balance with improved liver function was documented in all these studies. Phosphate, potassium, and magnesium supplementation should be ensured to avoid refeeding syndrome.

Alcoholic cirrhosis

The only study evaluating the role of parenteral nutrition in alcoholic cirrhotics was of jaundiced patients with alcoholic cirrhosis with serum bilirubin of greater than or equal to 5 mg/dL. Therefore, this study was included in the analysis of parenteral nutrition in AH. Although the group (N = 20) with 40 g IV amino acid supplementation showed improved bilirubin and nutritional status compared with group with standard diet alone (n = 20), there was no improvement in survival (5% vs 5%, P = .99).[104]

Branched-Chain Amino Acids

BCAAs, such as valine, leucine, and isoleucine, have a branched side chain instead of an aromatic group in AAAs, such as phenylalanine, histidine, and tryptophan. BCAAs help protein synthesis and turnover in the peripheral muscles with subsequent generation of energy. This leads to reduced BCAA levels in patients with cirrhosis.[108] Alternatively, increased levels of AAA due to reduced hepatic metabolism and shunting from portal hypertension result in their migration across the blood-brain barrier, leading to neurotransmitter imbalance and hepatic encephalopathy. These changes are potentially reversed with BCAA supplementation (**Fig. 3**).

An initial RCT of 37 cirrhotics showed that BCAA supplementation compared with conventional protein supplementation (80 g protein/d intake in both groups) was superior in improving hepatic encephalopathy without any effect on the serum ammonia levels.[109] Later, 2 randomized double-blind crossover studies failed to improve encephalopathy and survival despite increased BCAA/AAA ratio.[110,111] These differences could be related to small sample size (8 and 4 patients) and short-term use (11–12 days) of BCAAs. Yoshida and colleagues,[112] in a prospective nonrandomized study, showed improved survival with BCAAs given over 2 to 4 years among patients with hepatitis B virus cirrhosis and baseline BCAA/AAA ratio less than 1.8 compared with a matched control group of patients not receiving BCAAs. Based on these data, 2 large RCTs have been published with the long-term use of BCAAs among patients with alcoholic cirrhosis. In 1 study of 174 patients, use of BCAAs (14.4 g/d) for 1 year (n = 59) was beneficial for improvement in liver function and nutritional status compared with supplementation with lactalbumin (12.6 g/d; n = 56) or maltodextrin (14.4 g/d; n = 59).[113] These beneficial effects resulted in significantly lower hospital admission rates with BCAA supplementation compared with lactalbumin (P = .006) and maltodextrin (P = .0003).[113] Furthermore, combined event rate of deterioration or death was lower with BCAAs compared with lactalbumin (16% vs 32%; P = .039) and a lower trend compared with maltodextrin (16% vs 27%; P = .11).[113] Lower patient acceptance due to poor palatability of BCAAs resulted in dropout of 5 patients in this study.

Table 3
Randomized controlled trials with enteral or parenteral supplementation in patients with alcoholic liver disease

Author	Year	Intervention Treatment	N T	N C	Duration	Mortality (%) Treatment	Mortality (%) Control	P
Studies on alcoholic hepatitis using enteral nutrition								
Cabre et al[92]	2000	T: BCAA-enriched EN 2000 kcal + 72 g protein/d C: Prednisolone 40 mg/d	36	35	28 d	31%	25%	NS
Calvey et al[89]	1985	T: standard diet + 65 g protein (20 g BCAA + 45 g AA or 65 g protein) C: standard diet (1800–2400 kcal + 70–100 g protein/d)	42	22	21 d	37%	32%	NS
Mendenhall et al[90]	1985	T: diet + protein supplement hepatic acid C: 2500 kcal/d	18	34	30 d	17%	21%	NS
Mendenhall et al[91]	1993	T: oxandrolone + 1200 kcal and 45 g protein/d supplement C: placebo + 198–264 kcal and 5–7 g protein/d supplement	137	136	180 d	35%	39%	NS
Moreno et al[93]	2010	T: 27 kcal/kg/d + NAC IV 300 mg/kg/d C: EN 27 kcal/kg/d + 5% dextrose IV	28	24	14 d	30%	16%	NS
Studies on alcoholic hepatitis using parenteral nutrition								
Bonkovsky et al[127]	1991	T: standard diet + 70 g AA supplement ± oxandrolone 20 mg qid C: standard diet (30 kcal/kg IBW + 1 g protein/kg IBW/d)	27	12	21 d	NA	NA	NA
Achord[105]	1987	T: Standard diet + IV AA (42.5 g protein + 830 kcal/d) C: standard diet (2674 kcal + 100 g protein/d)	14	14	21 d	7%	20%	NS

Study	Year	Intervention	N	N	Duration	%	%	p
Nasrallah and Galambos[102]	1980	T: diet + 70–85 g IV AA/d C: diet (3000 kcal/d + 100 g protein/d)	18	17	28 d	0%	24%	<0.02
Diehl et al[103]	1985	T: standard diet + IV AA (51.6 g protein, 130 g glucose and 720 kcal)/d C: standard diet + IV glucose 130 g/d	5	10	30 d	0%	0%	NS
Mezey et al[107]	1991	T: standard diet + IV AA (51.6 g protein, 130 g glucose and 700 kcal)/d C: standard diet + 130 g glucose/d	28	26	30 d	21%	19%	NS
Simon and Galambos[106]	1988	T: diet + 70–85 g IV AA/d C: diet (3000 kcal/d + 100 g protein/d)	16	18	28 d	19%	22%	NS
Naveau et al[104]	1986	T: standard diet + IV supplement 40 kcal and 200 mg nitrogen/kg/d C: standard diet	20	20	28 d	5%	5%	NS
Studies on alcoholic cirrhosis using enteral nutrition								
Cabre et al[96]	1990	T: enteral tube feeding 2115 kcal and 71 g protein/d C: standard diet mean intake 1320 kcal/d	16	19	In patient	13%	47%	0.02
Hirsch et al[97]	1993	T: standard diet + supplement of 1000 kcal + 34 g protein/d C: standard diet + placebo capsule	26	25	30 d	12%	24%	0.33
Kearns et al[98]	1992	T: TF 167 kcal/kg/d + 1.5 g/k/d protein supplement C: standard diet 50% less calorie and protein intake	16	15	28 d	13%	27%	0.29
Bunout et al[95]	1989	T: 50 kcal/k/d + 1.5 g/k/d protein C: standard diet	17	19	28 d	12%	26%	0.25
Dupont et al[99]	2012	T: standard diet + supplement (30–35 kcal/k/d) C: standard diet (1800 cal and 60 g protein/d)	44	55	365 d	39%	35%	0.07

Abbreviations: N, number; T, treatment; C, controls; EN, enteric nutrition; NAC, n-acetyl cysteine.

Box 2
Indications for parenteral nutritional supplementation for patients with alcoholic liver disease

1. Gastrointestinal tract not functioning

    a. Paralytic ileus

    b. Small bowel obstruction

    c. Postoperative state

2. Intolerance to enteral nutrition

    a. Nausea and vomiting

    b. Malabsorption and diarrhea

3. Enteral route unsafe or not possible

    a. Encephalopathy and altered sensorium

    b. Compromised swallow and cough reflexes with risk of aspiration

    c. Acute pancreatitis

    d. Gastrointestinal fistulas

Despite this, quality of life improved with BCAA supplementation.[113] A much larger study 646 of patients showed benefit of BCAA granules supplementation (12 g/d for 2 y) in 314 patients to reduce the composite primary endpoint of death or transplantation compared with standard protein intake in 308 patients (21% vs 29%; P = .03; HR 0.67 [0.49–0.83]) due to reduced progression to liver failure (4% vs 8%; P = .04; HR 0.45 [0.23–0.88]). There was no difference, however, in the occurrence of rupture of varices (3% vs 3%), liver cancer (13% vs 16%), and death (2% vs 2%). Also, BCAA supplementation resulted in improved quality of life. The use of more palatable form of BCAAs as granules instead of powder form in the previous study resulted in improved patient compliance, with 86% of patients taking the full amount of recommended dose throughout the study.[114] Based on these data, BCAA supplementation is recommended for patients with hepatic encephalopathy.[71,115]

Dietary Supplements Used as Antioxidants

Because oxidative stress is a major component in the pathogenesis of alcoholic liver disease, antioxidant supplementation in cirrhosis has been evaluated.[56,57,116,117]

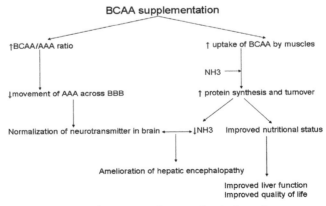

Fig. 3. Mechanisms of action of BCAA supplementation in liver disease.

Alcoholic hepatitis

Steroids and pentoxifylline are specific options to treat severe AH.[56,57,118] In 1 study, use of antioxidant cocktail as an adjuvant to steroids improved survival at 1 month but this benefit was lost at 1 year.[119] In another RCT, use of vitamin E alone did not improve survival despite improved serum hyaluronic acid levels.[120]

Alcoholic cirrhosis

In an RCT, use of vitamins E and C failed to improve biochemical parameters, hospitalization rates, and survival.[121] Polyenylphosphatidylcholine, used orally in a dose of 4.5 g/d in 3 divided doses in 789 veterans with biopsy-proved alcoholic cirrhosis, failed to reduce fibrosis by one stage. In a subgroup of patients, however, with concomitant hepatitis C virus infection, the drug was found useful in improvement of liver function.[122] Use of SAM has been tested with animal data, showing benefit in restoring glutathione levels. In the largest RCT from Europe, use of SAM in a dose of 1.2 g/d for 2 years in 123 alcoholic cirrhotics reduced the composite endpoint of death or liver transplantation compared with placebo-treated patients (30% vs 16%) when data were analyzed only for Child-Turcotte-Pugh stages A and B patients.[59] Other agents that have been tried and not found consistently useful are zinc, silymarin, and betaine.[117] Larger and better designed RCTs are suggested for evaluating the role of antioxidants, using a homogeneous population with earlier-stage disease and using antioxidants for a fair length of time before their routine use is recommended in clinical practice.

Oxandrolone

From the 2 RCTs of use of oxandrolone in veterans patients with alcoholic liver disease, this drug was found effective as an adjuvant to nutritional supplementation in patients with moderate malnutrition and lacked efficacy in those with severe malnutrition.[91]

Coffee Drinking

Drinking 2 or more cups of coffee daily has been shown protective for development of cirrhosis and HCC among chronic alcoholics by more than 50% compared with those who do not or drink less than 1 cup per day[123–125] Similar mortality benefit is also reported among patients with alcoholic cirrhosis.[126] In a large prospective study, coffee intake was associated with total and cause-specific mortality. Apart from liver disease, coffee drinking also protected from cardiopulmonary disease, stroke, injuries, diabetes, and infections.[125] The mechanisms and components of coffee that are protective are not clear.

REFERENCES

1. Mendenhall CL, Moritz TE, Roselle GA, et al. Protein energy malnutrition in severe alcoholic hepatitis: diagnosis and response to treatment. The VA Cooperative Study Group #275. JPEN J Parenter Enteral Nutr 1995;19:258–65.
2. Cheung K, Lee SS, Raman M. Prevalence and mechanisms of malnutrition in patients with advanced liver disease, and nutrition management strategies. Clin Gastroenterol Hepatol 2012;10:117–25.
3. McClain CJ, Barve SS, Barve A, et al. Alcoholic liver disease and malnutrition. Alcohol Clin Exp Res 2011;35:815–20.
4. Achord JL. Malnutrition and the role of nutritional support in alcoholic liver disease. Am J Gastroenterol 1987;82:1–7.

5. Mendenhall CL, Anderson S, Weesner RE, et al. Protein-calorie malnutrition associated with alcoholic hepatitis. Veterans administration cooperative study group on alcoholic hepatitis. Am J Med 1984;76:211–22.

6. DiCecco SR, Wieners EJ, Wiesner RH, et al. Assessment of nutritional status of patients with end-stage liver disease undergoing liver transplantation. Mayo Clin Proc 1989;64:95–102.

7. Hehir DJ, Jenkins RL, Bistrian BR, et al. Nutrition in patients undergoing orthotopic liver transplant. JPEN J Parenter Enteral Nutr 1985;9:695–700.

8. Roongpisuthipong C, Sobhonslidsuk A, Nantiruj K, et al. Nutritional assessment in various stages of liver cirrhosis. Nutrition 2001;17:761–5.

9. Sarin SK, Dhingra N, Bansal A, et al. Dietary and nutritional abnormalities in alcoholic liver disease: a comparison with chronic alcoholics without liver disease. Am J Gastroenterol 1997;92:777–83.

10. Lolli R, Marchesini G, Bianchi G, et al. Anthropometric assessment of the nutritional status of patients with liver cirrhosis in an Italian population. Ital J Gastroenterol 1992;24:429–35.

11. Carvalho L, Parise ER. Evaluation of nutritional status of nonhospitalized patients with liver cirrhosis. Arq Gastroenterol 2006;43:269–74.

12. Campillo B, Richardet JP, Scherman E, et al. Evaluation of nutritional practice in hospitalized cirrhotic patients: results of a prospective study. Nutrition 2003;19: 515–21.

13. Rissanen A, Sarlio-Lahteenkorva S, Alfthan G, et al. Employed problem drinkers: a nutritional risk group? Am J Clin Nutr 1987;45:456–61.

14. Simko V, Connell AM, Banks B. Nutritional status in alcoholics with and without liver disease. Am J Clin Nutr 1982;35:197–203.

15. Sam J, Nguyen GC. Protein-calorie malnutrition as a prognostic indicator of mortality among patients hospitalized with cirrhosis and portal hypertension. Liver Int 2009;29:1396–402.

16. Alvares-da-Silva MR, Reverbel da Silveira T. Comparison between handgrip strength, subjective global assessment, and prognostic nutritional index in assessing malnutrition and predicting clinical outcome in cirrhotic outpatients. Nutrition 2005;21:113–7.

17. Mendenhall C, Roselle GA, Gartside P, et al. Relationship of protein calorie malnutrition to alcoholic liver disease: a reexamination of data from two Veterans Administration Cooperative Studies. Alcohol Clin Exp Res 1995;19:635–41.

18. Stephenson GR, Moretti EW, El-Moalem H, et al. Malnutrition in liver transplant patients: preoperative subjective global assessment is predictive of outcome after liver transplantation. Transplantation 2001;72:666–70.

19. Merli M, Giusto M, Gentili F, et al. Nutritional status: its influence on the outcome of patients undergoing liver transplantation. Liver Int 2010;30:208–14.

20. Madden AM, Bradbury W, Morgan MY. Taste perception in cirrhosis: its relationship to circulating micronutrients and food preferences. Hepatology 1997;26: 40–8.

21. Verne GN, Soldevia-Pico C, Robinson ME, et al. Autonomic dysfunction and gastroparesis in cirrhosis. J Clin Gastroenterol 2004;38:72–6.

22. Aqel BA, Scolapio JS, Dickson RC, et al. Contribution of ascites to impaired gastric function and nutritional intake in patients with cirrhosis and ascites. Clin Gastroenterol Hepatol 2005;3:1095–100.

23. Galati JS, Holdeman KP, Dalrymple GV, et al. Delayed gastric emptying of both the liquid and solid components of a meal in chronic liver disease. Am J Gastroenterol 1994;89:708–11.

24. Kalaitzakis E, Bosaeus I, Ohman L, et al. Altered postprandial glucose, insulin, leptin, and ghrelin in liver cirrhosis: correlations with energy intake and resting energy expenditure. Am J Clin Nutr 2007;85:808–15.

25. Ockenga J, Bischoff SC, Tillmann HL, et al. Elevated bound leptin correlates with energy expenditure in cirrhotics. Gastroenterology 2000;119:1656–62.

26. Marchesini G, Bianchi G, Lucidi P, et al. Plasma ghrelin concentrations, food intake, and anorexia in liver failure. J Clin Endocrinol Metab 2004;89:2136–41.

27. Davcev P, Vanovski B, Sestakov D, et al. Protein-losing enteropathy in patients with liver cirrhosis. Digestion 1969;2:17–22.

28. Roggin GM, Iber FL, Kater RM, et al. Malabsorption in the chronic alcoholic. Johns Hopkins Med J 1969;125:321–30.

29. Witte MH, Dumont AE, Cole WR, et al. Lymph circulation in hepatic cirrhosis: effect of portacaval shunt. Ann Intern Med 1969;70:303–10.

30. Dumont AE, Witte CL, Witte MH. Protein content of liver lymph in patients with portal hypertension secondary to hepatic cirrhosis. Lymphology 1975;8:111–3.

31. Smadja C, Franco D. Portacaval shunts in the treatment of portal hypertension. Ann Gastroenterol Hepatol (Paris) 1988;24:357–61 [in French].

32. Georgopoulos P, Mowat C, McMillan DC, et al. Is portal hypertension associated with protein-losing enteropathy? J Gastroenterol Hepatol 2005;20:103–7.

33. Morgan MY. Enteral nutrition in chronic liver disease. Acta Chir Scand Suppl 1981;507:81–90.

34. Thuluvath PJ, Triger DR. Autonomic neuropathy and chronic liver disease. Q J Med 1989;72:737–47.

35. Rodrigo C, Antezana C, Baraona E. Fat and nitrogen balances in rats with alcohol-induced fatty liver. J Nutr 1971;101:1307–10.

36. Leevy CM, Moroianu SA. Nutritional aspects of alcoholic liver disease. Clin Liver Dis 2005;9:67–81.

37. Charlton MR, Adey DB, Nair KS. Evidence for a catabolic role of glucagon during an amino acid load. J Clin Invest 1996;98:90–9.

38. Petrides AS, De Fronzo RA. Failure of glucagon to stimulate hepatic glycogenolysis in well-nourished patients with mild cirrhosis. Metabolism 1994;43:85–9.

39. Caufriez A, Reding P, Urbain D, et al. Insulin-like growth factor I: a good indicator of functional hepatocellular capacity in alcoholic liver cirrhosis. J Endocrinol Invest 1991;14:317–21.

40. Wu JC, Daughaday WH, Lee SD, et al. Radioimmunoassay of serum IGF-I and IGF-II in patients with chronic liver diseases and hepatocellular carcinoma with or without hypoglycemia. J Lab Clin Med 1988;112:589–94.

41. Lieber CS. The influence of alcohol on nutritional status. Nutr Rev 1988;46:241–54.

42. Dudrick SJ, Kavic SM. Hepatobiliary nutrition: history and future. J Hepatobiliary Pancreat Surg 2002;9:459–68.

43. Cascino A, Cangiano C, Fiaccadori F, et al. Plasma and cerebrospinal fluid amino acid patterns in hepatic encephalopathy. Dig Dis Sci 1982;27:828–32.

44. Marchesini G, Zoli M, Dondi C, et al. Prevalence of subclinical hepatic encephalopathy in cirrhotics and relationship to plasma amino acid imbalance. Dig Dis Sci 1980;25:763–8.

45. McCullough AJ. Malnutrition in liver disease. Liver Transpl 2000;(4 Suppl 1):S85–96.

46. Cabre E, Hernandez-Perez JM, Fluvia L, et al. Absorption and transport of dietary long-chain fatty acids in cirrhosis: a stable-isotope-tracing study. Am J Clin Nutr 2005;81:692–701.

47. Changani KK, Jalan R, Cox IJ, et al. Evidence for altered hepatic gluconeogenesis in patients with cirrhosis using in vivo 31-phosphorus magnetic resonance spectroscopy. Gut 2001;49:557–64.

48. Petrides AS, Luzi L, Reuben A, et al. Effect of insulin and plasma amino acid concentration on leucine metabolism in cirrhosis. Hepatology 1991;14:432–41.

49. Merli M, Leonetti F, Riggio O, et al. Glucose intolerance and insulin resistance in cirrhosis are normalized after liver transplantation. Hepatology 1999;30:649–54.

50. Muller MJ, Lautz HU, Plogmann B, et al. Energy expenditure and substrate oxidation in patients with cirrhosis: the impact of cause, clinical staging and nutritional state. Hepatology 1992;15:782–94.

51. Reinus JF, Heymsfield SB, Wiskind R, et al. Ethanol: relative fuel value and metabolic effects in vivo. Metabolism 1989;38:125–35.

52. Lieber CS. ALCOHOL: its metabolism and interaction with nutrients. Annu Rev Nutr 2000;20:395–430.

53. Bjarnason I, Peters TJ, Wise RJ. The leaky gut of alcoholism: possible route of entry for toxic compounds. Lancet 1984;1:179–82.

54. McClain CJ, Barve S, Deaciuc I, et al. Cytokines in alcoholic liver disease. Semin Liver Dis 1999;19:205–19.

55. Braillon A, Gaudin C, Poo JL, et al. Plasma catecholamine concentrations are a reliable index of sympathetic vascular tone in patients with cirrhosis. Hepatology 1992;15:58–62.

56. Singal AK, Shah VH. Alcoholic hepatitis: prognostic models and treatment. Gastroenterol Clin North Am 2011;40:611–39.

57. Lucey MR, Mathurin P, Morgan TR. Alcoholic hepatitis. N Engl J Med 2009;360:2758–69.

58. Dolz C, Raurich JM, Ibanez J, et al. Ascites increases the resting energy expenditure in liver cirrhosis. Gastroenterology 1991;100:738–44.

59. Halsted CH. Nutrition and alcoholic liver disease. Semin Liver Dis 2004;24:289–304.

60. Detsky AS, McLaughlin JR, Baker JP, et al. What is subjective global assessment of nutritional status? JPEN J Parenter Enteral Nutr 1987;11:8–13.

61. Pikul J, Sharpe MD, Lowndes R, et al. Degree of preoperative malnutrition is predictive of postoperative morbidity and mortality in liver transplant recipients. Transplantation 1994;57:469–72.

62. DiCecco SR, Francisco-Ziller N. Nutrition in alcoholic liver disease. Nutr Clin Pract 2006;21:245–54.

63. Nielsen K, Kondrup J, Martinsen L, et al. Nutritional assessment and adequacy of dietary intake in hospitalized patients with alcoholic liver cirrhosis. Br J Nutr 1993;69:665–79.

64. Figueiredo FA, Dickson ER, Pasha TM, et al. Utility of standard nutritional parameters in detecting body cell mass depletion in patients with end-stage liver disease. Liver Transpl 2000;6:575–81.

65. Frisancho AR. New norms of upper limb fat and muscle areas for assessment of nutritional status. Am J Clin Nutr 1981;34:2540–5.

66. Schlussel MM, dos Anjos LA, de Vasconcellos MT, et al. Reference values of handgrip dynamometry of healthy adults: a population-based study. Clin Nutr 2008;27:601–7.

67. Andersen H, Borre M, Jakobsen J, et al. Decreased muscle strength in patients with alcoholic liver cirrhosis in relation to nutritional status, alcohol abstinence, liver function, and neuropathy. Hepatology 1998;27:1200–6.

68. Mendenhall CL, Chernausek SD, Ray MB, et al. The interactions of insulin-like growth factor I(IGF-I) with protein-calorie malnutrition in patients with alcoholic

liver disease: V.A. Cooperative Study on Alcoholic Hepatitis VI. Alcohol Alcohol 1989;24:319–29.

69. Englesbe MJ, Patel SP, He K, et al. Sarcopenia and mortality after liver transplantation. J Am Coll Surg 2010;211:271–8.

70. Prijatmoko D, Strauss BJ, Lambert JR, et al. Early detection of protein depletion in alcoholic cirrhosis: role of body composition analysis. Gastroenterology 1993; 105:1839–45.

71. Plauth M, Cabre E, Riggio O, et al. ESPEN guidelines on enteral nutrition: liver disease. Clin Nutr 2006;25:285–94.

72. Pirlich M, Schutz T, Spachos T, et al. Bioelectrical impedance analysis is a useful bedside technique to assess malnutrition in cirrhotic patients with and without ascites. Hepatology 2000;32:1208–15.

73. Selberg O, Bottcher J, Tusch G, et al. Identification of high- and low-risk patients before liver transplantation: a prospective cohort study of nutritional and metabolic parameters in 150 patients. Hepatology 1997;25:652–7.

74. Figueiredo F, Dickson ER, Pasha T, et al. Impact of nutritional status on outcomes after liver transplantation. Transplantation 2000;70:1347–52.

75. Mullen JL. Consequences of malnutrition in the surgical patient. Surg Clin North Am 1981;61:465–87.

76. Shanbhogue RL, Bistrian BR, Jenkins RL, et al. Resting energy expenditure in patients with end-stage liver disease and in normal population. JPEN J Parenter Enteral Nutr 1987;11:305–8.

77. Swart GR, Zillikens MC, van Vuure JK, et al. Effect of a late evening meal on nitrogen balance in patients with cirrhosis of the liver. BMJ 1989;299:1202–3.

78. Plank LD, Gane EJ, Peng S, et al. Nocturnal nutritional supplementation improves total body protein status of patients with liver cirrhosis: a randomized 12-month trial. Hepatology 2008;48:557–66.

79. Cordoba J, Lopez-Hellin J, Planas M, et al. Normal protein diet for episodic hepatic encephalopathy: results of a randomized study. J Hepatol 2004;41: 38–43.

80. Mullen KD, Dasarathy S. Protein restriction in hepatic encephalopathy: necessary evil or illogical dogma? J Hepatol 2004;41:147–8.

81. Teratani T, Tomita K, Suzuki T, et al. A high-cholesterol diet exacerbates liver fibrosis in mice via accumulation of free cholesterol in hepatic stellate cells. Gastroenterology 2012;142:152–164.e10.

82. Ioannou GN, Morrow OB, Connole ML, et al. Association between dietary nutrient composition and the incidence of cirrhosis or liver cancer in the United States population. Hepatology 2009;50:175–84.

83. Ekstedt M, Franzen LE, Mathiesen UL, et al. Statins in non-alcoholic fatty liver disease and chronically elevated liver enzymes: a histopathological follow-up study. J Hepatol 2007;47:135–41.

84. Battistella FD, Widergren JT, Anderson JT, et al. A prospective, randomized trial of intravenous fat emulsion administration in trauma victims requiring total parenteral nutrition. J Trauma 1997;43:52–8 [discussion: 8–60].

85. Stickel F, Kessebohm K, Weimann R, et al. Review of liver injury associated with dietary supplements. Liver Int 2011;31:595–605.

86. Lundbom N, Laurila O, Laurila S. Central pontine myelinolysis after correction of chronic hyponatraemia. Lancet 1993;342:247–8.

87. de Ledinghen V, Beau P, Mannant PR, et al. Early feeding or enteral nutrition in patients with cirrhosis after bleeding from esophageal varices? A randomized controlled study. Dig Dis Sci 1997;42:536–41.

88. Baltz JG, Argo CK, Al-Osaimi AM, et al. Mortality after percutaneous endoscopic gastrostomy in patients with cirrhosis: a case series. Gastrointest Endosc 2010;72:1072–5.

89. Calvey H, Davis M, Williams R. Controlled trial of nutritional supplementation, with and without branched chain amino acid enrichment, in treatment of acute alcoholic hepatitis. J Hepatol 1985;1:141–51.

90. Mendenhall C, Bongiovanni G, Goldberg S, et al. VA Cooperative Study on Alcoholic Hepatitis. III: changes in protein-calorie malnutrition associated with 30 days of hospitalization with and without enteral nutritional therapy. JPEN J Parenter Enteral Nutr 1985;9:590–6.

91. Mendenhall CL, Moritz TE, Roselle GA, et al. A study of oral nutritional support with oxandrolone in malnourished patients with alcoholic hepatitis: results of a Department of Veterans Affairs cooperative study. Hepatology 1993;17:564–76.

92. Cabre E, Rodriguez-Iglesias P, Caballeria J, et al. Short- and long-term outcome of severe alcohol-induced hepatitis treated with steroids or enteral nutrition: a multicenter randomized trial. Hepatology 2000;32:36–42.

93. Moreno C, Langlet P, Hittelet A, et al. Enteral nutrition with or without N-acetylcysteine in the treatment of severe acute alcoholic hepatitis: a randomized multicenter controlled trial. J Hepatol 2010;53:1117–22.

94. Alvarez MA, Cabre E, Lorenzo-Zuniga V, et al. Combining steroids with enteral nutrition: a better therapeutic strategy for severe alcoholic hepatitis? Results of a pilot study. Eur J Gastroenterol Hepatol 2004;16:1375–80.

95. Bunout D, Aicardi V, Hirsch S, et al. Nutritional support in hospitalized patients with alcoholic liver disease. Eur J Clin Nutr 1989;43:615–21.

96. Cabre E, Gonzalez-Huix F, Abad-Lacruz A, et al. Effect of total enteral nutrition on the short-term outcome of severely malnourished cirrhotics. A randomized controlled trial. Gastroenterology 1990;98:715–20.

97. Hirsch S, Bunout D, de la Maza P, et al. Controlled trial on nutrition supplementation in outpatients with symptomatic alcoholic cirrhosis. JPEN J Parenter Enteral Nutr 1993;17:119–24.

98. Kearns PJ, Young H, Garcia G, et al. Accelerated improvement of alcoholic liver disease with enteral nutrition. Gastroenterology 1992;102:200–5.

99. Dupont B, Dao T, Joubert C, et al. Randomised clinical trial: enteral nutrition does not improve the long-term outcome of alcoholic cirrhotic patients with jaundice. Aliment Pharmacol Ther 2012;35(10):1166–74.

100. Plauth M, Cabre E, Campillo B, et al. ESPEN Guidelines on parenteral nutrition: hepatology. Clin Nutr 2009;28:436–44.

101. Galambos JT, Hersh T, Fulenwider JT, et al. Hyperalimentation in alcoholic hepatitis. Am J Gastroenterol 1979;72:535–41.

102. Nasrallah SM, Galambos JT. Aminoacid therapy of alcoholic hepatitis. Lancet 1980;2:1276–7.

103. Diehl AM, Boitnott JK, Herlong HF, et al. Effect of parenteral amino acid supplementation in alcoholic hepatitis. Hepatology 1985;5:57–63.

104. Naveau S, Pelletier G, Poynard T, et al. A randomized clinical trial of supplementary parenteral nutrition in jaundiced alcoholic cirrhotic patients. Hepatology 1986;6:270–4.

105. Achord JL. A prospective randomized clinical trial of peripheral amino acid-glucose supplementation in acute alcoholic hepatitis. Am J Gastroenterol 1987;82:871–5.

106. Simon D, Galambos JT. A randomized controlled study of peripheral parenteral nutrition in moderate and severe alcoholic hepatitis. J Hepatol 1988;7:200–7.

107. Mezey E, Caballeria J, Mitchell MC, et al. Effect of parenteral amino acid supplementation on short-term and long-term outcomes in severe alcoholic hepatitis: a randomized controlled trial. Hepatology 1991;14:1090–6.

108. Charlton M. Branched-chain amino acid-enriched supplements as therapy for liver disease: Rasputin lives. Gastroenterology 2003;124:1980–2.

109. Horst D, Grace ND, Conn HO, et al. Comparison of dietary protein with an oral, branched chain-enriched amino acid supplement in chronic portal-systemic encephalopathy: a randomized controlled trial. Hepatology 1984;4: 279–87.

110. Christie ML, Sack DM, Pomposelli J, et al. Enriched branched-chain amino acid formula versus a casein-based supplement in the treatment of cirrhosis. JPEN J Parenter Enteral Nutr 1985;9:671–8.

111. McGhee A, Henderson JM, Millikan WJ Jr, et al. Comparison of the effects of Hepatic-Aid and a Casein modular diet on encephalopathy, plasma amino acids, and nitrogen balance in cirrhotic patients. Ann Surg 1983;197:288–93.

112. Yoshida T, Muto Y, Moriwaki H, et al. Effect of long-term oral supplementation with branched-chain amino acid granules on the prognosis of liver cirrhosis. Gastroenterol Jpn 1989;24:692–8.

113. Marchesini G, Bianchi G, Merli M, et al. Nutritional supplementation with branched-chain amino acids in advanced cirrhosis: a double-blind, randomized trial. Gastroenterology 2003;124:1792–801.

114. Muto Y, Sato S, Watanabe A, et al. Effects of oral branched-chain amino acid granules on event-free survival in patients with liver cirrhosis. Clin Gastroenterol Hepatol 2005;3:705–13.

115. Charlton M. Branched-chain amino-acid granules: can they improve survival in patients with liver cirrhosis? Nat Clin Pract Gastroenterol Hepatol 2006;3: 72–3.

116. Dey A, Cederbaum AI. Alcohol and oxidative liver injury. Hepatology 2006;43: S63–74.

117. Singal AK, Jampana SC, Weinman SA. Antioxidants as therapeutic agents for liver disease. Liver Int 2011;31:1432–48.

118. Singal AK, Walia I, Singal A, et al. Corticosteroids and pentoxifylline for the treatment of alcoholic hepatitis: current status. World J Hepatol 2011;3: 205–10.

119. Phillips M, Curtis H, Portmann B, et al. Antioxidants versus corticosteroids in the treatment of severe alcoholic hepatitis—a randomised clinical trial. J Hepatol 2006;44:784–90.

120. Mezey E, Potter JJ, Rennie-Tankersley L, et al. A randomized placebo controlled trial of vitamin E for alcoholic hepatitis. J Hepatol 2004;40:40–6.

121. de la Maza MP, Petermann M, Bunout D, et al. Effects of long-term vitamin E supplementation in alcoholic cirrhotics. J Am Coll Nutr 1995;14:192–6.

122. Lieber CS, Weiss DG, Groszmann R, et al. Veterans Affairs Cooperative Study of polyenylphosphatidylcholine in alcoholic liver disease. Alcohol Clin Exp Res 2003;27:1765–72.

123. Ruhl CE, Everhart JE. Coffee and tea consumption are associated with a lower incidence of chronic liver disease in the United States. Gastroenterology 2005; 129:1928–36.

124. Klatsky AL, Armstrong MA. Alcohol, smoking, coffee, and cirrhosis. Am J Epidemiol 1992;136:1248–57.

125. Freedman ND, Park Y, Abnet CC, et al. Association of coffee drinking with total and cause-specific mortality. N Engl J Med 2012;366:1891–904.

126. Tverdal A, Skurtveit S. Coffee intake and mortality from liver cirrhosis. Ann Epidemiol 2003;13:419–23.

127. Bonkovsky HL, Fiellin DA, Smith GS, et al. A randomized, controlled trial of treatment of alcoholic hepatitis with parenteral nutrition and oxandrolone. I. Short-term effects on liver function. Am J Gastroenterol 1991;86:1200–8.

Alcohol's Effect on Other Chronic Liver Diseases

Maximilian Lee, MD, MPH, Kris V. Kowdley, MD*

KEYWORDS

- Alcohol • Autoimmune hepatitis • Fatty liver disease • Hepatitis B • Hepatitis C
- Hemochromatosis • Fibrosis • Cirrhosis

KEY POINTS

- Alcohol consumption synergistically exacerbates liver injury in several major nonalcoholic chronic liver diseases.
- Alcohol's synergistic injury results in increased hepatic inflammation and accelerated rates of fibrosis.
- Alcohol also increases the risks of developing cirrhosis, liver cancer, and death.
- There does not seem to be a safe level of alcohol consumption in chronic liver diseases.

ALCOHOL AND FATTY LIVER DISEASE

Nonalcoholic fatty liver disease (NAFLD) is increasingly recognized as the downstream hepatic consequence of the metabolic syndrome. Well-known risk factors for NAFLD include obesity (especially with increased waist circumference), insulin resistance (with either elevated fasting glucose or frank type 2 diabetes), and hypertriglyceridemia, and these risk factors are also strongly associated with the development of metabolic syndrome.[1] Other risk factors for the metabolic syndrome such as hyperlipidemia and hypertension may also prompt suspicion for NAFLD; therefore, metabolic syndrome is a strong predictor for the development of NAFLD.[2] The absence of excessive alcohol consumption is a necessary prerequisite for the diagnosis of NAFLD from alcoholic liver disease, because the 2 conditions may be histologically indistinguishable[3]; however, recent studies indicate that alcohol may play a role in both the progression and pathogenesis of NAFLD, as reviewed later.

Most patients with NAFLD have hepatic steatosis in the absence of necroinflammatory features or fibrosis; however, a significant minority may have nonalcoholic steatohepatitis (NASH), which is characterized by hepatocellular inflammation, injury,

Liver Center of Excellence, Virginia Mason Medical Center, 1100 Ninth Avenue, Mailstop C3-GAS, Seattle, WA 98101, USA
* Corresponding author.
E-mail address: kris.kowdley@vmmc.org

Clin Liver Dis 16 (2012) 827–837
http://dx.doi.org/10.1016/j.cld.2012.08.010
liver.theclinics.com

and fibrosis.[4] Prolonged duration of NASH may ultimately lead to cirrhosis and many cases of "cryptogenic cirrhosis."[5] Obesity-related insulin resistance is one of the main pathogenic factors responsible for this progression, as hyperinsulinemia has been shown to increase the levels of free fatty acids and cholesterol[6] within the liver, resulting in cytotoxicity and oxidative stress, which then promote hepatic stellate cell activation and fibrosis.[7]

Like with other chronic liver diseases, alcohol seems to be an important risk factor for progressive fibrosis in NASH. One recent experimental animal model confirmed this effect by randomizing mice between a regular diet, a NASH-inducing high-fat diet, a regular diet with alcohol-laced drinking water (up to a concentration of 5%), and a combined high-fat and alcohol diet. The NASH-inducing high-fat diet significantly induced hepatic triglyceride accumulation and the expression of proinflammatory and profibrogenic genes compared with alcohol alone. However, in mice given a combined high-fat and alcohol diet, both proinflammatory and profibrogenic gene expressions were even more significantly elevated than with either diet alone, and there was a further marked induction of hepatic fibrosis.[8] Another recent study in rats also showed that moderate alcohol consumption, along with a high-fat diet, led to significantly more hepatic inflammation and cellular apoptosis, compared with a high-fat diet alone.[9] In humans, moderate alcohol consumption has also been associated with the progression of hepatic fibrosis in NAFLD.[10] On the other hand, light-to-moderate alcohol use has also been shown to decrease insulin resistance and the risks of both metabolic syndrome[11] and cardiovascular mortality.[12] Because the risk factors for NAFLD overlap with those of cardiovascular disease, patients may end up receiving contradictory recommendations[13] from different health care providers.

Recent studies have attempted to clarify whether there may be an optimal concentration of alcohol use in NAFLD patients. In a study of 132 morbidly obese Brazilian patients, light-to-moderate alcohol consumption (defined as between <20 g/d and 40 g/d) did not have an impact on the severity of steatosis and steatohepatitis,[14] although light-to-moderate alcohol consumption caused a decrease in insulin resistance in these patients. Several Japanese cohort studies have further examined whether alcohol consumption may actually be protective against NAFLD. In a large Japanese cohort of 4957 men and 2155 women, alcohol consumption was inversely associated with a lower prevalence of fatty liver compared with nondrinkers in both men (28% vs 40%) and women (10% vs 16%). Furthermore, light alcohol consumption (defined as <20 g/d for only 1–3 days per week) was associated with a lower prevalence of NAFLD with an odds ratio of 0.47, suggesting a protective effect against the development of NAFLD.[15] Two other large Japanese cohort studies have also examined whether this potential protective effect held true across broader categories of alcohol consumption, including moderate and heavy drinking. In 2009, Gunji and colleagues[16] found in 5599 Japanese men that both light (40–140 g/wk) and moderate (140–280 g/wk) alcohol consumption were significantly associated with a reduction in the risk of developing NAFLD (odds ratios of 0.824 and 0.754, respectively). In 2011, Hiramine and colleagues[17] found in 9886 Japanese men that the prevalence of fatty liver disease followed a U-shaped distribution across several categories of alcohol use among 44.7% of nondrinkers, 39.3% of light drinkers (<20 g/d), 35.9% of moderate drinkers (20–59 g/d), and 40.1% of heavy drinkers (>60 g/d). The prevalence of NAFLD was inversely associated with alcohol consumption, with odds ratios of 0.71 in light drinkers, 0.55 in moderate drinkers, and 0.44 in heavy drinkers. NAFLD prevalence was also inversely associated with the frequency of alcohol consumption (>21 d/mo) but not necessarily volume consumed, with an odds ratio of 0.62. In another large 2012 cohort study of 18,571 Japanese men and women, Hamaguchi and colleagues[18] also found gender differences in the potential protective effect of alcohol consumption on developing NAFLD; any level of alcohol consumption was protective in men, although only light to moderate consumption was protective in women. However, alcohol consumption was not protective against developing the metabolic syndrome in either men or women.

The potential protective effect of light-to-moderate alcohol consumption against the development of NAFLD is intriguing, especially when considering that recent microarray gene expression analysis found that gene expression of the known genes in the pathways of alcohol catabolism are increased in the liver of patients with NASH compared with those of normal patients.[19] Genes associated with liver inflammation and fibrosis, which are hypothesized to be downstream to these alcohol catabolic pathways, were also found to be upregulated in livers with NASH compared with normal livers. Therefore, in addition to insulin resistance, alcohol may play a crucial pathogenic role in the development of NAFLD and its progression to NASH; for example, in alcohol drinkers who already have NAFLD and/or NASH, alcohol may cause synergistic injury, and in nondrinkers, obesity-related intestinal overgrowth may produce endogenous alcohol. It remains unclear why certain patients who are at risk for NAFLD are apparently able to derive the protective effects of alcohol, whereas those who already have NAFLD suffer worsening injury from alcohol.

ALCOHOL AND CHRONIC HEPATITIS C

Hepatitis C virus (HCV) is the leading cause of chronic liver disease in the United States, with an estimated 4.1 million people containing serologic evidence of HCV infection, and 3.2 million people with active chronic HCV infection.[20] Worldwide, HCV infection affects approximately 170 million people. The natural history of untreated chronic hepatitis C results in the progression to cirrhosis with the complications of decompensated liver disease and development of hepatocellular carcinoma. Although the prevalence of chronic HCV infection in the United States is expected to decrease during the next few decades as a result of the aging of current patients, a recent multicohort natural history model by Davis and colleagues[21] also estimated that by 2040, the prevalence of chronic hepatitis C–related cirrhosis will increase to 39% of this population. This model was supported by a meta-analysis by Thein and colleagues[22] that found that duration of infection was the most consistent factor significantly associated with progression of fibrosis toward cirrhosis, with an estimated prevalence of cirrhosis of 16% after 20 years of chronic HCV infection. Based on different observational studies, alcohol consumption was present in 19% of these cohorts; however, the definition of excessive alcohol use varied by cohort, with a range of alcohol consumption from more than 20 g/d to more than 80 g/d.

Alcohol consumption is a common comorbidity in patients with chronic HCV infection. Multiple studies have shown that it results in synergistic injury, with accelerated rates of fibrosis and the development of cirrhosis and liver cancer, and several mechanisms have been proposed including: alcohol's effect on HCV viral replication, HCV-related cytotoxicity, hepatic oxidative stress, and immune modulation. In an HCV replicon study, Zhang and colleagues[23] showed that alcohol significantly increased HCV viral replication in a concentration-dependent fashion. Kim and colleagues[24] showed that alcohol potentiates HCV core protein induction of necrosis factor-κB, which is associated with promoting hepatic inflammation. Pianko and colleagues[25] demonstrated that Fas-mediated hepatocyte apoptosis was increased in alcoholic HCV-infected livers compared with HCV-infected livers from nonalcoholics. Alcohol can also induce hepatocyte apoptosis by glutathione depletion, which sensitizes HCV-infected hepatocytes to the action of tumor necrosis factor-α.[26] Although not directly cytotoxic, hepatitis C infection results in hepatocellular injury by increasing oxidative stress in the liver. This can occur via direct generation of reactive oxidative species by the production of HCV core protein,[27] induction of plasma membrane–associated oxidases in macrophages and neutrophils,[28] or secondary hepatic iron overload.[29] In hepatoma cells that expressed HCV core protein and cytochrome P450 2E1, Otani and colleagues[30] showed that oxidative stress was potentiated when treated with alcohol, which exacerbated oxidative species production and cell death. In transgenic mice expressing HCV core protein, Perlemuter and colleagues[31] also showed that alcohol increased lipid peroxidation and enhanced production of the cytokines tumor necrosis factor-α and hepatic transforming growth factor-β, which are associated with increased reactive oxidative species generation and stimulating hepatic fibrosis, respectively. In HCV patients, antibody markers of oxidative stress were also found to be increased with alcohol consumption, by up to 3-fold in moderate (up to 50 g/d) and 13- to 24-fold in heavy (>50 g/d) drinkers.[32] Furthermore, alcohol consumption was significantly associated with piecemeal necrosis, and this was 4-fold more frequent in those with antibody markers of oxidative stress. Additionally, alcohol may modulate and reduce host immune factors that aid in HCV infection clearance.[33] In vitro findings by Ye and colleagues[34] have shown that alcohol suppresses intracellular expression of interferon-α/β and that this significantly enhanced HCV viral replication, which may contribute to chronic infection and reduce interferon-based antiviral therapy. Alcohol has also been shown to reduce the ability of dendritic cells, which are specialized antigen presenting cells, in generating cytotoxic T-cell responses to HCV viral proteins.[35] Immunosuppression by alcohol also generates HCV quasi-species complexity,[36] although the clinical significance of this remains uncertain.

In patients with chronic HCV, multiple studies have shown that alcohol consumption of at least 50 g/d may be the threshold amount that results in accelerated liver injury with the rapid development of advanced fibrosis, cirrhosis, hepatocellular carcinoma, and death, but lesser amounts of alcohol consumption still increased the risk of these complications. An early study from 1998 by Wiley and colleagues[37] on liver biopsies from 176 patients with HCV infection showed that chronic alcohol consumption of more than 60 g/d was associated with a 2- to 3-fold increased risk of developing cirrhosis compared with nondrinkers; 58% of these patients were also found to have developed cirrhosis within 20 years of HCV infection versus 10% in nondrinkers. Another study from 1998 by Ostapowicz and colleagues[38] on 234 patients with HCV infection showed instead that greater total lifetime alcohol consumption was significantly associated with the development of cirrhosis, as opposed to average daily alcohol consumption. Average daily alcohol consumption was not significantly different between the patients who developed or did not develop cirrhosis, and these authors concluded that there was no "safe" amount of alcohol consumption in persons with chronic HCV. In a smaller study from 2002 based on serial liver biopsies from 78 patients with HCV infection, Westin and colleagues[39] also showed that even moderate alcohol consumption (<40 g/d) was associated with fibrosis progression. In their 2004 study of 800 patients with HCV infection, Monto and colleagues[40] found that there was a range in fibrosis within different categories of alcohol consumption (none, up to 20 g/d, up to 50 g/d, up to 80 g/d, and >80 g/d), but higher categories of alcohol consumption compared with lower categories were still associated with increased fibrosis. In a multivariate modeling of fibrosis progression, however, alcohol intake was not an independent predictor of fibrosis, and Monto and colleagues found that patient age, serum alanine aminotransferase, and histologic inflammation were independent predictors of fibrosis. Given the range in fibrosis within each category of alcohol intake, their model suggested that other host factors, possibly immunologic and/or genetic variables, had a more central role than alcohol intake. Taking into account the different definitions of heavy alcohol consumption across many studies, a 2005 meta-analysis by Hutchinson and colleagues[41] of 20 studies including more than 15,000 patients with HCV infection found that the pooled relative risk of cirrhosis from heavy alcohol intake, between at least 210 and 560 g/wk, was 2.33. The increased risk of cirrhosis also results in earlier rates of developing cirrhosis and death. From 2313 patients with HCV infection, Poynard and colleagues[42] determined that alcohol use of more than 50 g/d led to the earlier development of cirrhosis compared with nondrinkers at 29 years versus 43 years. From another large group of 2646 patients with HCV infection, Marcellin and colleagues[43] also determined that death occurred earlier in men who drank more than 50 g/d at 58 years versus 70 years in nondrinkers. Most patients with alcohol consumption (94.6%) had cirrhosis at the time of death, and 33.1% had liver cancer. In addition to its synergistic effect on the development of cirrhosis, alcohol consumption also promotes carcinogenesis in patients with HCV infection, and the combination of heavy alcohol consumption (>80 g/d) and chronic HCV infection has been estimated to increase the risk for liver cancer to greater than 100-fold.[44] A recent 2009 study has shown that a primary contributor to alcohol-induced liver cancer in HCV patients is the Toll-like receptor 4 (TLR4). In their study on ethanol-fed HCV-infected transgenic mice, Machida and colleagues[45] provided the first evidence that TLR4 is induced by the HCV nonstructural protein NS5A and that this induction mediated synergistic liver injury by alcohol-induced endotoxemia. TLR4 was also found to increase expression of a novel downstream gene and stem/progenitor cell marker, Nanog. This study suggested that alcohol-enhanced TLR4 activation in HCV disease may induce other tumor-driver genes and that a stem cell phenotype may have a role in oncogenesis in combined alcohol and HCV disease.

ALCOHOL AND CHRONIC HEPATITIS B

Hepatitis B virus (HBV) is the leading global cause of chronic liver disease, and HBV infection affects more than one third of the world's population, with more than 2 billion people containing serologic evidence of present or past HBV infection.[46] The natural history of untreated chronic hepatitis B includes progression to cirrhosis and the development of hepatocellular carcinoma, with or without the presence of cirrhosis.

Alcohol consumption in patients with chronic hepatitis B results in synergistic injury, with accelerated rates of fibrosis and the development of cirrhosis, and earlier rates of liver cancer and death. Experimental animal models have been used to study the interaction between alcohol and HBV infection. In HBV-infected transgenic mice that produce consistent levels of viral replication, chronic alcohol consumption led to increased levels of HBV surface antigen and viral replication compared with control mice that did not consume alcohol.[47] In transgenic mice overexpressing the HBV X protein, alcohol induced increased hepatocyte injury and apoptosis compared with controls.[48] In humans, similar interaction effects between alcohol and HBV infection have been found. Nomura and colleagues[49] found that the prevalence of abnormal liver function tests in 932 HBV carriers was increased in patients with light (<59 g/d) and heavy (≥60 g/d) alcohol consumption compared with nondrinkers, and that in 1113 patients with HBV infection, the prevalence of hepatitis B e antigen was also increased,[50] suggesting prolonged seroconversion. Poynard and colleagues[42] found that alcohol consumption rapidly accelerated fibrosis and the development of cirrhosis in 777 patients with HBV infection. In heavy alcohol drinkers, the

50% probability for cirrhosis occurred at an earlier age (46 years) compared nondrinkers and moderate alcohol drinkers (75 years). Marcellin and colleagues[43] also found that heavy alcohol use (>350 g/wk) in 1327 patients with HBV infection was associated with an earlier age of death (52 vs 64 years). The major cause of death in this study was cirrhosis (93%), and 35% had liver cancer. In a small series of 43 patients, Gelatti and colleagues[51] showed a slight, but insignificant, trend toward earlier presentation of liver cancer in patients with HBV and heavy alcohol use ($\geq$60 g/d) compared with nondrinkers, at 60.7 versus 63.4 years, respectively. In 2 large Asian cohort studies of more than 2000 patients with HBV infection each, heavy alcohol consumption was associated with an approximately 1.5-fold increased risk of liver cancer.[52,53] Two case-control studies, each with approximately 500 patients with HBV-related liver cancer, also showed a 1.5- to 2-fold increased risk as a result of heavy alcohol consumption.[54,55] In the setting of HBV cirrhosis, heavy alcohol users were reported to have a higher, 3-fold increased risk of liver cancer.[56]

ALCOHOL AND HEMOCHROMATOSIS

Hereditary hemochromatosis (HH) is an autosomal recessive gene disorder in which *HFE* gene mutations causes chronic intestinal hyperabsorption of iron, resulting in excessive iron deposition in various organs, especially the heart, pancreas, and liver.[57] This deposition can lead to cardiomyopathy, diabetes, and cirrhosis, respectively. The pathophysiology of liver disease in HH is the result of hepatic iron overload causing oxidative stress and increasing fibrosis,[58] ultimately leading to cirrhosis. In addition to being directly hepatotoxic itself, alcohol further promotes hepatic iron overload by increasing iron uptake through the upregulation of the transferrin receptor on hepatocytes,[59] decreasing hepcidin expression,[60] and dissociating iron from ferritin.[61] Together, alcohol and hepatic iron overload cause synergistic hepatotoxicity that has been well studied. In an early retrospective study by Adams and colleagues[62] on 105 putative homozygotes for HH, heavy alcohol consumption (>80 g/d) was found in 15% of these patients. Although histologic evidence of alcoholic liver disease was uncommon in these patients, there was an increased prevalence of cirrhosis compared with nondrinkers (44% vs 15%), suggesting an additive hepatotoxic effect. Scotet and colleagues[63] also studied the effects of heavy alcohol consumption in 378 patients with C282Y homozygous hemochromatosis, of whom 33 drank more than 80 g/d. These patients had significantly increased iron parameters and elevated liver enzymes. In a 2002 study based on liver biopsy data on 224 patients with C282Y homozygous hemochromatosis, Fletcher and colleagues[64] showed that a lower threshold of alcohol consumption (60 g/d) could result in severe fibrosis and cirrhosis. The prevalence of cirrhosis was significantly increased in patients with hemochromatosis who consumed more than 60 g/day compared with those who drank less than 60 g/day (66% vs 7%), and this represented an approximately 9-fold increased relative risk of developing cirrhosis. Excessive alcohol consumption was also associated with a 4.25-fold increased risk of accelerated hepatic fibrosis.[65] This explains the rapid development of cirrhosis, which occurs approximately 14 years earlier in patients with hemochromatosis with reported heavy alcohol use compared with patients who were moderate drinkers or nondrinkers (61 vs 75 years).[42]

ALCOHOL AND AUTOIMMUNE LIVER DISEASES

Autoimmune liver diseases include autoimmune hepatitis, primary biliary cirrhosis (PBC), primary sclerosing cholangitis, and autoimmune cholangitis. These are generally characterized by circulating elevations of autoantibodies associated with a specific histologic pattern of liver injury, such as lymphocyte-mediated attacks against either the hepatocytes or bile ducts in autoimmune hepatitis and PBC, respectively. Occasionally, an overlap syndrome can develop, in which the histologic features of liver injury do not correlate with the detected autoantibody.

The contribution of alcohol to autoimmune liver diseases remains unclear, but a recent mouse study showed that alcohol metabolites that were adducted to liver cytosolic proteins could induce autoimmune hepatitis, with elevated aminotransferase levels, hepatocyte injury, and detectable anti–smooth muscle antibodies, and IgG antibodies and T-lymphocytes that were directed toward these liver cytosolic proteins.[66] Transferring these immunized T-lymphocytes to naïve animals also reproduced biochemical and histologic patterns of liver damage. These data suggest that alcohol could be a pathogenic antigen in the development of autoimmune hepatitis.

Alcohol consumption in the presence of autoimmune liver diseases has not been extensively studied, but in a study of 274 patients with untreated PBC, Sorrentino and colleagues[67] determined that moderate alcohol consumption ($\geq$30 g/d) was an independent predictor of advanced PBC stage. In these patients, moderate alcohol consumption was also significantly correlated with increased oxidative stress and steatosis on their liver biopsies, which was thought to contribute to worsening of PBC stage.

SUMMARY

Alcohol has been shown to cause synergistic injury in combination with other chronic liver diseases, particularly NAFLD, chronic viral hepatitis, HH, and autoimmune liver diseases. Alcohol consumption, particularly in excess, rapidly accelerates the development of hepatic fibrosis and cirrhosis, and also increases the risk of liver cancer and death from liver disease. Despite the effect of light alcohol consumption on decreasing insulin resistance and cardiovascular mortality, there does not seem to be a "safe" limit for alcohol consumption in the setting of combined chronic liver disease.

REFERENCES

1. Grundy SM. Metabolic complications of obesity. Endocrine 2000;13(2):155–65.
2. Hamaguchi M, Kojima T, Takeda N, et al. The metabolic syndrome as a predictor of nonalcoholic fatty liver disease. Ann Intern Med 2005;143(10):722–8.
3. Diehl AM, Goodman Z, Ishak KG. Alcohollike liver disease in nonalcoholics. A clinical and histologic comparison with alcohol-induced liver injury. Gastroenterology 1988;95(4):1056–62.
4. Ludwig J, Viggiano TR, McGill DB, et al. Nonalcoholic steatohepatitis: Mayo Clinic experiences with a hitherto unnamed disease. Mayo Clin Proc 1980; 55(7):434–8.
5. Caldwell SH, Lee VD, Kleiner DE, et al. NASH and cryptogenic cirrhosis: a histological analysis. Ann Hepatol 2009;8(4):346–52.
6. Arteel GE. Beyond reasonable doubt: who is the culprit in lipotoxicity in NAFLD/NASH? Hepatology 2012;55(6):2030–2.
7. Chitturi S, Farrell GC. Etiopathogenesis of nonalcoholic steatohepatitis. Semin Liver Dis 2001;21(1):27–41.
8. Gabele E, Dostert K, Dorn C, et al. A new model of interactive effects of alcohol and high-fat diet on hepatic fibrosis. Alcohol Clin Exp Res 2011;35(7):1361–7.
9. Wang Y, Seitz HK, Wang XD. Moderate alcohol consumption aggravates high-fat diet induced steatohepatitis in rats. Alcohol Clin Exp Res 2010;34(3):567–73.

10. Ekstedt M, Franzen LE, Holmqvist M, et al. Alcohol consumption is associated with progression of hepatic fibrosis in non-alcoholic fatty liver disease. Scand J Gastroenterol 2009;44(3):366–74.

11. Alkerwi A, Boutsen M, Vaillant M, et al. Alcohol consumption and the prevalence of metabolic syndrome: a meta-analysis of observational studies. Atherosclerosis 2009;204(2):624–35.

12. Thun MJ, Peto R, Lopez AD, et al. Alcohol consumption and mortality among middle-aged and elderly U.S. adults. N Engl J Med 1997;337(24):1705–14.

13. Sozio MS, Chalasani N, Liangpunsakul S. What advice should be given to patients with NAFLD about the consumption of alcohol? Nat Clin Pract Gastroenterol Hepatol 2009;6(1):18–9.

14. Cotrim HP, Freitas LA, Alves E, et al. Effects of light-to-moderate alcohol consumption on steatosis and steatohepatitis in severely obese patients. Eur J Gastroenterol Hepatol 2009;21(9):969–72.

15. Moriya A, Iwasaki Y, Ohguchi S, et al. Alcohol consumption appears to protect against non-alcoholic fatty liver disease. Aliment Pharmacol Ther 2011;33(3): 378–88.

16. Gunji T, Matsuhashi N, Sato H, et al. Light and moderate alcohol consumption significantly reduces the prevalence of fatty liver in the Japanese male population. Am J Gastroenterol 2009;104(9):2189–95.

17. Hiramine Y, Imamura Y, Uto H, et al. Alcohol drinking patterns and the risk of fatty liver in Japanese men. J Gastroenterol 2011;46(4):519–28.

18. Hamaguchi M, Kojima T, Ohbora A, et al. Protective effect of alcohol consumption for fatty liver but not metabolic syndrome. World J Gastroenterol 2012;18(2): 156–67.

19. Baker SS, Baker RD, Liu W, et al. Role of alcohol metabolism in non-alcoholic steatohepatitis. PloS One 2010;5(3):e9570.

20. Armstrong GL, Wasley A, Simard EP, et al. The prevalence of hepatitis C virus infection in the United States, 1999 through 2002. Ann Intern Med 2006; 144(10):705–14.

21. Davis GL, Alter MJ, El-Serag H, et al. Aging of hepatitis C virus (HCV)-infected persons in the United States: a multiple cohort model of HCV prevalence and disease progression. Gastroenterology 2010;138(2):513–21, e511–6.

22. Thein HH, Yi Q, Dore GJ, et al. Estimation of stage-specific fibrosis progression rates in chronic hepatitis C virus infection: a meta-analysis and meta-regression. Hepatology 2008;48(2):418–31.

23. Zhang T, Li Y, Lai JP, et al. Alcohol potentiates hepatitis C virus replicon expression. Hepatology 2003;38(1):57–65.

24. Kim WH, Hong F, Jaruga B, et al. Additive activation of hepatic NF-kappaB by ethanol and hepatitis B protein X (HBX) or HCV core protein: involvement of TNF-alpha receptor 1-independent and -dependent mechanisms. FASEB J 2001;15(13):2551–3.

25. Pianko S, Patella S, Ostapowicz G, et al. Fas-mediated hepatocyte apoptosis is increased by hepatitis C virus infection and alcohol consumption, and may be associated with hepatic fibrosis: mechanisms of liver cell injury in chronic hepatitis C virus infection. J Viral Hepat 2001;8(6):406–13.

26. Colell A, Garcia-Ruiz C, Miranda M, et al. Selective glutathione depletion of mitochondria by ethanol sensitizes hepatocytes to tumor necrosis factor. Gastroenterology 1998;115(6):1541–51.

27. Piccoli C, Quarato G, Ripoli M, et al. HCV infection induces mitochondrial bioenergetic unbalance: causes and effects. Biochim Biophys Acta 2009;1787(5):539–46.

28. Thoren F, Romero A, Lindh M, et al. A hepatitis C virus-encoded, nonstructural protein (NS3) triggers dysfunction and apoptosis in lymphocytes: role of NADPH oxidase-derived oxygen radicals. J Leukoc Biol 2004;76(6):1180–6.

29. Miura K, Taura K, Kodama Y, et al. Hepatitis C virus-induced oxidative stress suppresses hepcidin expression through increased histone deacetylase activity. Hepatology 2008;48(5):1420–9.

30. Otani K, Korenaga M, Beard MR, et al. Hepatitis C virus core protein, cytochrome P450 2E1, and alcohol produce combined mitochondrial injury and cytotoxicity in hepatoma cells. Gastroenterology 2005;128(1):96–107.

31. Perlemuter G, Letteron P, Carnot F, et al. Alcohol and hepatitis C virus core protein additively increase lipid peroxidation and synergistically trigger hepatic cytokine expression in a transgenic mouse model. J Hepatol 2003;39(6):1020–7.

32. Rigamonti C, Mottaran E, Reale E, et al. Moderate alcohol consumption increases oxidative stress in patients with chronic hepatitis C. Hepatology 2003;38(1):42–9.

33. Szabo G, Wands JR, Eken A, et al. Alcohol and hepatitis C virus: interactions in immune dysfunctions and liver damage. Alcohol Clin Exp Res 2010;34(10): 1675–86.

34. Ye L, Wang S, Wang X, et al. Alcohol impairs interferon signaling and enhances full cycle hepatitis C virus JFH-1 infection of human hepatocytes. Drug Alcohol Depend 2010;112(1–2):107–16.

35. Encke J, Wands JR. Ethanol inhibition: the humoral and cellular immune response to hepatitis C virus NS5 protein after genetic immunization. Alcohol Clin Exp Res 2000;24(7):1063–9.

36. Takahashi K, Takahashi T, Takahashi S, et al. Difference in quasispecies of the hypervariable region 1 of hepatitis C virus between alcoholic and non-alcoholic patients. J Gastroenterol Hepatol 2001;16(4):416–23.

37. Wiley TE, McCarthy M, Breidi L, et al. Impact of alcohol on the histological and clinical progression of hepatitis C infection. Hepatology 1998;28(3):805–9.

38. Ostapowicz G, Watson KJ, Locarnini SA, et al. Role of alcohol in the progression of liver disease caused by hepatitis C virus infection. Hepatology 1998;27(6): 1730–5.

39. Westin J, Lagging LM, Spak F, et al. Moderate alcohol intake increases fibrosis progression in untreated patients with hepatitis C virus infection. J Viral Hepat 2002;9(3):235–41.

40. Monto A, Patel K, Bostrom A, et al. Risks of a range of alcohol intake on hepatitis C-related fibrosis. Hepatology 2004;39(3):826–34.

41. Hutchinson SJ, Bird SM, Goldberg DJ. Influence of alcohol on the progression of hepatitis C virus infection: a meta-analysis. Clin Gastroenterol Hepatol 2005; 3(11):1150–9.

42. Poynard T, Mathurin P, Lai CL, et al. A comparison of fibrosis progression in chronic liver diseases. J Hepatol 2003;38(3):257–65.

43. Marcellin P, Pequignot F, Delarocque-Astagneau E, et al. Mortality related to chronic hepatitis B and chronic hepatitis C in France: evidence for the role of HIV coinfection and alcohol consumption. J Hepatol 2008;48(2):200–7.

44. Mueller S, Millonig G, Seitz HK. Alcoholic liver disease and hepatitis C: a frequently underestimated combination. World J Gastroenterol 2009;15(28):3462–71.

45. Machida K, Tsukamoto H, Mkrtchyan H, et al. Toll-like receptor 4 mediates synergism between alcohol and HCV in hepatic oncogenesis involving stem cell marker Nanog. Proc Natl Acad Sci U S A 2009;106(5):1548–53.

46. Lavanchy D. Hepatitis B virus epidemiology, disease burden, treatment, and current and emerging prevention and control measures. J Viral Hepat 2004;11(2):97–107.

47. Larkin J, Clayton MM, Liu J, et al. Chronic ethanol consumption stimulates hepatitis B virus gene expression and replication in transgenic mice. Hepatology 2001; 34(4 Pt 1):792–7.

48. Kim WH, Hong F, Jaruga B, et al. Hepatitis B virus X protein sensitizes primary mouse hepatocytes to ethanol- and TNF-alpha-induced apoptosis by a caspase-3-dependent mechanism. Cell Mol Immunol 2005;2(1):40–8.

49. Nomura H, Kashiwagi S, Hayashi J, et al. An epidemiologic study of effects of alcohol in the liver in hepatitis B surface antigen carriers. Am J Epidemiol 1988;128(2):277–84.

50. Nomura H, Hayashi J, Kajiyama W, et al. Alcohol consumption and seroconversion from hepatitis B e antigen in the Okinawa Japanese. Fukuoka Igaku Zasshi 1996;87(11):237–41.

51. Gelatti U, Donato F, Tagger A, et al. Etiology of hepatocellular carcinoma influences clinical and pathologic features but not patient survival. Am J Gastroenterol 2003; 98(4):907–14.

52. Wang LY, You SL, Lu SN, et al. Risk of hepatocellular carcinoma and habits of alcohol drinking, betel quid chewing and cigarette smoking: a cohort of 2416 HBsAg-seropositive and 9421 HBsAg-seronegative male residents in Taiwan. Cancer Causes Control 2003;14(3):241–50.

53. Jee SH, Ohrr H, Sull JW, et al. Cigarette smoking, alcohol drinking, hepatitis B, and risk for hepatocellular carcinoma in Korea. J Natl Cancer Inst 2004;96(24): 1851–6.

54. Donato F, Tagger A, Gelatti U, et al. Alcohol and hepatocellular carcinoma: the effect of lifetime intake and hepatitis virus infections in men and women. Am J Epidemiol 2002;155(4):323–31.

55. Zhu GT, Lou GQ, Shi JP. To investigate the relationship of alcohol intake and hepatocellular carcinoma among patients with hepatitis B virus infection. Zhonghua Shi Yan He Lin Chuang Bing Du Xue Za Zhi 2011;25(5):328–30 [in Chinese].

56. Ikeda K, Saitoh S, Suzuki Y, et al. Interferon decreases hepatocellular carcinogenesis in patients with cirrhosis caused by the hepatitis B virus: a pilot study. Cancer 1998;82(5):827–35.

57. Siddique A, Kowdley KV. Review article: the iron overload syndromes. Aliment Pharmacol Ther 2012;35(8):876–93.

58. Nieto N, Friedman SL, Cederbaum AI. Stimulation and proliferation of primary rat hepatic stellate cells by cytochrome P450 2E1-derived reactive oxygen species. Hepatology 2002;35(1):62–73.

59. Suzuki Y, Saito H, Suzuki M, et al. Up-regulation of transferrin receptor expression in hepatocytes by habitual alcohol drinking is implicated in hepatic iron overload in alcoholic liver disease. Alcohol Clin Exp Res 2002;26(Suppl 8):26S–31S.

60. Harrison-Findik DD. Gender-related variations in iron metabolism and liver diseases. World J Hepatol 2010;2(8):302–10.

61. Valerio LG Jr, Parks T, Petersen DR. Alcohol mediates increases in hepatic and serum nonheme iron stores in a rat model for alcohol-induced liver injury. Alcohol Clin Exp Res 1996;20(8):1352–61.

62. Adams PC, Agnew S. Alcoholism in hereditary hemochromatosis revisited: prevalence and clinical consequences among homozygous siblings. Hepatology 1996;23(4):724–7.

63. Scotet V, Merour MC, Mercier AY, et al. Hereditary hemochromatosis: effect of excessive alcohol consumption on disease expression in patients homozygous for the C282Y mutation. Am J Epidemiol 2003;158(2):129–34.

64. Fletcher LM, Dixon JL, Purdie DM, et al. Excess alcohol greatly increases the prevalence of cirrhosis in hereditary hemochromatosis. Gastroenterology 2002; 122(2):281–9.
65. Wood MJ, Powell LW, Dixon JL, et al. Clinical cofactors and hepatic fibrosis in hereditary hemochromatosis: the role of diabetes mellitus. Hepatology 2012 Mar 15. http://dx.doi.org/10.1002/hep.25720 [Epub ahead of print].
66. Thiele GM, Duryee MJ, Willis MS, et al. Autoimmune hepatitis induced by syngeneic liver cytosolic proteins biotransformed by alcohol metabolites. Alcohol Clin Exp Res 2010;34(12):2126–36.
67. Sorrentino P, Terracciano L, D'Angelo S, et al. Oxidative stress and steatosis are cofactors of liver injury in primary biliary cirrhosis. J Gastroenterol 2010;45(10): 1053–62.

Liver Cancer and Alcohol

Priya Grewal, MD*, Vijay Anand Viswanathen, MD

KEYWORDS

- Alcohol • Liver cancer • Hepatitis C • Obesity • Diabetes mellitus • Smoking
- Pathogenesis

KEY POINTS

- Alcohol is an independent and strong risk factor for development of HCC though the real quantification of the association is difficult.
- Chronic alcohol use of more than 80 g/d for longer than 10 years increases the risk of HCC by 5-fold. The risk decreases significantly with complete abstinence from alcohol.
- The annual incidence of HCC in patients with decompensated alcoholic cirrhosis is 1% per year.
- Alcohol increases the risk of HCC in patients with other chronic liver disease such as viral hepatitis, fatty liver disease and genetic liver diseases.
- Alcohol along with other agents such as tobacco hasten liver damage by unique perturbation of several metabolic pathways leading DNA damage and impaired control of gene expression. Future treatments targeted against these relevant pathways will help reduce the risk of HCC.

INTRODUCTION

Annually, HCC is diagnosed is approximately a half-million people worldwide, predominantly in Africa and Southeast Asia, where hepatitis B is widely prevelant.[1–3] In the United States, approximately 7% of adults abuse alcohol, which is 5 times higher than the prevalence of hepatitis C.[4] Based on the strong association of alcohol with cancer, an International Agency for Research on Cancer working group recently deemed alcoholic beverages "carcinogenic to humans," being causally related to occurrence of malignant tumors of the oral cavity, pharynx, larynx, esophagus, liver, colorectum, and female breast.[5,6]

Alcohol acts synergistically with pre-existing chronic liver disease, such as hepatitis C, hepatitis B, and fatty liver disease, as well as lifestyle choices, such as smoking and obesity, to further increase the risk of HCC in these disease states.

Alcohol promotes the generation of reactive oxygen species (ROS), which are highly reactive, oxygen-containing molecules that can damage cellular molecules, such as

Division of Liver Diseases, Mount Sinai School of Medicine, One Gustave L. Levy Place, Box 1104, New York, NY 10029, USA
* Corresponding author.
E-mail address: Priya.Grewal@mountsinai.org

fats, proteins, or DNA. Alcohol metabolism in the liver leads to ROS production, induction of activity of cytochrome P450s, and reduction of antioxidants. ROS production and oxidative stress in hepatocytes play a crucial role in the development of alcoholic liver disease.[7]

This review attempts to analyze the epidemiology and pathogenesis of alcohol in HCC in both alcoholic liver disease and other chronic liver diseases where alcohol is a cofactor.

EPIDEMIOLOGY
Data for Alcohol as Carcinogen

Chronic alcohol use of more than 80 g/d for longer than 10 years increases the risk for HCC by 5-fold.[8] In a meta-analysis of alcohol drinking and cancer risk, increased trends in risk were observed for cancers of the liver (relative risk [RR] 1.86). Higher risks were found even for the lowest dose of alcohol (25 g/d) corresponding to approximately 2 drinks per day (**Fig. 1**).[9]

In an analysis of causes of 51,400 deaths from 1999 to 2006, in the United States, patients who died with a history of heavy alcohol use were more likely to die of HCC than from non–chronic liver diseases compared with those without heavy alcohol use.[10] The analysis of data collected from 1992 to 2006, which included 4,409,809 person-years in the European Prospective Investigation into Cancer and Nutrition, revealed that heavy alcohol intake (odds ratio [OR] 1.77; 95% CI, 0.73–4.27) was associated with HCC.[11] All patients diagnosed with HCC from 2007 to 2009 at the Mayo Clinic, Rochester, (n = 460), were analyzed for risk factors, and hepatitis C virus (HCV) (56%), alcohol use (29%), and nonalcoholic fatty liver disease (13%) were the most common causes.[12]

A study from the University of Michigan confirmed that alcohol consumption had a dose-dependent effect on the risk of HCC; the risk increased after 1500 g-years of alcohol exposure (60 g/d for at least 25 years). When HCC cases were compared with cirrhotics without HCC and healthy controls, the risk of HCC increased 6-fold

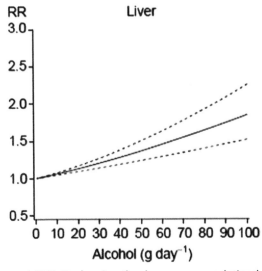

Fig. 1. RR functions and 95% CIs showing the dose-response relationship between alcohol consumption and the risk of liver cancer.

for alcohol (OR 5.7; 95% CI, 2.4–13.7), 5-fold for tobacco (OR 4.9; 95% CI, 2.2–10.6), and 4-fold with obesity (OR 4.3; 95% CI, 2.1–8.4).[13] Another meta-analysis showed dose-response relationship between alcohol intake and liver cancer with RRs of 1.19 (95% CI, 1.12–1.27), 1.40 (95% CI, 1.25–1.56), and 1.81 (95% CI, 1.50–2.19) for 25 g, 50 g, and 100 g of alcohol intake per day, respectively.[14]

There is no safety limit for the effects of alcohol on liver. In a study from Japan involving 804 HCC cases, the multivariate-adjusted HRs (95% CI) for alcohol intakes of 0.1–22.9, 23.0–45.9, 46.0–68.9, 69.0–91.9, and >92.0 g/d compared with occasional drinkers were 0.88 (0.57–1.36), 1.06 (0.70–1.62), 1.07 (0.69–1.66), 1.76 (1.08–2.87), and 1.66 (0.98–2.82), respectively. In women who drank more than 23.0 g/d, a significantly increased risk was noted when compared with social drinkers (hazard ratio [HR] 3.60; 95% CI, 1.22–10.66).[15]

A meta-analysis of 4 studies performed to assess the decline of liver cancer risk with time for former drinkers found that the risk of liver cancer falls after cessation by 6% to 7% a year, but an estimated time period of 23 years is required after drinking cessation, with a large 95% CI of 14 to 70 years, for the risk of liver cancer to be equal to that of nondrinkers.[16]

Synergy with Other Factors

Alcohol acts synergistically with pre-existing underlying chronic liver disease, such as hepatitis C, hepatitis B, and fatty liver disease, as well as life style choices, such as smoking and obesity, to further increase the risk of HCC in these disease states.

Alcohol and Hepatitis C

Several studies have reported high rates of HCV infection have been found in persons with alcohol abuse and with alcohol-induced liver disease.[17–22] In a landmark study on natural history of liver fibrosis progression in patients with chronic hepatitis C by Poynard and colleagues,[23] daily alcohol consumption of 50 g or more was 1 of 3 independent factors associated with an increased rate of fibrosis progression. In a retrospective cohort study by Berman and colleagues,[24] the patients with cirrhosis due to a combination of HCV and alcohol had a significantly higher risk of HCC than those with cirrhosis due to alcohol alone (HR 11.2; 95% CI, 2.3–55.0).

Miyakawa and colleagues[25] studied a total of 114 patients with hepatitis C due to blood transfusions; 29 of 94 (31%) patients with HCV without alcohol use developed HCC compared with 12 of 20 (60%, P<.05) with HCV and alcohol use. Because the duration of HCV infection was defined and well matched in both groups, HCC development was accelerated in the cohort with chronic HCV and heavy alcohol use. Patients with alcohol use and hepatitis C may develop HCC at a younger age. Shimauchi and colleagues[26] evaluated 18 of 648 patients less than 50 years of age with HCC and HCV. Statistical analysis suggested that heavy drinking and hepatitis B virus (HBV) were independently associated with the development of HCC in HCV patients younger than 50.

The HCC that develops in patients with HCV and alcohol may differ biologically from those with hepatitis C alone. Okada and colleagues[27] showed that patients who consumed more than 85 g/d alcohol for more than 5 years had a shorter tumor-free and overall survival after resection of the liver cancer. Kubo and colleagues[28] also compared the histology and survival after resection of HCC in 80 male patients with HCV infection. The proportion with well-differentiated HCC was lower (2 of 38 [5%]) among those who had consumed more than 86 g/d than in those without alcohol use (19 of 42 [45%], P<.0001). Patients with HCV and alcohol had reduced tumor-free survival compared with those with HCV alone (P<.05).

The risk of developing HCC after a negative contrast-enhanced CT scan was highest for patients with cirrhosis due to HCV and alcohol combined. Alcoholic Liver Disease (ALD) had the lowest risk of HCC during follow-up. This may be because of selection bias in patients with alcohol-related cirrhosis because they may not be referred to hepatologists until decompensation or cessation from alcohol use (**Fig. 2**).[24]

Alcohol and Hepatitis B

Multivariate analysis of 553 patients with HCC and 160 control subjects affected with HBV from China by Zhu and colleagues[29] revealed that heavy alcohol use, smoking, and positive family history of liver cancer are associated with HCC development among patients with HBV infection. In patients with HBV infection who also had history of heavy alcohol intake, however, most of the risk is due HBV infection, not alcohol.[29]

On the contrary, a study from Korea by Kwon and colleagues,[30] analyzed the effect of alcohol on development of HCC in hepatitis B-related cirrhosis and found that proportion with a lifetime alcohol intake of more than 292 kg (30.8% vs 34.9%) did not differ between cases (146 with HCC) and controls (146 without HCC). Both groups were matched for Child-Pugh class, HBV DNA levels, and hepatitis B e antigen sero-positivity. They concluded that alcohol intake might not increase the risk of HCC in patients with HBV infection.

Several earlier studies, before discovery of HCV, showing additive effects of alcohol on chronic hepatitis B in development of HCC need to be re-evaluated for the contribution of undiagnosed underlying chronic HCV in these cases.

Alcohol and Smoking

The interaction of alcohol and smoking in causation of HCC has been difficult to study due to high preponderance of their coexistence in the majority of patients. Some studies, however, have found interactive effects.

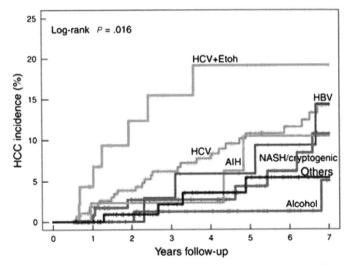

Fig. 2. Probability of HCC during follow-up by etiology of cirrhosis. Cumulative incidence curve demonstrating the risk of HCC stratified by etiology, after a negative contrast-enhanced CT. (*From* Berman K, Tandra S, Vuppalanch R, et al. Hepatic and extrahepatic cancer in cirrhosis: a longitudinal cohort study. Am J Gastroenterol 2011;106:899–906; with permission.)

An analysis of data from January 1995 to December 1998 of 333 cases of HCC (Kuper and colleagues)[31] showed a strong and statistically significant effect of heavy smoking and heavy drinking in the development of HCC (OR for both exposures 9.6). This interaction was most evident among individuals without hepatitis B and hepatitis C viral infections. A prospective case-control study of 210 subjects from the University of Michigan found that there was a dose-dependent relationship between alcohol and tobacco exposure with risk of HCC and synergistic index of 3.3.[13]

A prospective cohort study of 2273 HCC cases (1990 with viral hepatitis and 283 without) enrolled between 1997 and 2004 in Taiwan and followed-up through 2007 assessed the impact of smoking and alcohol on prognosis. A history of smoking and alcohol abuse worsened prognosis independent of each other especially in viral hepatitis-related and early HCC. Abstinence from either reduced HCC-specific mortality but only after 10 years of cessation.[32]

It is postulated that carcinogenic compounds in cigarette smoke have an increased effect in the presence of heavy alcohol use, because they exert their carcinogenicity in the context of liver injury. Cellular proliferation from injury and repair may predispose the liver to developing cancer. In addition, the liver plays an important role in metabolizing carcinogens absorbed from tobacco use.[33] CYP2E1 induction by alcohol may alter and enhance the carcinogenic potential of agents in tobacco.[31]

Alcohol and Obesity, Metabolic Syndrome, and Diabetes

Data linking obesity, metabolic syndrome, and diabetes to liver disease and HCC are well established. In Los Angeles County, a case-control study of HCC was conducted from 1984 to 2002 involving 295 HCC cases and 435 matched control subjects with assessment of lifestyle risk factors along with hepatitis B and HCV serologies. Heavy alcohol consumption was independently associated with a 2-fold to 3-fold increase in risk of HCC after adjustment for hepatitis B and hepatitis C status. A synergistic interaction on HCC risk was observed between heavy alcohol consumption and diabetes (OR 4.2; 95% CI, 2.6–5.8), heavy alcohol consumption, and viral hepatitis (OR 5.5; 95% CI, 3.9–7.0). It was concluded that heavy alcohol consumption, diabetes, and viral hepatitis were found to exert independent and synergistic effects on risk of HCC.[34]

A study from Italy enrolled 465 HCC patients and compared them with 618 cirrhotic patients without HCC and 490 healthy controls, evaluating the association among diabetes mellitus and alcohol abuse in HCC group versus both controls groups. This study showed that for alcohol abuse alone, OR for HCC was 3.7 (CI, 2.5–5.4; $P<.0001$) and 49.0 (CI, 21.5–111.8; $P<.0001$) in diabetics with significant alcohol intake.[35]

In a prospective case-control study of 210 patients enrolled in University of Michigan, the risk of HCC increased 6-fold for patients with lifetime alcohol exposure greater than 1500 g-years, equivalent to 60 g/d for 25 years; 5-fold with greater than 20 pack-years of smoking; and 4-fold with body mass index (BMI) greater than 30. There was significant interaction between alcohol, tobacco, and obesity, with synergistic indices for the interaction between alcohol and tobacco, tobacco and obesity, and alcohol and obesity if 3.3, 2.9, and 2.5, respectively.[13]

An analysis of 2260 Taiwanese men from the Risk Evaluation of Viral Load Elevation and Associated Liver Disease/Cancer–Hepatitis B Virus (REVEAL–HBV) study cohort showed that the risk of HCC increased synergistically in alcohol users who had extreme obesity compared with those without extreme obesity and with nonusers of alcohol (shown in **Fig. 3**).[36]

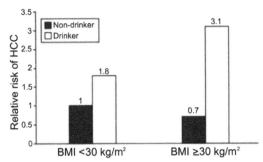

Fig. 3. Risk of incident HCC is 3.1 (95% CI, 1.1–8.3) times higher in alcohol users who have a BMI of 30 kg/m² or greater as compared with nonusers of alcohol with a BMI of less than 30 kg/m², which is suggestive of multiplicative effect. This figure shows that obesity significantly augments the risk of incident HCC in alcohol users but not in nonusers. (*From* Loomba R, Yang HI, Su J, et al. Obesity and alcohol synergize to increase the risk of incident hepatocellular carcinoma in men. Clin Gastroenterol Hepatol 2010;8(10):891–8; with permission.)

In a cohort of 771 patients with well-compensated alcohol (478), HCV (220), HCV and alcohol related cirrhosis (73) from France, who were screened prospectively for HCC and followed-up for a mean period of 4.2 ± 3 years, 220 patients developed HCC. BMI greater than or equal to 25 and diabetes were risk factors for development of HCC.[37]

Alcohol and Iron Overload Disorders

The role of iron overload and HFE gene mutations in HCC occurrence in patients with alcohol-related liver disease is controversial. In a study of 301 consecutive cirrhotic patients (162 alcoholics and 139 with HCV), iron overload on initial biopsy, according to modified Deugnier score,[38] and C282Y/H63D HFE gene mutation carriage were assessed and found independent risk factors for HCC in patients with alcohol-related but not HCV-related cirrhosis.[39]

A study from Spain noted that 9/43 (20.9%) patients with alcoholic cirrhosis and HCC were heterozygous for the C282Y mutation, compared with 6/136 (4.4%) patients without tumor ($P = .002$), suggesting that the presence of this mutation could be associated with an increased risk of developing HCC.[40] A retrospective analysis from France showed that C282Y-homozygous patients with alcohol consumption of more than 60 g/d presented significantly increased iron parameters and elevated liver enzymes, suggesting that alcohol accentuates disease expression and attendant risks.[41]

In another cohort, however, of 162 consecutive patients with HCC from Austria (36% with alcoholic etiology), C282Y and H63D allele frequencies did not differ significantly from previously published data in healthy subjects and no difference in the age at diagnosis was noted in patients with or without HFE gene mutations.[42] Researchers from France observed comparable proportions of the C282Y heterozygous state in 133 cirrhotic patients (of any etiology) with HCC and 100 without and concluded that these mutations do not seem associated with an increased risk of HCC in patients with cirrhosis.[43]

Hence, although C282 homozygosity may confer additional risk for HCC in patients with alcoholic cirrhosis, the contribution of HFE heterozygosity needs to be studied further.

Alcohol and Dietary Carcinogens

Aflatoxin B1 is a major hepatocarcinogen, which acts in part by causing mutations of codon 249, a mutational hotspot of the p53 tumor suppressor gene. Aflatoxin is metabolized by CYP2E1, which is induced by alcohol. Thus, alcohol may have an incremental genotoxic effect on aflatoxin B1. Epidemiologic evidence suggests that combining aflatoxin load and alcohol intake has a synergistic and a statistically significant effect on RR (RR 35).[44] Vinyl chloride is also metabolized by CYP 2E1 and its exposure is associated with the development of HCC, which is again increased several-fold by additional alcohol consumption.[45]

PATHOGENESIS - ALCOHOL AS A CARCINOGEN

The stomach absorbs 20% of alcohol, the rest absorbed by the duodenum and small intestine.[46,47] Alcohol dehydrogenase (ADH), located in the cytoplasm of hepatocytes, metabolizes the majority of alcohol.[46–52] ADH-dependent alcohol metabolism results in oxidation of alcohol to acetaldehyde.[46,52] Acetaldehyde is further oxidized to acetate by the mitochondrial form of aldehyde dehydrogenase. The resulting acetate is then incorporated to form acetylcoenzyme A and oxidized in the Krebs cycle.[52,53] Homan and colleagues[54] analyzed patients expressing the ADH1C*1/1 genotype and showed an increased RR for developing HCC (RR 3.56; CI, 1.33–9.53). The cytochrome P450 2E1 of microsomal ethanol oxidizing system in the hepatocytes also plays an important role in hepatic carcinogenesis.[55–58] In moderate alcohol consumption, the microsomal ethanol oxidizing system CYP2E1 pathway accounts for a small fraction of alcohol metabolism, ADH representing the more common pathway for alcohol oxidization.[59] Chronic alcohol abuse leads to the marked induction of CYP2E1, leading to increased hepatic acetaldehyde production.[50,60,61] CYP2E1-dependent alcohol metabolism results in increased hepatic oxidative stress and production of ROS, especially hydroxyethyl radicals.[56,58,60–62] The ROS can form DNA and protein adducts directly. They can also react with lipid molecules in the cell membrane, resulting in production of biologically reactive aldehyde molecules, such as 4-hydroxynonenal and malondialdehyde (MDA), compounds similar to acetaldehyde.[50,55,56,58,63–66]

The acetaldehyde can form DNA adducts mainly, N2-ethyl-20-deoxyguanosine and N2-propano-20-deoxyguanosine.[62,67] Acetaldehyde leads to formation of PdG adducts in DNA are in 2 forms. In the nucleoside or single-stranded DNA form, the PdG adduct exists in a closed ring, which is mutagenic due to its effects on base pair formation.[62] Chronic alcohol consumption leads to increased conversion of several procarcinogens, including nitrosamines and azo compounds to carcinogen derivatives through CYP2E1-dependent metabolism.[55,66,68–71] Chronic alcohol consumption alters the balance of bacterial flora within the gastrointestinal tract and increases the gut permeability to lipopolysaccharide.[72–74] The increased intrahepatic lipopolysaccharide levels lead to the activation of the liver's Kupffer cells (KCs), which in turn release proinflammatory cytokines, such as tumor necrosis factor α, prostaglandins, and interleukins.[62,73–78] The role of KCs in mediating the harmful effects of alcohol on the liver has been demonstrated through the use of antibiotics to reduce total gastrointestinal bacteria[73] and by the depletion of KCs (using gadolinium chloride).[79,80] These approaches significantly inhibit ethanol-related hepatic injury.

Ethanol leads to activation of hepatic stellate cells (HSCs) through the generation of ROS. Attenuation of oxidative stress may lead to improvement in alcohol-induced fibrosis/cirrhosis.[58,81,82] After cessation of alcohol, as liver regeneration occurs, the aberrations in this process become amplified in the setting of activated KCs and

HSCs and surrounded by cytokines and growth factors released by these cells. Previous studies have shown increased numbers of KCs and HSCs in the HCC, which is dependent on the chemokine, CCL2.[83] The number and size of tumor foci were decreased in mice that were deficient in the receptor for CCL2 (CCR2-deficient mice). Increased neovascularization results from attraction of HSCs to the tumor, leading to increased secretion of matrix metalloproteinase 2. These studies provide definitive evidence that attenuation of CCR2 signaling decreases HCC formation corresponding with a reduction in HSCs, KCs, and neovascularization.[83] Given the highly vascular nature of HCC and the effects of alcohol on blood vessels, continued alcohol consumption increases blood flow to the HCC mass.

SUMMARY

Alcohol is a leading cause of liver cancer and alcohol abuse is 5 times more prevalent than chronic hepatitis C in the United States. Epidemiologic evidence supports that alcohol is an independent and strong risk factor for HCC. Quantification of the association is difficult, however, because cirrhosis and other liver conditions antedating the HCC diagnosis invariably lead to a substantial decrease in alcohol drinking. The annual incidence of HCC in patients with decompensated alcohol-induced cirrhosis is approximately 1% per year. Although there are robust data, mostly retrospective in nature, that heavy alcohol use hastens the development of HCC in patients with chronic HCV and fatty liver disease, its role in chronic HBV infection and iron overload syndromes needs further study. Studying the role of alcohol in development of liver disease and progression to HCC is complex. Alcohol acts synergistically with a variety of other agents that increase the risk of HCC, partly by enhancing and hastening the damage caused to the liver and partly through its unique perturbation of several metabolic pathways, leading ultimately to DNA damage and impaired control of gene expression. Invariably, more pathways will be demonstrated in the future. The knowledge of these relevant pathogenetic mechanisms will enable reducing the risk of HCC developing in patients with alcoholic liver disease. In the meantime, early detection by surveillance of HCC using ultrasonography every 6 months in patients with alcoholic cirrhosis, as recommended by AASLD guidelines, will lead to improved outcomes with potential for subsequent curative treatment such as surgical resection or liver transplantation. Analysis of recent studies show that alpha-fetoprotein determination lacks adequate sensitivity and specificity for adequate surveillance and hence imaging with ultrasound or CT scan is recommended.[84]

REFERENCES

1. Ferlay J, Bray F, Pisani P, et al. GLOBOCAN 2000: cancer incidence, mortality and prevalence worldwide, version 1.0. International Agency for Research on Cancer CancerBase no. 5. Lyon (France): IARC Press; 2001.
2. Surveillance, epidemiology, and End results (SEER) Program. SEER*Stat database: incidence — SEER 9 Regs research data, Nov 2009 Sub (1973-2007). Bethesda (MD): National Cancer Institute; 2010.
3. World Health Organization, International Agency for Research on Cancer. GLOBOCAN 2008. Available at: http://globocan.iarc.fr.
4. Grant B, Harford T, Dawson D, et al. Prevalence of DSM-IV alcohol abuse and dependence United States, 1992. Alcohol Health Res World 1994;18:243–8.
5. Alcoholic beverage consumption and ethyl caramate (urethane). IARC monographs on the evaluation of carcinogenic risks to humans 96. Lyon: International Agency for Research on Cancer.

6. IARC. Preamble to the IARC monographs on the evaluation of carcinogenic risks to humans. Available at: http://monographs.iarc.fr/ENG/Preamble/Current Preamble.pdf.

7. Wu D, Cederbaum AI. Alcohol, oxidative stress, and free radical damage. Alcohol Res Health 2003;27(4):277–84.

8. Donato F, Tagger A, Gelatti U, et al. Alcohol and hepatocellular carcinoma the effect of lifetime intake and hepatitis virus infections in men and women. Am J Epidemiol 2002;155:323–31.

9. Bagnardi V, Blangiardo M, La Vecchia C, et al. A meta-analysis of alcohol drinking and cancer risk. Br J Cancer 2001;85(11):1700–5.

10. Dong C, Yoon YH, Chen CM, et al. Heavy alcohol use and premature death from hepatocellular carcinoma in the United States, 1999–2006. J Stud Alcohol Drugs 2011;72(6):892–902.

11. Trichopoulos D, Bamia C, Lagiou P, et al. Hepatocellular carcinoma risk factors and disease burden in a European cohort: a nested case–control study. J Natl Cancer Inst 2011;103(22):1686–95.

12. Yang JD, Harmsen WS, Slettedahl SW, et al. Factors that affect risk for hepatocellular carcinoma and effects of surveillance. Clin Gastroenterol Hepatol 2011;9:617–23.

13. Marrero JA, Fontana RJ, Fu S, et al. Alcohol, tobacco and obesity are synergistic risk factors for hepatocellular carcinoma. J Hepatol 2005;42:218–24.

14. Corrao G, Bagnardi V, Zambon A, et al. A meta-analysis of alcohol consumption and the risk of 15 diseases. Prev Med 2004;38:613–9.

15. Shimazu T, Sasazuki S, Wakai K, et al. Alcohol drinking and primary liver cancer: a pooled analysis of four Japanese cohort studies. Int J Cancer 2012;130(11): 2645–53.

16. Heckley GA, Jarl J, Asamoah BO, et al. How the risk of liver cancer changes after alcohol cessation: a review and meta-analysis of the current literature. BMC Cancer 2011;11:446.

17. Fong TL, Kanel GC, Conrad A, et al. Clinical significance of concomitant hepatitis C infection in patients with alcoholic liver disease. Hepatology 1994; 19:554–7.

18. Gonzalez-Quintela A, Alende R, Aguilera A, et al. Hepatitis C virus antibodies in alcoholic patients. Rev Clin Esp 1995;195:367–72.

19. Zignego AL, Foschi M, Laffi G, et al. "Inapparent" hepatitis B virus infection and hepatitis C virus replication in alcoholic subjects with and without liver disease. Hepatology 1994;19:577–82.

20. Oshita M, Hayashi N, Kasahara A, et al. Increased serum hepatitis C virus RNA levels among alcoholic patients with chronic hepatitis. Hepatology 1994;20:1115–20.

21. Befrits R, Hedman M, Blomquist L. Chronic hepatitis C in alcoholic patients: prevalence, genotypes, and correlation to liver disease. Scand J Gastroenterol 1995; 30:1113–8.

22. Mendenhall CL, Moritz T, Rouster S, et al. Epidemiology of hepatitis C among veterans with alcoholic liver disease. Am J Gastroenterol 1993;88:1022–6.

23. Poynard, Bedossa, Opolon. Natural history of liver fibrosis progression in patients with chronic hepatitis C; for the OBSVIRC, METAVIR, CLINIVIR, and DOSVIRC group. Lancet 1997;349:825–32.

24. Berman K, Tandra S, Vuppalanch R, et al. Hepatic and extrahepatic cancer in cirrhosis: a longitudinal cohort study. Am J Gastroenterol 2011;106:899–906.

25. Miyakawa H, Sato C, Tazawa J, et al. A prospective study on hepatocellular carcinoma in liver cirrhosis respective roles of alcohol and hepatitis C virus infection. Alcohol Alcohol Suppl 1994;29(1):75–9.

26. Shimauchi Y, Tanaka M, Koga K, et al. Clinical characteristics of patients in their 40s with HCV antibody-positive hepatocellular carcinoma. Alcohol Clin Exp Res 2000;24:64S–7S.

27. Okada S, Ishii H, Nose H, et al. Effect of heavy alcohol intake on long-term results after curative resection of hepatitis C virus-related hepatocellular carcinoma. Jpn J Cancer Res 1996;87:867–73.

28. Kubo S, Kinoshita H, Hirohashi K, et al. High malignancy of hepatocellular carcinoma in alcoholic patients with hepatitis C virus. Surgery 1997;121:425–9.

29. Zhu GT, Lou GQ, Shi JP. To investigate the relationship of alcohol intake and hepatocellular carcinoma among patients with hepatitis B virus infection. Zhonghua Shi Yan He Lin Chuang Bing Du Xue Za Zhi 2011;25(5):328–30 [in Chinese].

30. Kwon OS, Jung YK, Kim YS, et al. Effect of alcohol on the development of hepatocellular carcinoma in patients with hepatitis B virus-related cirrhosis: a cross-sectional case-control study. Korean J Hepatol 2010;16:308–14.

31. Kuper H, Tzonou A, Kaklamani E, et al. Tobacco smoking, alcohol consumption and their interaction in the causation of hepatocellular carcinoma. Int J Cancer 2000;85:498–502.

32. Shih WL, Chang HC, Liaw YF, et al. Influences of tobacco and alcohol use on hepatocellular carcinoma survival. Int J Cancer 2012. http://dx.doi.org/10.1002/ijc.27508.

33. Staretz ME, Murphy SE, Patten CJ, et al. Comparative metabolism of the tobacco-related carcinogens benzo[a]pyrene, 4-(methylnitrosamino)-1-(3-pyridyl)-1-butanone, 4-(methylnitrosamino)-1-(3-pyridyl)-1-butanol, and N'- nitrosonornicotine in human hepatic microsomes. Drug Metab Dispos 1997;25:154–62.

34. Yuan JM, Govindarajan S, Arakawa K, et al. Synergism of alcohol, diabetes, and viral hepatitis on the risk of hepatocellular carcinoma in blacks and whites in the U.S. Cancer 2004;101(5):1009–17.

35. Balbi M, Donadon V, Ghersetti M, et al. Alcohol and HCV chronic infection are risk cofactors of type 2 diabetes mellitus for hepatocellular carcinoma in Italy. Int J Environ Res Public Health 2010;7:1366–78.

36. Loomba R, Yang HI, Su J, et al. Obesity and alcohol synergize to increase the risk of incident hepatocellular carcinoma in men. Clin Gastroenterol Hepatol 2010; 8(10):891–8.

37. N'Kontchou G, Paries J, Htar MT, et al. Risk factors for hepatocellular carcinoma in patients with alcoholic or viral C cirrhosis. Clin Gastroenterol Hepatol 2006;4: 1062–8.

38. Ganne-Carrie N, Christidis C, Chastang C, et al. Liver iron is predictive of death in alcoholic cirrhosis: a multivariate study of 229 consecutive patients with alcoholic and/or hepatitis C virus cirrhosis: a prospective follow up study. Gut 2000;46: 277–82.

39. Nahon P, Sutton A, Rufat P, et al. Liver iron, HFE gene mutations, and hepatocellular carcinoma occurrence in patients with cirrhosis. Gastroenterology 2008;134: 102–10.

40. Lauret E, Rodríguez M, González S, et al. HFE gene mutations in alcoholic and virus-related cirrhotic patients with hepatocellular carcinoma. Am J Gastroenterol 2002;97:1016–21.

41. Scotet V, Mérour MC, Mercier AY, et al. Hereditary hemochromatosis: effect of excessive alcohol consumption on disease expression in patients homozygous for the C282Y mutation. Am J Epidemiol 2003;158:129–34.

42. Cauza E, Peck-Radosavljevic M, Ulrich-Pur H, et al. Mutations of the HFE gene in patients with hepatocellular carcinoma. Am J Gastroenterol 2003;98:442–7.

43. Boige V, Castéra L, de Roux N, et al. Lack of association between HFE gene mutations and hepatocellular carcinoma in patients with cirrhosis. Gut 2003;52: 1178–81.
44. Bulatao-Jayme J, Almero EM, Castro CA, et al. A case–control dietary study of primary liver cancer risk from aflatoxin exposure. Int J Epidemiol 1982;11: 112–9.
45. Tamburro CH, Lee HM. Primary hepatic cancer in alcoholics. Clin Gastroenterol 1981;10:457–77.
46. Gemma S, Vichi S, Testai E. Individual susceptibility and alcohol effects: biochemical and genetic aspects. Ann Ist Super Sanita 2006;42(1):8–16.
47. Norberg A, Jones AW, Hahn RG, et al. Role of variability in explaining ethanol pharmacokinetics: research and forensic applications. Clin Pharmacokinet 2003;42(1):1–31.
48. Crabb DW, Liangpunsakul S. Acetaldehyde generating enzyme systems: roles of alcohol dehydrogenase, CYP2E1 and catalase, and speculations on the role of other enzymes and processes. Novartis Found Symp 2007;285:4–16 [discussion: 16–22].
49. Eriksson CJ. The role of acetaldehyde in the actions of alcohol (update 2000). Alcohol Clin Exp Res 2001;25(Suppl):15S–32S.
50. Seitz HK, Becker P. Alcohol metabolism and cancer risk. Alcohol Res Health 2007;30(1):38–41.
51. Tuma DJ, Casey CA. Dangerous byproducts of alcohol breakdown–focus on adducts. Alcohol Res Health 2003;27(4):285–90.
52. Zakhari S. Overview: how is alcohol metabolized by the body? Alcohol Res Health 2006;29(4):245–54.
53. Deitrich RA, Petersen D, Vasiliou V. Removal of acetaldehyde from the body. Novartis Found Symp 2007;285:23–40 [discussion: 40–51].
54. Homann N, Stickel F, Konig IR, et al. Alcohol dehydrogenase 1C*1 allele is a genetic marker for alcohol-associated cancer in heavy drinkers. Int J Cancer 2006;118(8):1998–2002.
55. Cederbaum AI. CYP2E1–biochemical and toxicological aspects and role in alcohol-induced liver injury. Mt Sinai J Med 2006;73(4):657–72.
56. Das SK, Vasudevan DM. Alcohol-induced oxidative stress. Life Sci 2007;81(3): 177–87.
57. Konishi M, Ishii H. Role of microsomal enzymes in development of alcoholic liver diseases. J Gastroenterol Hepatol 2007;22(Suppl 1):S7–10.
58. Lu Y, Cederbaum AI. CYP2E1 and oxidative liver injury by alcohol. Free Radic Biol Med 2008;44(5):723–38.
59. Lieber CS, DeCarli LM. The role of the hepatic microsomal ethanol oxidizing system (MEOS) for ethanol metabolism in vivo. J Pharmacol Exp Ther 1972; 181(2):279–87.
60. Badger TM, Ronis MJ, Seitz HK, et al. Alcohol metabolism: role in toxicity and carcinogenesis. Alcohol Clin Exp Res 2003;27(2):336–47.
61. Koop DR. Oxidative and reductive metabolism by cytochrome P450 2E1. FASEB J 1992;6(2):724–30.
62. Zima T, Kalousova M. Oxidative stress and signal transduction pathways in alcoholic liver disease. Alcohol Clin Exp Res 2005;29(Suppl 11):110S–5S.
63. Baan R, Straif K, Grosse Y, et al. Carcinogenicity of alcoholic beverages. Lancet Oncol 2007;8(4):292–3.
64. Brooks PJ, Theruvathu JA. DNA adducts from acetaldehyde: implications for alcohol-related carcinogenesis. Alcohol 2005;35(3):187–93.

65. Lenaz G. The mitochondrial production of reactive oxygen species: mechanisms and implications in human pathology. IUBMB Life 2001;52(3–5):159–64.

66. Tanaka E, Terada M, Misawa S. Cytochrome P450 2E1: its clinical and toxicological role. J Clin Pharm Ther 2000;25(3):165–75.

67. Vaca CE, Fang JL, Schweda EK. Studies of the reaction of acetaldehyde with deoxynucleosides. Chem Biol Interact 1995;98(1):51–67.

68. Lieber CS. Cytochrome P-4502E1: its physiological and pathological role. Physiol Rev 1997;77(2):517–44.

69. Lieber CS. ALCOHOL: its metabolism and interaction with nutrients. Annu Rev Nutr 2000;20:395–430.

70. Guengerich FP, Shimada T, Yun CH, et al. Interactions of ingested food, beverage, and tobacco components involving human cytochrome P4501A2, 2A6, 2E1, and 3A4 enzymes. Environ Health Perspect 1994;102(Suppl 9):49–53.

71. Yang CS, Yoo JS, Ishizaki H, et al. Cytochrome P450IIE1: roles in nitrosamine metabolism and mechanisms of regulation. Drug Metab Rev 1990;22(2–3): 147–59.

72. Nagata K, Suzuki H, Sakaguchi S. Common pathogenic mechanism in development progression of liver injury caused by non-alcoholic or alcoholic steatohepatitis. J Toxicol Sci 2007;32(5):453–68.

73. Thurman RG II. Alcoholic liver injury involves activation of Kupffer cells by endotoxin. Am J Physiol 1998;275(4 Pt 1):G605–11.

74. Bode C, Bode JC. Activation of the innate immune system and alcoholic liver disease: effects of ethanol per se or enhanced intestinal translocation of bacterial toxins induced by ethanol. Alcohol Clin Exp Res 2005;29(Suppl):166S–71S.

75. Hoek JB, Pastorino JG. Ethanol, oxidative stress, and cytokine-induced liver cell injury. Alcohol 2002;27(1):63–8.

76. Hoek JB, Pastorino JG. Cellular signaling mechanisms in alcohol-induced liver damage. Semin Liver Dis 2004;24(3):257–72.

77. Roberts RA, Ganey PE, Ju C, et al. Role of the Kupffer cell in mediating hepatic toxicity and carcinogenesis. Toxicol Sci 2007;96(1):2–15.

78. Thakur V, McMullen MR, Pritchard MT, et al. Regulation of macrophage activation in alcoholic liver disease. J Gastroenterol Hepatol 2007;22(Suppl 1):S53–6.

79. Ruttinger D, Vollmar B, Wanner GA, et al. In vivo assessment of hepatic alterations following gadolinium chloride-induced Kupffer cell blockade. J Hepatol 1996;25(6):960–7.

80. Vollmar B, Ruttinger D, Wanner GA, et al. Modulation of Kupffer cell activity by gadolinium chloride in endotoxemic rats. Shock 1996;6(6):434–41.

81. Albano E. Oxidative mechanisms in the pathogenesis of alcoholic liver disease. Mol Aspects Med 2008;29(1–2):9–16.

82. Lirussi F, Azzalini L, Orando S, et al. Antioxidant supplements for non-alcoholic fatty liver disease and/or steatohepatitis. Cochrane Database Syst Rev 2007;(1):CD004996.

83. Yang X, Lu P, Ishida Y, et al. Attenuated liver tumor formation in the absence of CCR2 with a concomitant reduction in the accumulation of hepatic stellate cells, macrophages and neovascularization. Int J Cancer 2006;118(2):335–45.

84. Bruix J, Sherman M. AASLD practice guideline for management of HCC. Hepatology 2011;53(3):1020–2.

Evaluation and Selection of the Patient with Alcoholic Liver Disease for Liver Transplant

Jennifer Leong, MD*, Gene Y. Im, MD

KEYWORDS

- Alcoholic liver disease • Alcoholic hepatitis • Liver transplantation • Relapse
- Evaluation

KEY POINTS

- Outcomes of those transplanted for ALD are comparable to those transplanted for non-alcoholic liver disease.
- Studies have demonstrated that patients with ALD are under-referred for liver transplant evaluation.
- The evaluation for liver transplant for those with ALD should be conducted in a multi-disciplinary manner and include a thorough medical evaluation, as well as the evaluation of a psychiatrist or addiction specialist in order to identify those at high risk of relapse.
- Requiring a 6-month period of abstinence does not ensure sobriety, and runs the risk of penalizing those who may remain sober despite maintaining abstinence for a shorter period of time prior to liver transplant.
- Recent studies demonstrate similar outcomes for liver transplantation for acute alcoholic hepatitis and should not be considered an absolute contraindication to liver transplant - these patients should be evaluated for liver transplant on a case-by-case basis.

INTRODUCTION

It is now commonly accepted that liver transplantation is a viable option for patients with end-stage liver disease (ESLD) secondary to alcoholic liver disease (ALD). Between 1988 and 2006, ALD was the second most common indication for liver transplantation (LT) in the United States, accounting for greater than 17.1% of all cases.[1-3] Studies have shown that these patients do as well as those transplanted for nonalcoholic liver disease.[4-6] Despite excellent outcomes, LT for alcoholic cirrhosis still generates significant controversy. Studies estimate that up to 20% to 50% of patients

The authors have no financial disclosures to make.
Recanati/Miller Transplantation Institute, Mount Sinai School of Medicine, One Gustave Levy Place, Box 1104, New York, NY 10029, USA
* Corresponding author.
E-mail address: Jennifer.leong@mountsinai.org

Clin Liver Dis 16 (2012) 851–863
http://dx.doi.org/10.1016/j.cld.2012.08.012
1089-3261/12/$ – see front matter © 2012 Elsevier Inc. All rights reserved.

who receive a liver transplant will admit to some alcohol use within 5 years, and about 10% to 15% resume heavy drinking.[7–11] Alcohol consumption after transplant can lead to harmful outcomes, resulting in compromise of the graft, whether indirectly through affecting medical compliance or through harmful alcohol intake.[12,13] Given the risk of relapse and loss of graft, many question whether these patients should be given lower priority, as many view the disease as being self inflicted. Studies have repeatedly shown that the general public, and even some physicians, would give alcoholics lower priority when it comes to allocating scarce resources such as a liver transplant.[14–16] Until recently, those presenting with acute alcoholic hepatitis were declined for LT because it was seen as a contraindication, largely because these patients were generally imbibing alcohol up until they decompensated.[17] Mathurin and colleagues[18] demonstrated that with careful selection, these patients should be transplanted and have comparable survival outcomes, thus leading to a renewed debate in the selection and evaluation of those with liver disease attributable to alcohol. This article reviews the literature and data on the evaluation and selection of patients with alcoholic cirrhosis for liver transplant, including in those with acute alcoholic hepatitis. The impact of ALD on other comorbid liver diseases is not discussed, nor are the outcomes of transplantation in affected individuals.

REFERRAL OF THE PATIENT

Evaluation of the patient for liver transplant often begins with referral of the patient for LT. At present, the United Network of Organ Sharing (UNOS) allocation policy gives equal priority to those whose liver disease is due to alcohol as for those with other liver diseases. However, some studies have shown that patients are being underreferred for LT evaluation when the culprit for cirrhosis is alcohol. It has been estimated that fewer than 3.5% to 5% of those with decompensated ALD in the United States will eventually be listed for a liver transplant.[19]

A study performed in the United Kingdom found that in a remote district hospital, only 5% of patients with alcoholic liver disease who were admitted were actually referred for a liver transplant.[20] Although one can perhaps lay the blame for this on the fact that when the study was conducted LT for ALD was still relatively new, these data were later supported in a study performed in a Veterans cohort by Julapalli and colleagues[21] published in 2005. These investigators found that LT was mentioned in only 20% of encounters in patients with ALD, and only in 21% of those who satisfied American Association of Liver Diseases (AASLD) guidelines for referral. In both these studies, nonreferral was generally due to most patients not fulfilling the criterion of being abstinent. However, it was also found that in the majority of these cases the mention of liver transplant as a life-saving measure was not discussed with these patients. It is conceivable that the hope of being a candidate for a life-saving measure such as a liver transplant could motivate an individual to attempt to modify their harmful behavior.

EVALUATION

Once the patient is referred for a liver transplant, the individual is then subject to the same rigorous evaluation that is expected of all those who are referred. However, there are a few additional issues that should be addressed in the evaluation of the patient with ALD, as long-term alcohol abuse can lead to damage of other organs as well as the liver. While certain conditions that are alcohol-related may be reversible, some of these issues can actually affect an individual's candidacy for LT. These issues include alcoholic cardiomyopathy, dementia due to Wernicke-Korsakoff syndrome, pancreatitis, malnutrition, and comorbid psychiatric conditions or other substance abuse aside from alcohol.

Medical Evaluation

A cardiac evaluation is required of all individuals being evaluated for a liver transplant. Severe cardiomyopathy is generally considered a contraindication to LT, although what is considered "too sick for transplant" may differ between centers. The diagnosis of alcoholic cardiomyopathy requires the presence of alcohol dependence or abuse as well as specific cardiac findings. It is important to keep in mind that the cardiomyopathy may be underestimated in those with cirrhosis. However, alcoholic cardiomyopathy is generally reversible if alcohol is stopped before the onset of severe heart failure. Given that most patients are abstinent from alcohol by the time they are referred, significant cardiomyopathy caused by alcohol abuse is generally an uncommon finding.[22,23]

As opposed to alcoholic cardiomyopathy, which can improve with abstinence, there are certain neurologic diseases that can be found in alcoholics that are not reversible, but can be difficult to distinguish from hepatic encephalopathy. These include Wernicke-Korsakoff syndrome and alcoholic cerebellar degeneration.[22–24] A full neurologic evaluation may be helpful in these situations in determining etiology as well as reversibility.

Acute or chronic pancreatitis will rarely affect the candidacy of a patient for liver transplant; however, it can delay a patient receiving a liver transplant in the setting of acute pancreatitis, as surgery in these patients is associated with high mortality.[22] Moreover, there is an increased risk of portal-vein thrombosis in these patients, which can affect the technical surgical feasibility of a liver transplant. Chronic pancreatitis can also influence a patient's use of narcotics in the transplant setting and contribute to the nutritional status of the patient before LT.[22,23,25]

Although malnutrition does not necessarily influence the candidacy of a patient for liver transplant, it can affect the outcome after transplant, as several studies have shown that such patients have a higher risk of posttransplant morbidity and mortality.[22–24] Kearns and colleagues[26] have shown that nutrition is vital in the care of patients with ALD and can lead to significant improvement in their condition.

Psychosocial Evaluation

A formal psychosocial evaluation should be performed in all patients being referred for liver transplant who have a history of alcohol abuse. It is probably the most crucial and, likewise, most controversial part of the evaluation process. Having a psychiatrist or addiction specialist, as well as a social worker, involved in the patient's evaluation is extremely beneficial in trying to predict who is at high risk for relapse but also in identifying those who need more aggressive management and monitoring in attempting to prevent a relapse.

The first step in evaluating these patients is determining whether alcohol dependence or alcohol abuse is present. A prospective study by Day and colleagues[27] demonstrated that in patients referred for liver transplant for nonalcoholic liver disease, a diagnosis of alcohol abuse or alcohol dependence was often missed by the referring physician. A detailed assessment may not be undertaken if the main cause of liver disease is not considered to be secondary to alcohol. The missed diagnosis may also be due to the fact that many people are now aware that a history of substance abuse can negatively affect their candidacy for a liver transplant, and thus may be less forthcoming.[28] Trying to obtain collateral information from family members, friends, or significant others helps in providing a more accurate assessment of the patient's drinking history and whether prior attempts had been made to stop drinking. It is also important to distinguish between alcohol abuse and dependence, as many studies have identified those with alcohol dependence as at a higher risk of relapse.[29–32] The *Diagnostic and Statistical Manual of Mental Disorders*, fourth edition (DSM-IV) characterizes both by excessive alcohol intake, but dependence is defined by evidence of tolerance, withdrawal, and compulsive use of alcohol, whereby drinking is continued despite harmful consequences.[33]

Numerous variables have been evaluated in trying to predict those who are at high risk of relapse after transplant. Psychosocial factors that have been studied include comorbid underlying psychiatric conditions, other substance abuse, age, gender, support, and a prior history of relapse. Factors such as age, gender, and even family history have been shown in some studies to predict relapse, whereas others have shown no association at all.[30,34–36] However, lack of social support, whether through marital status, having a significant other, or some other form of stability, has consistently been shown to increase the risk of relapse.[7,13,36,37] A prior history of relapse has been a problematic variable in trying to determine risk attributable to issues in definition leading to contradictory results.[7,35,38,39] Some studies looked at a prior history of alcohol rehabilitation, whereas others looked at whether patients listened to the advice of their doctors. A lack of prior relapse may indicate that an attempt had never been made because of a lack of insight, whereas a prior relapse might indicate that while the patient did relapse, the patient actually was motivated in trying to become abstinent.

A high prevalence of other substance abuse of up to 40% has been reported to exist in those with ALD.[30] Some studies have shown an increased risk of relapse, whereas others have found the absence of any other substance abuse to be a positive predictor of abstinence after transplant. Most studies show no correlation between a history of other substance abuse and risk of relapse for alcoholism.[8,35,40]

Similarly, a large percentage of alcoholics are often found to have comorbid underlying psychiatric conditions.[41,42] Certain psychiatric disorders may predispose an individual to a higher risk of relapse as well as to noncompliance with immunosuppression and follow-up appointments in the posttransplant setting. Axis I disorders such as anxiety and depression have been found to have a much higher risk of alcohol dependence and relapse.[29,43] However, others have shown that when depression is adequately treated, the risk of relapse is decreased.[8,35] Axis II disorders, such as personality and psychotic disorders, in particular have been found to be independent predictors of recidivism.[7,23,29,44] Although a diagnosis of a personality disorder is not an absolute contraindication for liver transplant, a period of abstinence along with a period of observation to ensure compliance may be necessary in making a decision on candidacy for these patients.

THE 6-MONTH RULE

Until recently, more than 85% of liver transplant programs and up to 43% of third-party payors in the United States required 6 months of abstinence before transplantation, commonly referred to as the 6-month rule.[28,45] This period of abstinence became a general requirement in 1997, when the UNOS cosponsored a national meeting to develop minimal criteria for placement of adults on the liver transplant waiting list.[1,46] This report was the first to specifically discuss the 6-month rule by stating that there was a "strong consensus" for this requirement, although UNOS stopped short of making it an absolute, formal requirement and recommended "exceptional" cases (good candidates with <6 months abstinence) for referral to regional review boards for consideration.[1,29] Current AASLD guidelines also recommend 6 months' abstinence before transplantation, but they also reinforce that this requirement alone is not sufficient for being accepted as a liver transplant candidate.[47]

The 6-month rule assists in achieving 2 goals: (1) to allow time for the liver to recover from the acute inflammatory effects of recent alcohol exposure without undergoing an unnecessary liver transplant, and (2) to examine the patient's commitment to sobriety while implementing preventive strategies against future recidivism.[28,48] Because decompensation often results from acute alcoholic hepatitis superimposed on preexisting liver disease, removing the harmful effects of alcohol by abstinence can result in improvement and possibly negate the need for a liver transplant.[48–53]

Many studies have been published that support the 6-month rule. In the largest retrospective study of European alcoholic transplant recipients published to date, Pfitzmann and colleagues[13] found that abstinence of less than 6 months before transplantation was significantly associated with an increased risk of recidivism. These investigators reported an overall recidivism rate of 19%, with 8% exhibiting "abusive drinking." Survival rates of patients who resumed abusive drinking were significantly lower than survival rates of abstinent patients or patients with minor lapses. A 2008 meta-analysis of 50 studies evaluating predictors of recidivism in alcoholic transplant recipients also identified pretransplant abstinence of less than 6 months as one of the significant risk factors for relapse.[54]

Conversely, numerous cohorts of apparently well-selected recipients with ALD have shown that even with adherence to the 6-month rule, there are high alcohol recidivism rates.[13,34–36,39,55,56] A well-cited prospective study on this topic by DiMartini and colleagues[30] examined the outcomes of 167 alcoholic transplant recipients who all had a minimum abstinence period of 6 months. In their multivariate analysis, duration of pretransplant sobriety was significantly associated with time to first drink and to binge use; 22% had used some alcohol at 1 year and 42% by 5 years posttransplantation, of whom 26% had a binge-drinking pattern. Their data also demonstrated that each additional month of pretransplant sobriety lowered the risk of posttransplant drinking by 33%. However, they were unable to identify a specific length of time that could reliably ensure posttransplant abstinence.

Furthermore, Yates and colleagues[57] showed that strict adherence to the 6-month rule can penalize those who are low risk for relapse. In this study, they compared the high-risk alcoholism relapse (HRAR) model, which predicts risk of relapse based on 3 variables (number of years of heavy drinking, usual daily number of alcoholic beverages, number of previous alcoholism treatment), to the 6-month rule and risk of relapse. The study found that while relapse risk rates declined with increasing duration of sobriety, the relapse risk rates were low even for those with no period of abstinence in the low-risk HRAR group. Conversely, in the high-risk HRAR group, 6 months of abstinence did not reliably predict lack of relapse.

A review by Tan and colleagues[56] encapsulates the conflicting evidence for the 6-month rule. These investigators identified 25 studies with a minimum of 30 patients that examined the value of the 6-month rule in alcoholic transplant recipients, with only 9 of 25 (36%) concluding that it was predictive of relapse after transplantation. By itself, 6 months of sobriety cannot reliably predict posttransplant abstinence from alcohol. However, it is generally accepted that the longer the period of abstinence, the lower the risk of relapse. Some studies suggest that an even longer period of sobriety is required. In a study by Gedaly and colleagues,[58] abstinence of less than 12 months was associated with relapse to any alcohol use. If one were to look for the best marker of maintaining abstinence, studies in alcoholics have shown that 5 years of abstinence can be the best predictor of no relapse of sustained sobriety, but this is an unrealistic expectation to achieve for patients with decompensated ALD before a liver transplant.[32,59]

DEFINING RELAPSE

One of the difficulties in trying to reliably identify risk factors for relapse, including duration of sobriety, comes from the ambiguity in the definition of relapse. Not all relapse events are equal. Most transplant centers consider any alcohol consumption after orthotopic LT as relapse and grounds for removing a person from the waiting list, whereas addiction specialists distinguish a relapse (prolonged and harmful drinking behavior) from a minor lapse or "slip" (sporadic drinking event followed by reestablishment of abstinence).[13] It is important to be able to identify a true relapse, as these different drinking patterns have been shown to be qualitatively different and can influence the prognosis of addictive behavior as well as affect graft function and survival.[11,60]

Two recent studies looked at risk factors that predicted risk of relapse to harmful drinking posttransplant. Kelly and colleagues[8] looked specifically at risk factors predicting relapse to harmful drinking as defined by "drinking with recorded medical or social harm, or drinking above 140 g of ethanol per week." In their multivariate analysis they found 6 variables, namely amount of daily alcohol intake before assessment for transplant, diagnosis of mental illness, stable relationship, family or friends support, tobacco use per day, and insight, which correctly classified the outcome of 89% of patients. It is interesting that the duration of abstinence before transplant did not predict recidivism, nor did it predict who became a harmful drinker in contrast to a "low-level" drinker. However, most of the patients in this study did have at least 6 months of abstinence.

In a large retrospective study of 387 patients, DeGottardi and colleagues[61] were able to identify 3 factors that were independently associated with a risk of relapse to "harmful alcohol consumption," which was defined as alcohol consumption of greater than 40 g daily along with the presence of alcohol-related damage, either physical (including histologic features on biopsy) or mental. The risk factors identified included a pretransplant diagnosis of a psychiatric disorder (anxiety or depression), an HRAR score of greater than 3, and a period of abstinence of less than 6 months at the time of listing. In the absence of these 3 risk factors, only 5% of patients returned to harmful drinking. If 1 factor was present this increased to 18% of patients, if 2 were present there was a relapse rate of 64%, and if all 3 were present 100% resumed harmful drinking, although only 3 patients met this criteria. In this study, only 11.9% of patients relapsed to harmful drinking in the mean follow-up period of 5 years.

MONITORING FOR RELAPSE

The patient should be monitored continuously for relapse during the evaluation process, up until the liver transplant, and even after transplantation. For those candidates who are able to participate in a rehabilitation program, the transplant team should obtain regular updates regarding the patient's progress. Random screening for blood or breath alcohol levels or urine toxicology should be obtained during visits as well, while keeping in mind that a false negative can occur because alcohol can be detectable only for a short period. Studies have looked at carbohydrate-deficient transferrin levels as a marker of heavy alcohol use, but this can be falsely elevated purely from severe liver disease.[62] Because of these limitations, monitoring for relapse relies heavily on the candidate's candor in answering routine questioning regarding alcohol use, which can be impeded by fears of being removed from the waiting list.

It is important to try to establish a balance between supporting patients in their efforts to maintain abstinence and honesty, so that the transplant team can identify those who may need more aggressive treatment and management while adhering to the abstinence policy.[28]

TRANSPLANT FOR ACUTE ALCOHOLIC HEPATITIS

The 1996 UNOS report recognized that the 6-month rule excludes patients with alcoholic hepatitis from consideration for LT.[1] Patients with mild to moderate alcoholic hepatitis (discriminant function [DF] <32) are likely to respond to conservative management and abstinence, with 90% survival at 1 month.[63,64] However, patients with severe disease (DF $\geq$32 or Model for End-stage Liver Disease [MELD] $\geq$21) have an overall mortality of about 40% within 6 months.[65] Corticosteroids may reduce mortality by up to 25% in these patients, but mortality remains high and is even higher in the approximately 40% of patients unresponsive to corticosteroids.[64] In this subset of severely ill patients, the 6-month rule essentially excludes transplant as the last therapeutic option available.

Two studies have examined the impact of superimposed histologic acute alcoholic hepatitis in the explanted recipient liver on outcomes after transplantation. It can be presumed histologically that these patients had recent alcohol use, often unsuspected, at the time of transplant. In 36 patients with these characteristics, Tome and Lucey[11] demonstrated no difference in the recidivism rate or survival compared with patients with alcoholic cirrhosis alone. In a similarly designed study, Wells and colleagues[66] identified 32 patients with acute alcoholic hepatitis in the explanted liver. Because the presence of histologic acute alcoholic hepatitis was significantly associated with pretransplant abstinence of less than 12 months, but not of less than 6 months, it is unclear whether these histologic changes represented clandestine drinking or persistent footprints of past injury. Again, there was no difference in the recidivism rate or survival compared with patients with alcoholic cirrhosis alone. These studies suggest that patients with alcoholic hepatitis (although mostly subclinical) in violation of the 6-month rule have the same outcomes as those with alcoholic cirrhosis meeting the rule, and thus should be considered as potential candidates for transplantation.

Given the high risk of early death and lack of other effective therapies in patients with severe alcoholic hepatitis not responding to medical therapy, an investigation into all available treatment options, including early LT, is necessary.[18,67] In recognition of this, the 2005 French Consensus Conference recommended pilot studies of early liver transplantation for severe alcoholic hepatitis in carefully selected patients.[68] Castel and colleagues[69] reported such a prospective, multicenter pilot study at the 2009 AASLD Meeting. Eighteen patients with severe alcoholic hepatitis unresponsive to steroids (Lille score $\geq$0.45) underwent LT an average 9 days after steroid nonresponse determination. Each case was matched to a control patient (medical management only) for age, sex, DF, and Lille score. Patient survival in the transplanted group was higher compared with controls at 1 year (83% vs 44%, $P = .009$). Among the nontransplanted patients, 50% to 90% of deaths occurred within the first 2 months, and only one patient relapsed about 2.5 years after transplant without any impact on graft function.

The promising results reported by Castel and colleagues led to the recent study by Mathurin and colleagues[18] published in the November 2011 issue of the *New England Journal of Medicine*. This study aimed to determine whether early LT improved survival among patients with severe alcoholic hepatitis unresponsive to medical therapy, to evaluate posttransplant recidivism in patients selected without meeting the 6-month rule, and to evaluate the impact of early transplantation on the overall transplantation activity of the participating centers. Seven centers in France participated in enrolling patients from 2006 to 2010 with severe alcoholic hepatitis defined as new-onset jaundice for less than 3 months and DF >32 unresponsive to medical therapy, defined as Lille score $\geq$0.45 after 7 days of 40 mg of prednisolone with standard medical care or a continuous increase in MELD. In addition, inclusion criteria included severe alcoholic hepatitis as the first liver-decompensating event, presence of "close supportive family members," absence of severe coexisting or psychiatric disorders (due to the very rapid selection process), and agreement by patients to adhere to lifelong complete abstinence. Four team circles comprising nurses and house staff, an addiction specialist, senior hepatologists, an anesthesiologist, and transplant surgeons were required to reach complete consensus on selection. Assessment of posttransplantation recidivism consisted of informal interviews with patient and family during clinical follow-up according to established protocols by a psychiatrist.

The 6-month survival rate was significantly higher among the 26 patients undergoing transplantation (77% vs 23%, P<.001) than among matched controls (and similar to responder controls), with a 90% mortality in the control group at 2 months after identification of nonresponse to medical therapy. In the Lille and Brussels centers, the most important reason for exclusion from early transplantation was a predisposition to addiction or unfavorable social or familial profiles, followed by the presence of a severe comorbidity. There was no recidivism at 6 months, but 3 of 26 patients relapsed at 720, 740, and 1140 days after transplantation. In this study, 2 patients remained daily consumers (30 g/d and >50 g/d), despite counseling by an addiction specialist, although none have had graft dysfunction.

The study's selection process was intentionally multidisciplinary and rigorous because of the likelihood that accepted patients with severe alcoholic hepatitis would have very high MELD scores and rank at the top of the waiting list. Patients presenting with their first liver-decompensating event and who were unaware of their underlying liver disease were deemed by the investigators to represent the most urgent clinical scenario. However, a prior history of liver decompensation suggested a lack of insight, and these subjects were therefore excluded. Overall, the study's selection process resulted in the selection of a very small number of patients with alcoholic hepatitis for early transplantation. Fewer than 2% of patients with severe alcoholic hepatitis presenting directly to the Lille and Brussels centers were selected. Overall, 12 (6.6%) of 181 patients in the Lille center were selected. Of note, nearly all (11 out of 12) were referred by community hospitals.

The findings of Mathurin and colleagues effectively challenged the value of the 6-month rule and the opinion of experts that alcoholic hepatitis is a contraindication for transplantation.[17] Despite the very brief median times from end of prednisolone therapy to listing of 13 days (range, 6–17 days) and from listing to LT of 9 days (range, 3–11 days), only 3 (11.5%) patients relapsed more than 2 years after transplantation without graft dysfunction. This result compares favorably with recidivism rates in transplantation for alcoholic cirrhosis without alcoholic hepatitis adhering to the 6-month rule as discussed previously. This study marks an important advancement in the field of LT, and may serve to loosen the rigidity of the 6-month rule by fostering emphasis on case-by-case evaluations by transplant centers and opening the door for potentially life-saving early transplantations in a very select group of the sickest patients with alcoholic hepatitis.

The results by Mathurin and colleagues[70] have been supported by a recent retrospective analysis of the UNOS database. This study showed that the 5-year graft and patient survival were similar for those transplanted for acute alcoholic hepatitis in comparison with those undergoing LT for alcoholic cirrhosis. Furthermore, the causes of graft loss and mortality were not found to be alcohol related in any patient.

SUMMARY

Liver transplant should be seen as only one component of the medical care in the patient with ALD. These patients should be treated in a multidisciplinary manner that addresses not only the medical needs of the patient but also the psychosocial and addiction issues that occur in the majority of these patients. The evaluation of the patient by a psychiatrist or addiction specialist is crucial in the evaluation process for identifying those at high risk of relapse, and those who may require aggressive intervention to prevent relapse. All of the authors' patients are required to sign a contract agreeing to abstinence from alcohol and any other substance abuse. The importance of a written behavioral contract is that it provides the patient with clearly delineated expectations regarding their substance abuse. It enables the transplant team to ensure that the patient has been fully informed of expectations to meet LT requirements, and clarifies any ambiguity that the patient may have regarding those expectations.

The recent publication of data regarding transplant for acute alcoholic hepatitis by Mathurin and colleagues forces us to reevaluate our methods of evaluating any alcoholic for a liver transplant. It is clear that trying to determine the risk of relapse during the evaluation of any patient with ALD cannot be reliably identified by a single parameter or score. The authors believe that many different factors contribute to an individual's risk of relapse and that each case must be considered on an individual basis, as there are obvious psychosocial measures that cannot be measured or to which a score can be assigned. Factors that are identified as placing the individual at risk of relapse should be addressed and managed if possible in the pretransplant evaluation. However, the process of maintaining abstinence for the majority of individuals requires time, and is unlikely to be achieved within a short period. This process must continue after transplantation to ensure sobriety.

REFERENCES

1. United Network for Organ Sharing (UNOS). Available at: http://optn.transplant. hrsa.gov. Accessed April 1, 2012.
2. Lucey MR. Liver transplantation in patients with alcoholic liver disease. Liver Transpl 2011;17(7):751–9.
3. DiMartini A, Crone C, Dew MA. Alcohol and substance use in liver transplant patients. Clin Liver Dis 2011;15(4):727–51.
4. Lucey MR, Schaubel DE, Guidinger MK, et al. Effect of alcoholic liver disease and hepatitis C infection on waiting list and posttransplant mortality and transplant survival benefit. Hepatology 2009;50(2):400–6.
5. Poynard T, Naveau S, Doffoel M, et al. Evaluation of efficacy of liver transplantation in alcoholic cirrhosis using matched and simulated controls: 5-year survival. Multi-centre group. J Hepatol 1999;30(6):1130–7.
6. Starzl TE, Van Thiel D, Tzakis AG, et al. Orthotopic liver transplantation for alcoholic cirrhosis. JAMA 1988;260(17):2542–4.
7. Gish RG, Lee A, Brooks L, et al. Long-term follow-up of patients diagnosed with alcohol dependence or alcohol abuse who were evaluated for liver transplantation. Liver Transpl 2001;7(7):581–7.

8. Kelly M, Chick J, Gribble R, et al. Predictors of relapse to harmful alcohol after orthotopic liver transplantation. Alcohol Alcohol 2006;41(3):278–83.

9. Lim JK, Keeffe EB. Liver transplantation for alcoholic liver disease: current concepts and length of sobriety. Liver Transpl 2004;10(10 Suppl 2):S31–8.

10. Pageaux GP, Bismuth M, Perney P, et al. Alcohol relapse after liver transplantation for alcoholic liver disease: does it matter? J Hepatol 2003;38(5):629–34.

11. Tome S, Lucey MR. Timing of liver transplantation in alcoholic cirrhosis. J Hepatol 2003;39(3):302–7.

12. Cuadrado A, Fabrega E, Casafont F, et al. Alcohol recidivism impairs long-term patient survival after orthotopic liver transplantation for alcoholic liver disease. Liver Transpl 2005;11(4):420–6.

13. Pfitzmann R, Schwenzer J, Rayes N, et al. Long-term survival and predictors of relapse after orthotopic liver transplantation for alcoholic liver disease. Liver Transpl 2007;13(2):197–205.

14. Dixon J, Welch HG. Priority setting: lessons from Oregon. Lancet 1991;337(8746): 891–4.

15. Neuberger J, Adams D, MacMaster P, et al. Assessing priorities for allocation of donor liver grafts: survey of public and clinicians. BMJ 1998;317(7152):172–5.

16. Ubel PA. Transplantation in alcoholics: separating prognosis and responsibility from social biases. Liver Transpl Surg 1997;3(3):343–6.

17. Bathgate AJ. Recommendations for alcohol-related liver disease. Lancet 2006; 367(9528):2045–6.

18. Mathurin P, Moreno C, Samuel D, et al. Early liver transplantation for severe alcoholic hepatitis. N Engl J Med 2011;365(19):1790–800.

19. Kotlyar DS, Burke A, Campbell MS, et al. A critical review of candidacy for orthotopic liver transplantation in alcoholic liver disease. Am J Gastroenterol 2008; 103(3):734–43 [quiz: 744].

20. Davies MH, Langman MJ, Elias E, et al. Liver disease in a district hospital remote from a transplant centre: a study of admissions and deaths. Gut 1992;33(10): 1397–9.

21. Julapalli VR, Kramer JR, El-Serag HB. Evaluation for liver transplantation: adherence to AASLD referral guidelines in a large Veterans Affairs center. Liver Transpl 2005;11(11):1370–8.

22. Keeffe EB. Comorbidities of alcoholic liver disease that affect outcome of orthotopic liver transplantation. Liver Transpl Surg 1997;3(3):251–7.

23. Watt KD, McCashland TM. Transplantation in the alcoholic patient. Semin Liver Dis 2004;24(3):249–55.

24. Neuberger J, Schulz KH, Day C, et al. Transplantation for alcoholic liver disease. J Hepatol 2002;36(1):130–7.

25. Neuberger J, James O. Guidelines for selection of patients for liver transplantation in the era of donor-organ shortage. Lancet 1999;354(9190):1636–9.

26. Kearns PJ, Young H, Garcia G, et al. Accelerated improvement of alcoholic liver disease with enteral nutrition. Gastroenterology 1992;102(1):200–5.

27. Day E, Best D, Sweeting R, et al. Detecting lifetime alcohol problems in individuals referred for liver transplantation for nonalcoholic liver failure. Liver Transpl 2008;14(11):1609–13.

28. Weinrieb RM, Van Horn DH, McLellan AT, et al. Interpreting the significance of drinking by alcohol-dependent liver transplant patients: fostering candor is the key to recovery. Liver Transpl 2000;6(6):769–76.

29. Beresford TP. Predictive factors for alcoholic relapse in the selection of alcohol-dependent persons for hepatic transplant. Liver Transpl Surg 1997;3(3):280–91.

30. DiMartini A, Day N, Dew MA, et al. Alcohol consumption patterns and predictors of use following liver transplantation for alcoholic liver disease. Liver Transpl 2006;12(5):813–20.
31. Grant BF. Alcohol consumption, alcohol abuse and alcohol dependence. The United States as an example. Addiction (Abingdon, England) 1994;89(11):1357–65.
32. Vaillant GE. The natural history of alcoholism and its relationship to liver transplantation. Liver Transpl Surg 1997;3(3):304–10.
33. Diagnostic and statistical manual for mental disorders. 4th edition. Washington, DC: American Psychiatric Association; 1994.
34. Foster PF, Fabrega F, Karademir S, et al. Prediction of abstinence from ethanol in alcoholic recipients following liver transplantation. Hepatology 1997;25(6):1469–77.
35. Jauhar S, Talwalkar JA, Schneekloth T, et al. Analysis of factors that predict alcohol relapse following liver transplantation. Liver Transpl 2004;10(3):408–11.
36. Mackie J, Groves K, Hoyle A, et al. Orthotopic liver transplantation for alcoholic liver disease: a retrospective analysis of survival, recidivism, and risk factors predisposing to recidivism. Liver Transpl 2001;7(5):418–27.
37. Dawson DA, Grant BF, Stinson FS, et al. Recovery from DSM-IV alcohol dependence: United States, 2001-2002. Addiction (Abingdon, England) 2005;100(3):281–92.
38. DiMartini A, Day N, Dew MA, et al. Alcohol use following liver transplantation: a comparison of follow-up methods. Psychosomatics 2001;42(1):55–62.
39. McCallum S, Masterton G. Liver transplantation for alcoholic liver disease: a systematic review of psychosocial selection criteria. Alcohol Alcohol (Oxford, Oxfordshire) 2006;41(4):358–63.
40. Coffman KL, Hoffman A, Sher L, et al. Treatment of the postoperative alcoholic liver transplant recipient with other addictions. Liver Transpl Surg 1997;3(3):322–7.
41. Howard LM, Williams R, Fahy TA. The psychiatric assessment of liver transplant patients with alcoholic liver disease: a review. J Psychosom Res 1994;38(7):643–53.
42. Ewusi-Mensah I, Saunders JB, Wodak AD, et al. Psychiatric morbidity in patients with alcoholic liver disease. Br Med J (Clin Res Ed) 1983;287(6403):1417–9.
43. Regier DA, Farmer ME, Rae DS, et al. Comorbidity of mental disorders with alcohol and other drug abuse. Results from the Epidemiologic Catchment Area (ECA) Study. JAMA 1990;264(19):2511–8.
44. Karman JF, Sileri P, Kamuda D, et al. Risk factors for failure to meet listing requirements in liver transplant candidates with alcoholic cirrhosis. Transplantation 2001;71(9):1210–3.
45. Everhart JE, Beresford TP. Liver transplantation for alcoholic liver disease: a survey of transplantation programs in the United States. Liver Transpl Surg 1997;3(3):220–6.
46. Lucey MR, Brown KA, Everson GT, et al. Minimal criteria for placement of adults on the liver transplant waiting list: a report of a national conference organized by the American Society of Transplant Physicians and the American Association for the Study of Liver Diseases. Liver Transpl Surg 1997;3(6):628–37.
47. Murray KF, Carithers RL Jr. AASLD practice guidelines: evaluation of the patient for liver transplantation. Hepatology 2005;41(6):1407–32.
48. Varma V, Webb K, Mirza DF. Liver transplantation for alcoholic liver disease. World J Gastroenterol 2010;16(35):4377–93.

49. Alexander JF, Lischner MW, Galambos JT. Natural history of alcoholic hepatitis. II. The long-term prognosis. Am J Gastroenterol 1971;56(6):515–25.

50. Borowsky SA, Strome S, Lott E. Continued heavy drinking and survival in alcoholic cirrhotics. Gastroenterology 1981;80(6):1405–9.

51. Chedid A, Mendenhall CL, Gartside P, et al. Prognostic factors in alcoholic liver disease. VA Cooperative Study Group. Am J Gastroenterol 1991;86(2):210–6.

52. Marbet UA, Bianchi L, Meury U, et al. Long-term histological evaluation of the natural history and prognostic factors of alcoholic liver disease. J Hepatol 1987;4(3):364–72.

53. Powell WJ Jr, Klatskin G. Duration of survival in patients with Laennec's cirrhosis. Influence of alcohol withdrawal, and possible effects of recent changes in general management of the disease. Am J Med 1968;44(3):406–20.

54. Dew MA, DiMartini AF, Steel J, et al. Meta-analysis of risk for relapse to substance use after transplantation of the liver or other solid organs. Liver Transpl 2008; 14(2):159–72.

55. Berlakovich GA, Steininger R, Herbst F, et al. Efficacy of liver transplantation for alcoholic cirrhosis with respect to recidivism and compliance. Transplantation 1994;58(5):560–5.

56. Tan HH, Virmani S, Martin P. Controversies in the management of alcoholic liver disease. Mt Sinai J Med 2009;76(5):484–98.

57. Yates WR, Martin M, LaBrecque D, et al. A model to examine the validity of the 6-month abstinence criterion for liver transplantation. Alcohol Clin Exp Res 1998; 22(2):513–7.

58. Gedaly R, McHugh PP, Johnston TD, et al. Predictors of relapse to alcohol and illicit drugs after liver transplantation for alcoholic liver disease. Transplantation 2008;86(8):1090–5.

59. Campbell DA Jr, Punch JD. Monitoring for alcohol use relapse after liver transplantation for alcoholic liver disease. Liver Transpl Surg 1997;3(3):300–3.

60. Fuller RK. Definition and diagnosis of relapse to drinking. Liver Transpl Surg 1997; 3(3):258–62.

61. DeGottardi A, Spahr L, Gelez P, et al. A simple score for predicting alcohol relapse after liver transplantation: results from 387 patients over 15 years. Arch Intern Med 2007;167(11):1183–8.

62. DiMartini A, Day N, Lane T, et al. Carbohydrate deficient transferrin in abstaining patients with end-stage liver disease. Alcohol Clin Exp Res 2001;25(12): 1729–33.

63. Carithers RL Jr, Herlong HF, Diehl AM, et al. Methylprednisolone therapy in patients with severe alcoholic hepatitis. A randomized multicenter trial. Ann Intern Med 1989;110(9):685–90.

64. Mathurin P, Mendenhall CL, Carithers RL Jr, et al. Corticosteroids improve short-term survival in patients with severe alcoholic hepatitis (AH): individual data analysis of the last three randomized placebo controlled double blind trials of corticosteroids in severe AH. J Hepatol 2002;36(4):480–7.

65. Whitfield K, Rambaldi A, Wetterslev J, et al. Pentoxifylline for alcoholic hepatitis. Cochrane Database Syst Rev (Online) 2009;(4):CD007339.

66. Wells JT, Said A, Agni R, et al. The impact of acute alcoholic hepatitis in the explanted recipient liver on outcome after liver transplantation. Liver Transpl 2007;13(12):1728–35.

67. Louvet A, Diaz E, Dharancy S, et al. Early switch to pentoxifylline in patients with severe alcoholic hepatitis is inefficient in non-responders to corticosteroids. J Hepatol 2008;48(3):465–70.

68. Consensus conference: indications for liver transplantation, January 19 and 20, 2005, Lyon Palais Des Congres: text of recommendations (long version). Liver Transpl 2006;12(6):998–1011.
69. Castel H, Moreno C, Antonini TM, et al. Early transplantation improves survival of non-responders to steroids in severe alcoholic hepatitis: a challenge to the 6 month rule of abstinence. Hepatology 2009;50(Suppl 4):307A–8A.
70. Singal AK, Bashar H, Anand BS, et al. Outcomes after liver transplantation for alcoholic hepatitis are similar to alcoholic cirrhosis: exploratory analysis from the UNOS database. Hepatology 2012;55(5):1398–405.

Complications in Patients with Alcohol-Associated Liver Disease Who Undergo Liver Transplantation

Paul J. Gaglio Jr[a], Paul J. Gaglio Sr, MD[b],*

KEYWORDS

• Alcoholism • Alcoholic hepatitis • Liver transplantation • Liver failure

KEY POINTS

- Liver transplantation in appropriately selected patients with alcohol associated liver disease is associated with excellent short and long term survival.
- Recognition and treatment of alcohol associated cardiac issues is critical in the pre, intra, and perioperative phases of transplantation.
- Maximizing the patients nutrition and level of physcial conditioning pre-transplantation will improve post-transplantation outcomes.
- De Novo head and neck malignancies occur at a higher rate following transplantation in patients with alcoholism.
- Careful patient selection, as well as pre and post transplantation counselling may minimize alcohol recidivism post liver transplantation.

INTRODUCTION

Cirrhosis caused by alcohol-associated liver disease is a common indication for liver transplantation worldwide. Patients with end-stage liver disease caused by alcoholism that require liver transplantation present several challenges because of multiple pretransplantation, intratransplation, and posttransplantation issues, many of which are induced by or exacerbated by alcohol use. In this regard, patients with alcohol-associated liver disease are unique when compared with the general population of patients undergoing liver transplantation. This article reviews important posttransplantation problems in patients transplanted for alcohol-associated liver disease.

Funding/support: n/a.
Financial disclosures/conflict of interest: The authors have nothing to disclose.
[a] Rutgers University College of Arts and Sciences, New Brunswick, NJ 08901, USA;
[b] Department of Medicine, Montefiore Einstein Liver Center, Albert Einstein College of Medicine, 111 East 210th Street, Rosenthal 2 Red Zone, Bronx, NY 01467, USA
* Corresponding author.
E-mail address: pgaglio@montefiore.org

Clin Liver Dis 16 (2012) 865–875
http://dx.doi.org/10.1016/j.cld.2012.08.013
1089-3261/12/$ – see front matter © 2012 Elsevier Inc. All rights reserved.

liver.theclinics.com

THE SCOPE OF THE PROBLEM

A review of data from the Organ Procurement and Transplantation Network Database indicates that alcohol-related cirrhosis is currently the second most common indication for liver transplantation in the United States.[1] Alcohol-associated liver disease is also a common indication for liver transplantation in Europe[2]; alcoholism may also accelerate progression to cirrhosis in patients with other etiologies of liver injury, including hepatitis C. The effects of alcohol on pretransplantation physiology, candidacy for liver transplantation, and other issues have been discussed elsewhere in this issue; however, several of these pretransplantation issues dramatically influence posttransplantation outcomes.

CARDIAC DISEASE

The increased prevalence of cardiac disease in patients with alcoholic cirrhosis has been recognized for many years. In general, alcoholic cardiomyopathy (ACM) is more prevalent in individuals with active alcohol abuse compared with patients who are abstinent. In a recent review, patients consuming greater than 90 g of alcohol a day (representing approximately seven to eight alcoholic beverages in a 24-hour period) for more than 5 years were at risk for the development of this complication.[3] ACM is usually associated with an increase in myocardial mass and dilation of the ventricles. These changes can result in diastolic and systolic dysfunction, inducing hypotension and heart failure. The pathophysiology of ACM may involve alcohol-induced cell death (possibly caused by apoptosis) with resultant myocardial dysfunction, with further resultant negative effects on cardiac function after liver transplantation.

In addition to ACM, chronic cardiac dysfunction in patients with cirrhosis, termed "cirrhotic cardiomyopathy," has recently garnered significant attention. Cirrhotic cardiomyopathy is characterized by impaired contractility or altered diastolic relaxation, an increased cardiac output, and diminished ventricular response to stress associated with electrophysiologic abnormalities in the absence of other known cardiac disease.[4] Cirrhotic cardiomyopathy has been identified before liver transplantation in many patients with cirrhosis including those with alcohol-related liver disease. Cirrhotic cardiomyopathy is problematic post–liver transplantation because patients may develop heart failure and other cardiac complications because of the dramatically increased cardiovascular stress that patients face in the immediate postoperative period. Posttransplant reperfusion after implantation of the new liver may result in cardiac death from a multitude of causes, including arrhythmias, acute heart failure, and myocardial infarction. In addition, chronic manifestations of cirrhotic cardiomyopathy may compromise cardiac function long term. In a recent review, pulmonary edema and other manifestations of diastolic dysfunction were present in up to 25% of patients after liver transplantation.[5]

Based on concern about pre-existing cardiac disease and the potential for perioperative complications, all patients considered for liver transplantation undergo a complete pretransplantation cardiac assessment. This is usually achieved by a noninvasive assessment of cardiac structure, performed by the use of Doppler echocardiography with a "bubble study" to assess right-to-left cardiac shunting and the presence of hepatopulmonary syndrome. In cases where either atherosclerotic heart disease or pulmonary hypertension are a concern, formal right and left heart catheterization with assessment of pulmonary arterial pressures, pulmonary vascular resistance, and coronary arteriography may be required.[6,7] A preoperative algorithm used at the senior author's liver transplantation center to assess patients for cardiovascular disease appears in **Fig. 1**.

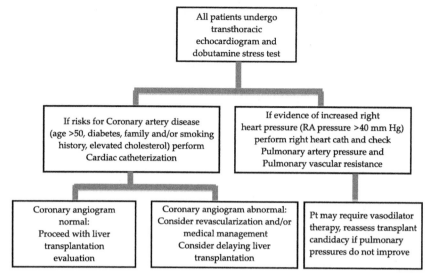

All patients undergo transthoracic echocardiogram and dobutamine stress test

If risks for Coronary artery disease (age >50, diabetes, family and/or smoking history, elevated cholesterol) perform Cardiac catheterization

If evidence of increased right heart pressure (RA pressure >40 mm Hg) perform right heart cath and check Pulmonary artery pressure and Pulmonary vascular resistance

Coronary angiogram normal: Proceed with liver transplantation evaluation

Coronary angiogram abnormal: Consider revascularization and/or medical management Consider delaying liver transplantation

Pt may require vasodilator therapy, reassess transplant candidacy if pulmonary pressures do not improve

Fig. 1. Preoperative cardiac assessment in patients with alcohol-associated liver disease.

Identification of preoperative cardiac dysfunction in a patient with alcoholic cirrhosis is critical; perioperative therapy targeted at the pathophysiologic processes that induce this complication is required to allow transplantation to occur. Several of the processes that induce cardiac dysfunction may be ameliorated by judicious use of β-blockers, angiotensin-converting enzyme inhibitors, and aldosterone-blocking agents.[5]

MALNUTRITION

Malnutrition is present in many patients with alcohol-associated liver disease before liver transplantation, and may portend a poor prognosis. Previously published studies indicate that in patients with acute alcoholic hepatitis, 30-day mortality increased from 2% in patients with mild malnutrition to 52% in patient with severe malnutrition.[8]

Malnutrition in this setting has many etiologies including impaired absorption of nutrients caused by cholestasis or pancreatitis; inadequate caloric intake; a hypermetabolic state associated with increased catabolism of proteins, lipids, and carbohydrates; and fat-soluble and B vitamin deficiency. Protein calorie malnutrition in this setting has additional ramifications, because this may enhance the toxicity of alcohol in patients who continue to consume it.[9] Hypocholesterolemia is also more common in patients with alcohol-associated liver disease, and may be associated with a greater risk of neurotoxicity caused by immunosuppression (specifically calcineurin inhibitors) in the postoperative period.

Most liver transplantation programs require repletion of calories in cirrhotics before liver transplantation, usually by enhancing enteral nutrition by supplementing the patient's diet or by nasogastric tube feeding, because malnutrition has been associated with diminished survival after liver transplantation. In general, most patients with a functioning liver graft recover their nutritional function after liver transplantation.

DECONDITIONING

Deconditioning in patients with alcoholic hepatitis is common and may be caused by multiple factors including malnutrition, muscle wasting defined as "sarcopenia," and the hypermetabolic effect of cirrhosis. Deconditioning and sarcopenia have been associated with significantly worse outcomes after liver transplantation. In a recently published prospective review, sarcopenia defined as decrease in psoas muscle area was assessed by pretransplantation CT scans; in patients with the most significant sarcopenia, 1- and 3-year posttransplantation survival was significantly decreased (49.7% and 26.4%) when compared with patients with minimal sarcopenia (87% and 77.2%) (**Fig. 2**). Sarcopenia was also identified as an independent risk factor for mortality after liver transplantation.[10]

Patients with alcohol-associated liver disease are also particularly vulnerable to the development of muscle injury, because alcohol has direct effects on muscle cell structure, causing skeletal myopathy, which may manifest as muscle weakness, muscle pain, and abnormal muscle enzymes on serologic assessment.

NEUROLOGIC ISSUES

The pathophysiologic effects of alcohol on the central nervous system have been well documented. Chronic, excessive alcohol consumption directly injures the brain and nerve fibers, and can be associated with structural damage. Alcohol has also been directly linked to neuropathy, because of injury to nerves. In patients with chronic alcohol abuse, neurologic consequences may also include hepatic encephalopathy, Wernicke encephalopathy, Korsakoff syndrome, Marchiafava-Bignami disease, central pontine myelinolysis, and neuropathy (reviewed in[11]).

A major complication of alcohol use is alcohol-related brain damage (ARBD). This process, induced by alcohol-associated loss of neurons, can result in enlargement of the ventricles with shrinking of the surrounding normal brain, and is often evident on noninvasive imaging modalities including magnetic resonance imaging (**Fig. 3**). In the setting of ARBD, if brain volume loss is caused by decrease in neurons, recovery of brain volume may be incomplete with alcohol abstinence.

An additional neurologic complication, hepatic encephalopathy, is common in patients with liver disease as a result of portal hypertension shunting of blood flow away from the liver and failure to clear substances which induce encephalopathy. Hepatic encephalopathy has been associated with direct damage to the brain by a mechanism that is different than ARBD; in contradistinction to ARBD, which leads to direct neuronal injury, the neuropathologic features of hepatic encephalopathy primarily include changes in the morphology and function of glial cells, specifically astroglial cells resulting in cell swelling, mimicking Alzheimer type II astrocytosis.[12]

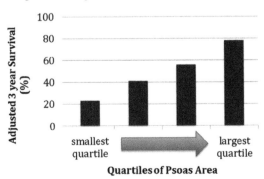

Fig. 2. Survival in patients with sarcopenia. (*Adapted from* Englesbe MJ, Patel SP, He K, et al. Sarcopenia and mortality after liver transplantation. J Am Coll Surg 2010;211:271–8; with permission.)

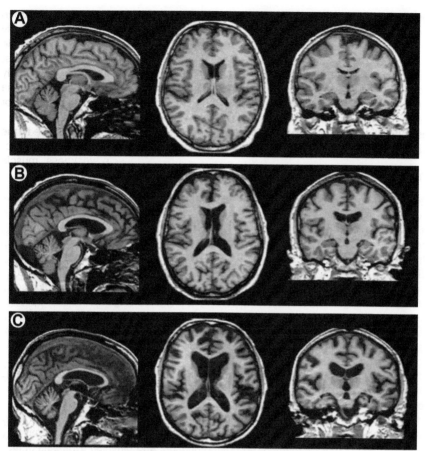

Fig. 3. Magnetic resonance imaging examples. (*A*) Normal 63-year-old man. (*B*) A 59-year-old male alcoholic. (*C*) A 63 year old with Wernicke-Korsakoff syndrome. (*Modified from* Welch KA. Neurologic complications of alcohol and misuse of drugs. Pract Neurol 2011;11:206–19; with permission.)

Alcohol-Related Dementia

In certain individuals undergoing pre–liver transplantation evaluation, alcohol-related dementia cannot be differentiated from hepatic encephalopathy. This distinction is exceptionally important, because alcohol-related dementia is often irreversible, unlike hepatic encephalopathy, which is largely reversible after liver transplantation. Patients with alcohol-related dementia may suffer from significant cognitive impairment with neuropsychologic syndromes, such as spastic paraparesis, seizures, and myoclonic convulsions, and language and visuospatial dysfunction. Many transplant centers struggle with the task of differentiating alcohol-associated dementia from hepatic encephalopathy, relying on difficult to perform neurocognitive testing, which may include the assessment of executive skills (planning, initiating, monitoring complex behavior), fine motor skills, general intelligence, learning and memory, postural stability, processing speed, and visuospatial skills.[13]

Based on the multitude of potential alcohol-related neurologic complications, it is apparent that significant neurologic defects may influence a patient's candidacy for liver transplantation, particularly because these complications effect adherence to the complicated medication and physical rehabilitation regimen required post–liver transplantation. After liver transplantation, seizures and neurologic complications caused by immunosuppression, particularly calcineurin inhibitiors, are more common in patients with alcoholic liver disease, especially in malnourished, hypocholesterolemic alcoholics.[14] Neuropathy may also be problematic; it may limit the patient's ability to participate in rehabilitation because of balance and coordination issues. In a recent review, 17% of patients developed a neurologic complication after transplantation; these complications occurred in 42% of patients with alcohol-associated liver disease and included hepatic encephalopathy (47.6% of patients) and seizures (9.5%).[15]

OSTEOPOROSIS

Patients with alcohol-associated liver disease are at significant risk of bone loss with resultant osteopenia or osteoporosis. In some series, osteopenia and osteoporosis has been reported in greater than 40% of patients.[16] Alcohol has a direct effect on osteoblasts and bone production, and induces a decrease in testosterone and estrogen, effecting bone formation. Recent data have suggested that bone loss in patients who consume significant amounts of alcohol is multifactorial, and may be associated not only with direct injury to osteoblasts and osterocytes, but also the thyroid, adrenal glands, kidney, and parathyroid glands (**Fig. 4**).[17] Bone density is routinely assessed in patients being evaluated for liver transplantation, and may be treated in appropriate cases with calcium and vitamin D replacement, or bisphosphonates in selected patients.

Identification of diminished bone density is imperative in the pretransplantation period, because during the post–liver transplantation period, osteopenia and osteoporosis often worsen, influenced by immunosuppression required to prevent immune recognition and rejection of the newly transplanted organ. In the immediate posttransplantation period and for several months after liver transplantation, glucocorticoids are used. These agents have several direct effects on bone because they directly inhibit bone formation by decreasing osteoblast recruitment and differentiation, and diminish synthesis of type I collagen. Glucocorticoids also increase bone resorption by enhancing osteoclast activity, and indirectly by reducing testosterone and estrogen production and altering the sensitivity of osteoclasts to parathyroid hormone. These effects contribute to rapid loss of bone density after liver transplantation[18] and may exacerbate the pre-existent osteoporosis often seen in patients with alcohol-associated liver disease.

Therapy of osteoporosis in the peritransplantation setting includes an attempt at preventing further bone loss, and techniques to increase bone density. In general, this includes vitamin D supplementation, judicious use of hormone-replacement therapy in appropriate patients, and bisphosphonates.[19]

CANCER AFTER LIVER TRANSPLANTATION

De novo malignancies after liver transplantation occur frequently, and represent one of the leading causes of "late death" after liver transplantation. In patients transplanted for alcohol-associated liver disease, concern has existed regarding a greater incidence of head and neck cancer, and esophageal cancer, particularly of the squamous cell variety.[20] A recently published study that evaluated malignancy after liver transplantation revealed 10 esophageal cancers in more than 1900 transplanted patients; in nine of these cases, alcohol-associated cirrhosis was the indication for liver transplantation.[21] Because many patients with alcohol-associated liver disease also smoke cigarettes, it is difficult to differentiate which risk factor contributed to oncogenesis,

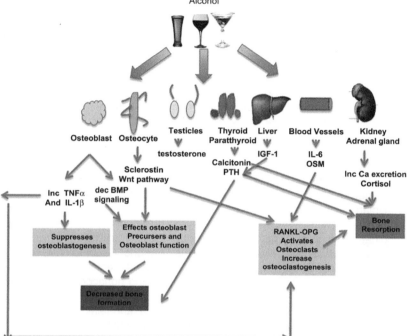

Fig. 4. Effect of alcohol on bone formation. BMP, bone morphogenic protein; IGF-1, insulin-like growth factor; IL-1β, interleukin 1β; IL-6, interleukin 6; OSM, oncostatin M; PTH, parathyroid hormone; RANKL OPG, receptor activator of nuclear factor κB ligand osteoprotegerin; TNF-α, tumor necrosis factor-α; WnT, canonical wingless. (*Adapted from* Maurel DB, Boisseau N, Benhamou CL, et al. Alcohol and bone: review of dose effects and mechanisms. Osteoporos Int 2012;23:1–16; with permission.)

because alcohol use and smoking can lead to increased risk of malignancy in the post-transplantation period.[22–24]

There are currently no national guidelines related to screening for head, neck, or esophageal neoplasia in a posttransplant patient population, although many liver transplant centers including those of the senior author have incorporated head and neck and esophageal cancer screening protocols for smokers, especially if they have a history of alcohol abuse. This includes annual evaluation by an ear, nose, and throat surgeon and annual upper endoscopy.

ALCOHOL USE BEFORE AND RECIDIVISM AFTER LIVER TRANSPLANTATION

Historically, liver transplantation in patients with alcohol-associated liver disease was contentious because of the perception that the patient's liver disease was self-inflicted and concerns related to alcohol recidivism after transplantation. However, it is clear that outcomes in appropriately selected patients with alcohol-associated liver disease who undergo liver transplantation meet or exceed those of other indications.[25] In a recent report in 123 patients, 1-, 5-, and 7-year patient survival was 84, 72, and 63, respectively, in individuals transplanted for alcohol-associated liver disease.[26] These excellent results must be contrasted against dismal survival outcomes in patients with decompensated alcohol-associated liver disease who do not undergo liver transplantation. Given the possibility of excellent posttransplantation outcomes in appropriately selected patients, liver transplantation professionals face the difficult ethical struggle of appropriate patient selection to "save the patient's life" while assessing the patient's future risk of alcohol recidivism and the possibility of graft failure.

In most liver transplantation programs worldwide, patients with alcohol-associated liver disease are required to be abstinent for more than 6 months before liver transplantation (reviewed in[25]). However, data from studies analyzing the efficacy of the "6-month rule" to predict freedom from posttransplantation alcohol recidivism are contentious, because many experienced transplant professionals note limited correlation with the length of pretransplant alcohol abstinence to predict return to alcohol use posttransplantation.[27–29] In addition, despite psychosocial intervention initiated by liver transplantation programs designed to diminish pretransplantation and posttransplantation return to alcohol use, alcohol consumption in patients accepted for liver transplantation is also common.[30,31] A recent study that assessed pretransplantation substance abuse by "anonymous urinalysis" in patients listed for liver transplantation indicated that 20% of patients had positive tests for alcohol.[32]

Based on the difficulty of relying on 6 months of sobriety to predict freedom from posttransplantation alcohol recidivism, many transplant centers have used other predictors to gauge risk for alcohol recidivism including nonacceptance of the use of alcohol as the cause of liver disease,[33] poor social support and family history of alcohol abuse, medical noncompliance, elicit drug use, and failed alcohol rehabilitation.[34] However, factors that predict freedom from alcohol recidivism include the acknowledgment by the patient of his or her addiction; strong social support; the ability to substitute alternative activities that diminish temptation to return to alcohol use, including pursuits that improve self-esteem or hope; a rehabilitative relationship with a healthcare professional, friend, or family member; and a perception by the drinker of the negative consequences of alcoholic relapse (reviewed in[25]).

Despite rigorous attempts to select appropriate patients for liver transplantation with a diagnosis of alcohol-associated liver disease, return to alcohol use after liver transplantation is common, ranging between 10% and 90%.[25,29] Analysis of recurrent alcohol use after transplantation has revealed distinct patterns, as published by DiMartini and colleagues.[35] These investigators noted that 80% of their posttransplantation patient population was abstinent or consumed only small amounts of alcohol occasionally, whereas the remaining 20% exhibited two patterns of alcohol recidivism: early onset moderate-to-heavy consumption, or late-onset moderate use (**Fig. 5**).

Despite a return to alcohol use in most patients after liver transplantation, outcomes are in general excellent in individuals who consume small amounts of alcohol. A recent analysis of patients meeting this description indicated that most remained compliant with their immunosuppressive regimens with only a small number developing significant histologic injury on liver biopsy.[36] In contradistinction, significant and excessive alcohol consumption after liver transplantation may be associated with rapidly progressive liver injury and alcoholic hepatitis[37] and reduced survival.[38] In a recent study of 316 patients transplanted in Italy, 23% reported "problem alcohol drinking" (any score >1 on CAGE criteria) with associated alcohol-related graft injury in more than 50% of patients.[39]

Another potential complication in patients with alcohol recidivism after transplantation is nonadherence to immunosuppression. Despite older publications that imply a high rate of adherence to immunosuppression in patients transplanted for alcoholic cirrhosis who consume small amounts of alcohol, a recent publication indicated that

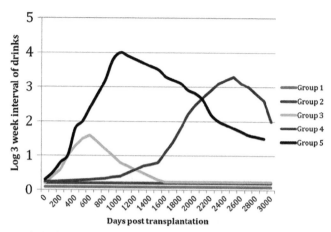

Fig. 5. Patterns of alcohol use after liver transplantation. Groups 1 and 2: minimal alcohol use. Groups 3 and 5: early moderate/heavy alcohol use. Group 4: late return to alcohol use. (*Adapted from* DiMartini A, Dew MA, Day N, et al. Trajectories of alcohol consumption following liver transplantation. Am J Transplant 2010;10:2305–12; with permission.)

up to 61% of patients transplanted for alcohol-associated liver disease reported non-adherence to immunosuppression.[40] Although posttransplantation outcomes were not documented in this publication, strategies to enhance compliance with immuno-suppression should be associated with improved outcomes posttransplantation.

Unfortunately, despite recognition of the nearly universal incidence of posttrans-plantation alcohol recidivism, recommendations regarding the treatment of this complication are limited. A recent review from Sweden indicated that a structured post–liver transplantation treatment program to prevent alcohol recidivism was valuable in decreasing alcohol relapse. This strategy included follow-up by telephone or in person by the transplant unit's social worker and transplant coordinator 3 months posttransplantation, and an interview conducted by an addiction psychologist or social worker at 1, 3, and 5 years after the transplantation. When compared with 48% of historical controls who returned to alcohol use, only 22% of patients who participated in this intervention program manifested alcohol recidivism.[41] Other trans-plantation programs follow similar strategies; follow-up by an addiction psychology/psychiatry team is common in the United Kingdom.[42] Many liver transplantation programs including the program directed by the senior author have adopted similar support and interventional methodologies designed to minimize alcohol recidivism post–liver transplantation.

SUMMARY

Patients with alcohol-associated liver disease who undergo liver transplantation face multiple challenging comorbid medical issues that enhance the potential for perioper-ative and postoperative complications. Awareness of these issues and appropriate therapeutic intervention may minimize the negative effect of these complications on posttransplantation survival.

REFERENCES

1. Available at: http://optn.transplant.hrsa.gov/.

2. Burra P, Senzolo M, Adam R, et al. Liver transplantation for alcoholic liver disease in Europe: a study from the ELTR (European Liver Transplant Registry). Am J Transplant 2010;10:138–48.

3. Piano MR. Alcoholic cardiomyopathy: incidence, clinical characteristics, and pathophysiology. Chest 2002;121:1638–50.

4. Wong F. Cirrhotic cardiomyopathy. Hepatol Int 2009;3:294–304.

5. Garcia-Tsao G, Lim JK. Management and treatment of patients with cirrhosis and portal hypertension: recommendations from the Department of Veterans Affairs hepatitis C resource center program and the national hepatitis C program. Am J Gastroenterol 2009;104:1802–29.

6. Russo MW. Current concepts in the evaluation of patients for liver transplantation. Expert Rev Gastroenterol Hepatol 2007;1:307–20.

7. Raval Z, Harinstein ME, Skaro AI, et al. Cardiovascular risk assessment of the liver transplant candidate. J Am Coll Cardiol 2011;58:223–31.

8. Mendenhall CL, Tosch T, Weesner RE, et al. VA cooperative study on alcoholic hepatitis; prognostic significance of protein-calorie malnutrition. Am J Clin Nutr 1986;43:213–8.

9. Schenker S, Halff GA. Nutritional therapy in alcoholic liver disease. Semin Liver Dis 1993;13:196–209.

10. Englesbe MJ, Patel SP, He K, et al. Sarcopenia and mortality after liver transplantation. J Am Coll Surg 2010;211:271–8.

11. Welch KA. Neurological complications of alcohol and misuse of drugs. Pract Neurol 2011;11:206–19.

12. Butterworth RF. Hepatic encephalopathy: a central neuroinflammatory disorder? Hepatology 2011;53:1372–6.

13. Durazzo TC, Rothlind J, Gazdzinski S, et al. A comparison of neurocognitive function in non-smoking and chronically smoking short-term abstinent alcoholics. Alcohol 2006;39:1–11.

14. Ghaus N, Bohlega S, Rezeig M. Neurological complications in liver transplantation. J Neurol 2001;248:1042–8.

15. Saner FH, Gensicke J, Olde Damink SW, et al. Neurologic complications in adult living donor liver transplant patients: an underestimated factor? J Neurol 2010; 257:253–8.

16. Turner RT. Skeletal response to alcohol. Alcohol Clin Exp Res 2000;24: 1693–701.

17. Maurel DB, Boisseau N, Benhamou CL, et al. Alcohol and bone: review of dose effects and mechanisms. Osteoporos Int 2012;23:1–16.

18. Rodino MA, Shane E. Osteoporosis after organ transplantation. Am J Med 1998; 104:459–69.

19. Kulak CA, Borba VZ, Kulak J Jr, et al. Osteoporosis after transplantation. Curr Osteoporos Rep 2012;10:48–55.

20. Diaz de Liano A, Artieda C, Yarnoz C, et al. Esophageal squamous cell carcinoma after liver transplantation. Clin Transl Oncol 2005;7:518–20.

21. Presser SJ, Schumacher G, Neuhaus R, et al. De novo esophageal neoplasia after liver transplantation. Liver Transpl 2007;13:443–50.

22. Benedetti A, Parent ME, Siemiatycki J. Lifetime consumption of alcoholic beverages and risk of 13 types of cancer in men: results from a case-control study in Montreal. Cancer Detect Prev 2009;32:352–62.

23. Herrero JI, Pardo F, D'Avola D, et al. Risk factors of lung, head and neck, esophageal, and kidney and urinary tract carcinomas after liver transplantation: the effect of smoking withdrawal. Liver Transpl 2011;17:402–8.

24. Leithead JA, Ferguson JW, Hayes PC. Smoking-related morbidity and mortality following liver transplantation. Liver Transpl 2008;14:1159–64.
25. Lucey M. Liver transplantation in patients with alcoholic liver disease. Liver Transpl 2011;17:751–9.
26. Bellamy CO, DiMartini AM, Ruppert K, et al. Transplantation for alcoholic cirrhosis: long term follow-up and impact of disease recurrence. Transplantation 2001;72:619–23.
27. Kotlyar DS, Burke A, Campbell MS, et al. A critical review of candidacy for orthotopic liver transplantation in alcoholic liver disease. Am J Gastroenterol 2008;103: 734–43.
28. Karim Z, Intaraprasong P, Scudamore CH, et al. Predictors of relapse to significant alcohol drinking after liver transplantation. Can J Gastroenterol 2010;24: 245–50.
29. Tome S, Lucey MR. Timing of liver transplantation in alcoholic cirrhosis. J Hepatol 2003;39:302–7.
30. Carbonneau M, Jensen LA, Bain VG, et al. Alcohol use while on the liver transplant waiting list: a single-center experience. Liver Transpl 2010;16:91–7.
31. Weinrieb RM, Van Horn DH, Lynch KG, et al. A randomized, controlled study of treatment for alcohol dependence in patients awaiting liver transplantation. Liver Transpl 2011;17:539–47.
32. Webzell I, Ball D, Bell J, et al. Substance use by liver transplant candidates: an anonymous urinalysis study. Liver Transpl 2011;17:1200–4.
33. Hartl J, Scherer MN, Loss M, et al. Strong predictors for alcohol recidivism after liver transplantation: non-acceptance of the alcohol problem and abstinence of <3 months. Scand J Gastroenterol 2011;46:1257–66.
34. Vaillant GE. A 60-year follow-up of alcoholic men. Addiction 2003;98:1043–51.
35. DiMartini A, Dew MA, Day N, et al. Trajectories of alcohol consumption following liver transplantation. Am J Transplant 2010;10:2305–12.
36. Fábrega E, Crespo J, Casafont F, et al. Alcoholic recidivism after liver transplantation for alcoholic cirrhosis. J Clin Gastroenterol 1998;26:204–6.
37. Pageaux GP, Bismuth M, Perney P, et al. Alcohol relapse after liver transplantation for alcoholic liver disease: does it matter? J Hepatol 2003;38:629–34.
38. Pfitzmann R, Schwenzer J, Rayes N, et al. Long-term survival and predictors of relapse after orthotopic liver transplantation for alcoholic liver disease. Liver Transpl 2007;13:197–205.
39. De Simone P, De Geest S, Ducci J, et al. Alcohol drinking after liver transplantation is associated with graft injury. Minerva Gastroenterol Dietol 2011;57:345–59.
40. Lamba S, Nagurka R, Desai KK, et al. Self-reported non-adherence to immunesuppressant therapy in liver transplant recipients: demographic, interpersonal, and intrapersonal factors. Clin Transplant 2011;26:328–35.
41. Björnsson E, Olsson J, Rydell A, et al. Long-term follow-up of patients with alcoholic liver disease after liver transplantation in Sweden: impact of structured management on recidivism. Scand J Gastroenterol 2005;40:206–16.
42. Bathgate AJ, UK Liver Transplant Units. Recommendations for alcohol-related liver disease. Lancet 2006;367:2045–6.

Index

Note: Page numbers of article titles are in **boldface** type.

Clin Liver Dis 16 (2012) 877–890
http://dx.doi.org/10.1016/S1089-3261(12)00117-1
1089-3261/12/$ – see front matter © 2012 Elsevier Inc. All rights reserved.

liver.theclinics.com

United States
Postal Service

Statement of Ownership, Management, and Circulation
(All Periodicals Publications Except Requestor Publications)

1. Publication Title	2. Publication Number	3. Filing Date
Clinics in Liver Disease	0 1 6 - 7 5 4	9/14/12

4. Issue Frequency	5. Number of Issues Published Annually	6. Annual Subscription Price
Feb, May, Aug, Nov	4	$271.00

7. Complete Mailing Address of Known Office of Publication (Not printer) (Street, city, county, state, and ZIP+4®)

Elsevier Inc.
360 Park Avenue South
New York, NY 10010-1710

Contact Person
Stephen R. Bushing

Telephone (Include area code)
215-239-3688

8. Complete Mailing Address of Headquarters or General Business Office of Publisher (Not printer)

Elsevier Inc., 360 Park Avenue South, New York, NY 10010-1710

9. Full Names and Complete Mailing Addresses of Publisher, Editor, and Managing Editor (Do not leave blank)

Publisher (Name and complete mailing address)

Kim Murphy, Elsevier, Inc., 1600 John F. Kennedy Blvd. Suite 1800, Philadelphia, PA 19103-2899

Editor (Name and complete mailing address)

Kerry Holland, Elsevier, Inc., 1600 John F. Kennedy Blvd. Suite 1800, Philadelphia, PA 19103-2899

Managing Editor (Name and complete mailing address)

Sarah Barth, Elsevier, Inc., 1600 John F. Kennedy Blvd. Suite 1800, Philadelphia, PA 19103-2899

10. Owner (Do not leave blank. If the publication is owned by a corporation, give the name and address of the corporation immediately followed by the names and addresses of all stockholders owning or holding 1 percent or more of the total amount of stock. If not owned by a corporation, give the names and addresses of the individual owners. If owned by a partnership or other unincorporated firm, give its name and address as well as those of each individual owner. If the publication is published by a nonprofit organization, give its name and address.)

Full Name	Complete Mailing Address
Wholly owned subsidiary of	1600 John F. Kennedy Blvd, Ste. 1800
Reed/Elsevier, US holdings	Philadelphia, PA 19103-2899

11. Known Bondholders, Mortgagees, and Other Security Holders Owning or Holding 1 Percent or More of Total Amount of Bonds, Mortgages, or Other Securities. If none, check box   ☐ None

Full Name	Complete Mailing Address
N/A	

12. Tax Status (For completion by nonprofit organizations authorized to mail at nonprofit rates) (Check one)
The purpose, function, and nonprofit status of this organization and the exempt status for federal income tax purposes:
☐ Has Not Changed During Preceding 12 Months
☐ Has Changed During Preceding 12 Months (Publisher must submit explanation of change with this statement)

PS Form 3526, September 2007 (Page 1 of 3 (Instructions Page 3)) PSN 7530-01-000-9931 PRIVACY NOTICE: See our Privacy policy in www.usps.com

---

13. Publication Title			14. Issue Date for Circulation Data Below
Clinics in Liver Disease			August 2012

15. Extent and Nature of Circulation			Average No. Copies Each Issue During Preceding 12 Months	No. Copies of Single Issue Published Nearest to Filing Date
a. Total Number of Copies (Net press run)			444	357
b. Paid Circulation (By Mail and Outside the Mail)	(1)	Mailed Outside-County Paid Subscriptions Stated on PS Form 3541. (Include paid distribution above nominal rate, advertiser's proof copies, and exchange copies)	170	161
	(2)	Mailed In-County Paid Subscriptions Stated on PS Form 3541 (Include paid distribution above nominal rate, advertiser's proof copies, and exchange copies)		
	(3)	Paid Distribution Outside the Mails Including Sales Through Dealers and Carriers, Street Vendors, Counter Sales, and Other Paid Distribution Outside USPS®	89	102
	(4)	Paid Distribution by Other Classes Mailed Through the USPS (e.g. First-Class Mail®)		
c. Total Paid Distribution (Sum of 15b (1), (2), (3), and (4))		▶	259	263
d. Free or Nominal Rate Distribution (By Mail and Outside the Mail)	(1)	Free or Nominal Rate Outside-County Copies Included on PS Form 3541	70	75
	(2)	Free or Nominal Rate In-County Copies Included on PS Form 3541		
	(3)	Free or Nominal Rate Copies Mailed at Other Classes Through the USPS (e.g. First-Class Mail)		
	(4)	Free or Nominal Rate Distribution Outside the Mail (Carriers or other means)		
e. Total Free or Nominal Rate Distribution (Sum of 15d (1), (2), (3) and (4))		▶	70	75
f. Total Distribution (Sum of 15c and 15e)		▶	329	338
g. Copies not Distributed (See instructions to publishers #4 (page #3))		▶	115	19
h. Total (Sum of 15f and g)		▶	444	357
i. Percent Paid (15c divided by 15f times 100)		▶	78.72%	77.81%

16. Publication of Statement of Ownership

☐ If the publication is a general publication, publication of this statement is required. Will be printed in the November 2012 issue of this publication.   ☐ Publication not required.

17. Signature and Title of Editor, Publisher, Business Manager, or Owner	Date
Stephen R. Bushing Stephen R. Bushing – Inventory Distribution Coordinator	September 14, 2012

I certify that all information furnished on this form is true and complete. I understand that anyone who furnishes false or misleading information on this form or who omits material or information requested on the form may be subject to criminal sanctions (including fines and imprisonment) and/or civil sanctions (including civil penalties).

PS Form 3526, September 2007 (Page 2 of 3)

Printed and bound by CPI Group (UK) Ltd, Croydon, CR0 4YY

03/10/2024

01040461-0007